# Contested Ground

# CONTESTED GROUND

*Public Purpose and Private Interest*
*in the Regulation of Prescription Drugs*

EDITED BY

## Peter Davis

New York    Oxford
OXFORD UNIVERSITY PRESS
1996

Oxford University Press

Oxford   New York
Athens   Auckland   Bangkok   Bombay
Calcutta   Cape Town   Dar es Salaam   Delhi
Florence   Hong Kong   Istanbul   Karachi
Kuala Lumpur   Madras   Madrid   Melbourne
Mexico City   Nairobi   Paris   Singapore
Taipei   Tokyo   Toronto

and associated companies in
Berlin   Ibadan

Library of Congress Cataloging-in-Publication Data
Contested ground : public purpose and private interest
in the regulation of prescription drugs / edited by Peter Davis.
p.   cm. Includes bibliographical references and index.
ISBN 0-19-509120-5
1. Pharmaceutical policy.
I. Davis, Peter, 1942–     .
RA401.A1C655   1996
362.1'782–dc20      95-47819

1 2 3 4 5 6 7 8 9

Printed in the United States of America
on acid-free paper

# Preface

This book arises out of a happy coincidence of events. First, I have had the opportunity over the last five years to develop an interest in public policy and therapeutic drugs, using as my field setting the institutional microcosm of the New Zealand health system. New Zealand is a small country that has recently undergone major economic, political, and health system change, and this has allowed me to study at first hand rapid institutional developments in the pharmaceutical sector. A summary of just some of these experiences was presented in an earlier volume published by the New Zealand branch of Oxford University Press. Second, I came due for an extended sabbatical leave from the Auckland Medical School and was fortunately able, through the good offices of my friend and colleague, John McKinlay, to take up a position for six months as Visiting Scholar at the Boston University Center for Health and Advanced Policy Studies. Finally, and again through a suggestion of John McKinlay's, I had the good fortune to meet Jeffrey House, Vice President of Oxford University Press, at the 1992 Conference of the American Public Health Association. He encouraged me to put my ideas down on paper as a formal publication proposal and he has continued to make useful suggestions that have contributed significantly to the coherence and direction of the book.

Why a book on public policy and therapeutic drugs? There is a strong public interest in this area that, at times, generates considerably more heat than light. This book is intended to channel that concern into what I hope will be useful and constructive policy debate. Pharmaceuticals are also an area of considerable public investment. A book of this kind should assist in the rational and better deployment of those resources. Also, there are good theoretical reasons for studying public policy and therapeutic drugs. It is an area where the debate over the regulation of economic activity in the public interest is keenly contested. And this is an area in great need of institutional development. The pharmaceutical industry has grown into a highly profitable and increasingly muscular giant of modern enterprise. The pace of change elsewhere on the institutional landscape has been much slower. New and powerful commercial pressures beset the workings of science. The caring professions still adhere to the individualistic philosophies of the nineteenth century, despite sharply altered working conditions. A heady mix of commercial, scientific, and political influences buffets our regulatory bodies in the areas of safety, information, pricing, and efficacy. All these changes require close academic scrutiny and urgently invite proposals for institutional development.

This book owes everything to the contributors. It has been one of the joys of preparing the volume to have had such positive dealings with the group of gifted, committed and hard-working colleagues around the world that make up the list of contributors. My sabbatical leave allowed me to make personal contact with practically all the authors, scattered as they are across three continents. That opportunity for personal contact has contributed greatly to the quality and promptness of the work the contributors have done, often under trying circumstances. Technology has also helped. I have managed to maintain a close personal dialogue with my authors, courtesy of the Internet and the fax. It would be invidious of me to single out any one contributor by name. Some I count as personal friends. All have shown enthusiasm for the project.

One thing that preparing this book has brought home to me is the uncanny mix of technology, personal contact, and confusing juxtapositions of time and place that are required to make a project like this work. The final manuscript, when I despatched it to Oxford, fitted onto a single computer disk. In its entirety it was edited on a computer probably not much bigger than the final publication itself. The computer sat on my dining table at home and I worked on the editing task surrounded by the benign temperatures, odors and sounds of a New Zealand garden, as the seasons passed in reverse of those experienced by my northern hemisphere colleagues. Meanwhile, my contributors around the world were being assailed by snowstorms (in Boston and New York), floods (in the Netherlands), heat waves (Chicago and England), and bushfires (Australia) – all conveyed to me at a glance from my work station by global television news!

Final acknowledgements must go to the University of Auckland (for funding my sabbatical leave), to my friend and colleague John McKinlay of the New England Research Institutes (for facilitating the project in various ways), to Jeffrey House of Oxford (for being stalwart and good-humoured in shepherding the book through to the publication stage), and above all to my partner, Helen Clark, for tolerating an academic hobby that at times threatened to become an obsession.

September 1995                                                    Peter Davis
Auckland, New Zealand

# Contents

## III    The Regulatory Framework: International Innovation

# Contributors

MICHAEL ARISTIDES
Director
Medical Technology Assessment Group
Chatswood NSW, Australia

ROBERT H. BALLANCE
Head, Industrial Statistics and Sectoral
  Surveys Branch
UNIDO
Vienna, Austria

BECKY A. BRIESACHER
Institute for Pharmaceutical Economics
Philadelphia College of Pharmacy and
  Science
Philadelphia, Pennsylvania

MICHAEL BURY
Department of Social Policy and Social
  Science
Royal Holloway University of London
London, England

PETER CONRAD
Department of Sociology
Brandeis University
Waltham, Massachusetts

PETER DAVIS
Department of Community Health
Auckland School of Medicine
Auckland, New Zealand

PETRA DENIG
Department of Health Sciences
University of Groningen
Groningen, The Netherlands

W. MICHAEL DICKSON
University of South Carolina
School of Pharmacy
Charleston, South Carolina

JONATHAN GABE
Department of Social Policy and Social
  Science
Royal Holloway University of London
London, England

DAVID J. GROSS
Barents Group, LLC of KPMG
Washington, DC

FLORA M. HAAIJER-RUSKAMP
Department of Health Sciences
University of Groningen
Groningen, The Netherlands

LEIGH HANCHER
Department of Constitutional Law
Erasmus University
Rotterdam, The Netherlands

DAVID A. HENRY
The University of Newcastle
Faculty of Medicine
Newcastle Mater Misericordiae Hospital
Waratah, Australia

CATHERINE HODGKIN
Health Action International
HAI-Europe
Amsterdam, The Netherlands

KENNETH I. KAITIN
Associate Director
Tufts Center for the Study of Drug
    Development
Tufts University
Boston, Massachusetts

ICHIRO KAWACHI
Department of Health and Social Behavior
Harvard School of Public Health
Boston, Massachusetts

JOSEPH KILE
U.S. General Accounting Office
Washington, DC

HUBERT LEUFKENS
Department of Pharmacoepidemiology and
    Pharmacotherapy
Utrecht University, Utrecht
and Institute for Pharmaceutical
Business Administration,
Laren, The Netherlands

JOEL LEXCHIN
Department of Family and Community
    Medicine
University of Toronto
Toronto, Canada

BARBARA MINTZES
Health Action International
HAI-Europe
Amsterdam, The Netherlands

ANDREW S. MITCHELL
Pharmaceutical Evaluation Section
Pharmaceutical Benefits Branch
Commonwealth Department of Human
    Services and Health
Canberra, Australia

MICHAEL MONTAGNE
Department of Pharmaceutical Sciences
Massachusetts College of Pharmacy and
    Allied Health Professions
Boston, Massachusetts

NEIL PEARCE
Wellington Asthma Research Group
Wellington School of Medicine
Wellington, New Zealand

JONATHAN RATNER
U.S. General Accounting Office
Washington, DC

J. WARREN SALMON
Department of Pharmacy Administration
The University of Illinois at Chicago
College of Pharmacy
Chicago, Illinois

CHRISTINE THOER
Département de Santé Communautaire
University of Montreal
Montreal, Canada

CELIA THOMAS
U.S. General Accounting Office
Washington, DC

PAULINE VAILLANCOURT ROSENAU
University of Texas
School of Public Health
Houston, Texas

ALBERT WERTHEIMER
First Health Services Corporation
Glen Allen, Virginia

Contested Ground

# Introduction:
# Medicines in a Postmodern World

PETER DAVIS

Pharmaceuticals are therapeutic drugs that are available either by prescription from a physician or over-the-counter from a pharmacist. A distinctive set of institutional and regulatory arrangements has grown up around their production and use. We include here the industry that creates and distributes medicines, the professions that prescribe and dispense them, the users who consume them, the media and other cultural agencies that shape them, and the state that arbitrates, regulates, and funds access to them (Davis, 1992). It is the structure, dynamics, and future evolution of these arrangements that provide the subject matter for this book.

Although medications have always been central to healing practices in traditional societies, it was only with the advent of allopathic Western medicine that pharmacology—the science of drugs—emerged as an entity distinct from what was, until then, a predominantly holistic pattern of therapy (World Health Organization, 1988: 1). Furthermore, it was not until early in this century that an identifiably modern pharmaceutical sector started to emerge with the application of scientific principles to the creation of new drugs and the use of industrial and commercial methods in their production and distribution (Lilja, 1988: 50–57). The industry that we now recognize as the modern pharmaceutical sector dates, in the first instance, from the therapeutic discoveries of the 1930s, but more especially from the period since World War II that has seen the rapid expansion of research in the biological sciences and of their application in the practice of modern scientific medicine.

While the industry does continue to grow, it now appears to be entering a phase that is much more contingent and uncertain, even postmodern, in character. The sector is characterized by almost constant global shaping and reshaping, there are dramatic research developments in molecular modeling and genetic manipulation, and, as companies aggressively promote themselves and their products to the professions and to the community at large, a complex and interactive relationship between the industry and the wider culture is rapidly evolving.

## Issues and Contentions

The pharmaceutical industry is unique in a number of respects: it operates in a highly politicized and regulated environment involving sensitive relations with state authorities; it combines outstanding success in fundamental research with a powerful marketing arm, exploiting to the full the commercial potential of its intellectual property rights; and it demonstrates the attributes of one of the few truly internationalized industries, with a global division of labor, a world market, and a dynamic and diverse infrastructure (Ballance et al., 1992: 1–2). It also has as its foundation an unusual market—the market for medicines—in which purchasing decisions are generally made on behalf of the user (the patient) by professional advisers (doctor and pharmacist), funded by a third party (public or private insurer).

Perhaps the most distinctive feature of the industry is its commitment to research and development (R&D). Investment in this area is costly and risky, yet it has paid off handsomely. According to estimates of the Office of Technology Assessment (OTA), for the United States in the 1980s the average after-tax R&D outlay was about $65 million for each new drug over an average of 12 years. Nevertheless, each new drug returned at least $36 million after taxes, once the initial outlay had been recouped. This was reflected in returns to the pharmaceutical sector, which exceeded those to corporations in other industries by 2 to 3% per year, and in growth of investment in R&D through the 1980s (about 10% per year). All this could change, however, with any moves towards greater price competition in the industry (OTA, 1993: 1–2).

There is, of course, very much more to pharmaceuticals than their industrial and market characteristics. The social dimension is all-important. There are fundamental issues about social definitions of health and ill health and about social conceptions of normality and deviance that need to be considered. Payer (1992) provides a popularized version of this concern in her critique of "disease-mongering"—the accelerated social manufacture of new diseases in contemporary American society. This quickening process of medicalization is problematic, not only because of its short-term iatrogenic impact, but also because of a range of longer-term ill effects of a financial, social and, ultimately, political nature. Among the causes she identifies for this apparent increase in medicalization are the growing number of physicians (and the greater fear of litigation), expanded media coverage and advertising for health products and services, hospital-induced cost escalation, and the pharmaceutical industry's greatly increased role in postgraduate medical education (Payer, 1992: 9–18).

Finally, it should be noted that, despite its undoubted commercial and therapeutic successes, the pharmaceutical industry remains an object of controversy. There are four areas in particular where public controversy has been significant and long-standing: safety (with a series of well-publicized disasters and adverse reactions), expenditure (particularly aggressive marketing and high profits), the volume of drug consumption (perceived to be high and increasing), and dubious industry practices in the developing world (Burstall and Reuben, 1990).

Allied to these more diffuse concerns has been the close attention directed by state authorities to the issue of cost containment. Although pharmaceuticals account for only about 10% of total health expenditure, a proportion that has remained remarkably stable for decades, they attract a considerable amount of attention from governments (Dickson and Poullier, 1992: 110). There are a number of reasons for this: costs are increasing and, as a budgetary item, lie close to the trigger threshold for policy intervention; there is evidence of inappropriate and wasteful use of drugs; and such controls in health care seem to be more readily justified where they involve an overtly commercial and highly profitable sector like the pharmaceutical industry.

Predicting the future course of the industry against this dynamic and somewhat turbulent background is difficult. Nevertheless, some trends can be discerned (Ballance et al., 1992: 201–220). Demographically, the growth and aging of populations in affluent countries is set to expand the market. In policy terms, governments are likely to pursue cost containment, using a mix of competitive and regulatory strategies, and there are prospects for the greater international harmonization of standards and procedures. Furthermore, it can be predicted that the major restructuring, integration, and transformation of the industry will continue. Finally, if countervailing action is not taken, there is the very real prospect of a growing mismatch, particularly in the developing world, between the needs of the population and the market priorities of the industry.

## Analytical Perspectives

In the chapters that follow the institutional arrangements governing prescription medicines are subjected to the scrutiny of a range of social and policy sciences. These analytical pieces are grouped into three parts: the broader social and cultural context of pharmaceuticals; the economic, technological, and industrial dimension of this sector; and a policy and regulatory focus, with emphasis on international innovation.

Part I locates prescription medicines within their social and cultural context. It begins with a review by Michael Montagne in which he seeks to unravel the cultural and conceptual underpinnings of the pharmaceutical sector and of the different interests within it. A key cultural process is that of medicalization, and it is this process that the chapter by Ichiro Kawachi and Peter Conrad addresses. Taking the special case of hypertension, they explore the relationship between the expansion of pharmacological treatment and broader institutional processes associated with the medical profession, the pharmaceutical industry, and wider cultural definitions. The role of the media in such issues of social definition and cultural elaboration is developed further in the third chapter, by Jonathan Gabe and Michael Bury. These authors address the controversy surrounding the use of the benzodiazepines in the treatment of anxiety, identifying the activities of a range of groups and the influence on their claims of the mass media. The activities of such actors are also crucial in determining the course of another controversy, the treatment of asthma. In Chapter 4, Neil Pearce demonstrates the complex interweaving of scientific, commercial, and bureaucratic interests as this issue threads through to a conclusion. The key element absent from these case studies is an active role for the consumer. Therefore, in the final chapter in Part I, Barbara Mintzes and Catherine Hodgkin establish the link between pharmaceutical controversies and the development of a strong and vibrant consumer movement.

Part II pieces together the principal market and industrial characteristics of pharmaceuticals, using the product cycle as an organizing theme. Chapter 6 is a broad-ranging review by Robert H. Ballance of the special features of the pharmaceutical industry and its likely future prospects, emphasizing the distinctive character of economic analysis in this sector. The fundamental dynamic force of the industry is research and development, and this is evaluated by Ken I. Kaitin of the Center for the Study of Drug Development. He concludes that there are conflicting tendencies in the scientific, commercial, and regulatory influences shaping the future of pharmaceutical innovation and that much depends on the future profitability of the industry. A key influence on profitability is pricing, which is the subject of the chapter written by David Gross and his colleagues from the U.S. General Accounting Office. They attempt to identify the relative influences of market forces and regulatory powers in shaping international price differences. The last two chapters in Part II address the professional and organizational context in which pharmaceuticals are distributed. For J. Warren Salmon, there is a powerful dynamic between the commercial, corporate, and competitive forces that drive health care in the United States, forces that seem to threaten the professional autonomy of both pharmacy and medicine. Chapter 10, by Albert Wertheimer and his colleagues, places these trends in a wider perspective, considering them in an international dimension and within the broader delivery system. It is evident from this chapter that the state plays a crucial role in most societies in managing the organization, funding, and distribution of prescription drugs.

Part III considers issues in the regulation and management of medicines in society, with an emphasis on international policy innovation. In Chapter 11, Leigh Hancher reviews the range of initiatives being introduced in the European Union to harmonize the diversity of legal codes, illustrating this with examples from the pharmaceutical sector. There are implications here for regulatory strategies at both national and international levels of intervention. One area in which such regulatory issues affect consumers in a very direct way is access to medication. In Chapter 12, Pauline Vaillancourt Rosenau and Christine Thoer consider the pressures in both Europe and North America toward deregulation and liberalization of access to medication. It is against this backdrop of general liberalization that the full range of regulatory measures has to be considered. One of the imperatives in the regulatory debate is economic, and Michael Aristides and his colleagues outline the initiatives undertaken in Australia and, increasingly, elsewhere to ensure that drugs introduced to the market and subject to state subsidy are not only safe but cost effective as well. Clearly, the state can directly manipulate subsidy levels in order to manage price and access to care, but it is less clear what instruments are available for shaping the flow of information to doctors and influencing the quality of the prescribing decisions they make. For both purposes, more subtle regulatory strategies are required, and it is to these issues that the final two chapters are devoted. Joel Lexchin and Ichiro Kawachi assess the effectiveness of industry self-regulation in ensuring adherence to marketing codes. They make the case for structural reform. Flora Haaijer-Ruskamp and Petra Denig review the research on educational interventions designed to influence the prescribing decisions of doctors, outlining a recent study in this field and concluding with a plea for a more practice-based approach.

## Contested Ground

The underlying theme of this book is the contested nature of the institutional arrangements that have been established around the production, distribution, and consumption of pharmaceuticals. At one level this does no more than give recognition to the fact that any such system of economic, social, and political relationships is bound to harbor divergent interests. In the case of the pharmaceutical industry, however, there is much more at stake. Because of their powerful healing and symbolic properties, medicines cannot be contained within the tight parameters of a straightforward market transaction; inevitably they are viewed in the broader context of political and social concern. This is exemplified by the activities in the pharmaceutical sector of both the state and the consumer movement.

At the heart of governmental regulatory tension is the requirement to reconcile three potentially conflicting policy goals: retaining access to health care for low-income citizens (social solidarity), restricting public-sector expenditure (cost containment), and maintaining an innovative and competitive industry (industrial development) (Redwood, 1992: 13–19). For the consumer movement, the areas of concern have been safety, expenditure (particularly marketing), the volume of drug consumption, dubious industry practices in the developing world, and, to a lesser extent, issues of national sovereignty and corruption (Burstall and Reuben, 1990).

Tensions are inevitable because of the complicated moral and symbolic character of pharmaceuticals. Medicines are profitable commodities that are potentially toxic, but that also have the power to heal. In this respect they possess a distinctly postmodern aspect (Rosenau, 1992) with moral and symbolic ambiguity. Competing discourses of commercial endeavor and lofty social and political purpose swirl around them. The marketing activities of the industry associate their products with the fundamental cultural narratives of health, healing, sexuality, mind, and body. The media spin each new pharmaceutical controversy, whether a scientific breakthrough or a safety scandal, according to more or less standard set of moral formulae. And over it all plays a constant cultural shaping and reshaping of medicines in imagery and metaphor, a restless organizational restructuring of the industry in the search for profit, and, at its source, a boundless scientific inventiveness.

## References

Ballance R, Pogany J and Forstner H (1992) *The World's Pharmaceutical Industries. An International Perspective on Innovation, Competition and Policy*. London: Edward Elgar.

Burstall ML and Reuben BG (1990) *Critics of the Pharmaceutical Industry. A Report by REMIT Consultants*. London: REMIT Consultants Ltd.

Davis P (1992) Pharmaceuticals and public policy. In: Davis P (ed.) *For Health or Profit? Medicine, the Pharmaceutical Industry, and the State in New Zealand*. Auckland, NZ: Oxford University Press, pp. 1–17.

Dickson M and Poullier J-P (1992) Prescription reimbursement systems in selected European countries. In: Huttin C and Bosanquet N (eds.) *The Prescription Drug Market. International Perspectives and Challenges for the Future*. Amsterdam: Elsevier Science Publishers B.V., pp. 109–37.

Lilja J (1988) *Theoretical Social Pharmacy – The Drug Sector from a Social Science Perspective*. Kuopio, Finland: Kuopio University Publications.

Payer L (1992) *Disease-Mongers. How Doctors, Drug Companies, and Insurers are Making You Feel Sick*. New York: John Wiley.

Redwood H (1992) *The Dynamics of Drug Pricing and Reimbursement in the European Community*. Suffolk UK: Oldwicks Press Ltd.

Rosenau PM (1992) *Post-Modernism and the Social Sciences. Insights, Inroads, and Intrusions*. Princeton NJ: Princeton University Press.

US Congress, Office of Technology Assessment (OTA) (1993) *Pharmaceutical R&D: Costs, Risks and Rewards*. OTA-H-522. Washington, DC: US Government Printing Office.

World Health Organisation (WHO) (1988) *The World Drug Situation*. Geneva: WHO.

# I

# THE SOCIAL AND CULTURAL CONTEXT

# 1

# The Pharmakon Phenomenon: Cultural Conceptions of Drugs and Drug Use

## MICHAEL MONTAGNE

Drugs are cultural entities as well as chemical compounds. Our knowledge, attitudes and behavior towards them are powerfully influenced by the conceptions we hold about them. Consumers want substances to help them achieve health and well-being; health professionals seek safe and effective medications; and pharmaceutical scientists search for new compounds. Each has a different perspective.

Yet there is a single concept that encompasses our response to the drugs we give and take. It is expressed in the original Greek term for drug, *pharmakon*. In classic times the word had three meanings: remedy, poison, and magical charm (Jonsen, 1988). Its relevance is that, while chemical substances used for medical purposes are thought of as remedies, many are also potentially toxic and can produce side effects and adverse reactions. Thus, the drug as remedy can also be at times poison or toxin. In earlier times such remedies were imbued with magical qualities as well. Hence, the drug as charm. Indeed, medicine and society today still represent many drugs in this way, viewing them as "magic bullets."

Thus, the boundaries of what constitutes drugs and drug use are largely cultural. They reflect our culturally influenced conceptions about these substances. Distinctions vary between the different domains of medicine, law, public debate, and personal action. The approach in this chapter is to define drugs and drug use in metaphorical terms. It will be argued that there is a range, or continuum, of substances and that their distinction as drugs or medicines is created and formed culturally through metaphors (Montagne, 1988). The nature and extent of this continuum will be noted throughout this discussion of cultural conceptions of drugs and drug use.

What does this all mean for everyday life in which drugs are given and taken for a variety of reasons? If such conceptions about drugs and their metaphorical associations structure and guide decisions to develop, prescribe, and use them, then variations in these conceptions are highly important and worthy of study. For example, individual or group needs for power, status, and material gain can exacerbate differences in conceptions (to the domination of one over the others), or they can distract from the pursuit of health goals. These different conceptions often collide in the contested ground between patients, health professionals, policy makers, and the pharmaceutical industry.

## The Creation of Social Knowledge

These conceptions are defined here as social knowledge. That is, they are viewed in this chapter as accumulations of information and past experiences that exist uniquely in individuals and collectively in societies (Berger and Luckmann, 1966). Social knowledge is expanded and refined with successive experiences. Therefore, what an individual or group of drug consumers knows about drugs—their social knowledge—will affect the actual use of drugs, and it will influence the experiences they have with drugs (Cooperstock and Lennard, 1979; Arluke, 1980; Montagne, 1984). Such knowledge also has a symbolic component, and the symbolic nature of drug giving and taking is extensive and powerfully influential.

How are we to assess social knowledge? There are two related approaches, one philosophical, one sociological. *Epistemology* is the study of the nature and scope of knowledge. As used here, epistemology is essentially a "way of knowing" (Kuhn, 1970; Wuketits, 1983). A closely related concept, *ideology*, also refers to social knowledge and human ideals, but these are viewed in a sociopolitical context and seen as reflecting class power and social order (Mannheim, 1968; Habermas, 1984; 1987). Consideration of the epistemologies, or ideologies, of various groups of drug givers and takers is important in understanding different perspectives, identifying the nature and boundaries, and clarifying policy debates about drugs and drug use. These "ways of knowing" about drug effects and drug use are also strongly related to the conceptual focus of different individuals and groups. There are different levels of experience or response that reflect the predominant emphasis of a particular group's interest in, or involvement with, drugs. These levels range from the molecular-cellular through the organal to the behavioral and social-cultural.

Scientists and health professionals focus on the pharmacological activity of drugs and believe that biological components are the basis for the physical and psychological effects of drugs. Scientists with a focus of study at the cellular level may be able to identify a specific drug action. But whether and how this cellular action equates to a particular drug effect at the human level is more problematic. Drug users, by contrast, are rarely concerned about drug activity at the cellular level. Instead, they focus on drug effects at the level of the organ—specific tissues and organ systems—or of behavior (for example, everyday life functioning). Arguably, for most drug consumers the predominant focus is the behavioral one, as reflected in the drug experience itself (Arluke, 1980; Conrad, 1985). Drug effects at the social or cultural level are unlikely to be noticed by individual users. Rather, these effects tend to be detected through broad assessments made by people who focus at this level, such as epidemiologists, social scientists, or the media. The pharmaceutical industry, government agencies, and consumer advocacy groups also often view drugs as social commodities.

## Pharmacomythologies and Cultural Conceptions

An important component of social knowledge is mythology. Hence, there are bound to be pharmacomythologies. These are cultural conceptions about drugs that are illusory, yet are regarded as fundamental principles. For example, most people believe that a drug produces one effect that is referred to as its main effect. This generally has a positive connotation. If other effects are experienced, they are considered to be side effects (with a negative connotation). In fact, drugs produce a great array of physiological and psychological changes, but these occur in the biological system of the organism itself.

There also is a related belief that a drug produces the same main effect every time it is taken, and in each person who takes it. These drug effects are seen to be caused by the chemical compound that is ingested, and by extension, drug effects are attributed to that chemical compound, rather than being viewed as a function of some change within the living organism. Yet, as Albert Hofmann (1995) and some pharmacologists have noted, "we can say of many drugs that we know *how* they act and in what way, but we are still quite unable to say *why* they act as they do."

From a very different perspective, cross-cultural studies have improved our understanding of the social norms and cultural beliefs that influence drug use (Rubin, 1975; DeRios, 1976; Everett et al., 1976; Montagne, 1991). In some situations metaphors for drug use have been important in culturally defining certain patterns of use as constituting social problems, thus making them open to social control; examples are alcohol, tranquillizers, oral contraceptives, asthma medications, and drugs. In these examples, partial, qualified, and fragile knowledge is continually transformed into certain and consistent fact. This facilitates the creation of technical and moral realities that are given form and meaning through culturally shared facts and beliefs, and are invoked to control behavior (Gusfield, 1981).

Cross-cultural studies of drugs also show the importance of beliefs, rituals, and social sanctions (DeRios, 1976). Rituals, stylized and prescribed behaviors surrounding the use of a drug, and social sanctions, norms regarding whether or not a particular drug should be used, work in a number of ways. They help to: define and approve controlled drug use, limit or prevent uncontrolled drug use, confine drug use to those settings that are more conducive to a beneficial effect or a therapeutic result, incorporate specific principles of appropriate use, identify possible ill-effects and the precautions to be taken against them, and assist drug users in interpreting and giving meaning to their drug experiences (Du Toit, 1977; Zinberg, 1984).

Thus, cultural belief systems give meaning and description to a drug taking experience. Indeed, the lack of relevant cultural beliefs can lead to difficulties in interpreting a particular episode, thus limiting the potential to benefit from the drug (Wallace, 1959). Many cultures attempt to control drug use—and thus limit problems—by ritual rather than by legal means, guiding drug taking towards specific cultural goals, with culturally valued reasons for use. Thus, definitions of use or misuse become cultural, not biomedical (DeRios and Smith, 1977). Cultural controls are also important in the prevention and treatment of drug use problems (Edwards and Arif, 1980).

Thinking more schematically, there is obviously a considerable range of cultural conceptions about drugs and drug use in society. For the purpose of exposition we can represent these different conceptions in simplified form, as in Table 1-1. Usually, a particular conceptual approach examines only one specific aspect of drug taking. This depends on epistemological orientation, type of knowledge used, focus of inquiry, and many other factors. Therefore each conception is relatively singular and narrow in orientation. Yet, these specific sets of images and metaphors of drugs manage to connect particular "ways of knowing" to the wider culture.

As suggested by Table 1-1, the focus of almost any given research study or drug development activity, of any patient education program, and of public policies on drug taking, is likely to be intimately connected to a specific perspective. The danger in this is that it can lead to the exclusion of other ideas, the attachment to a single epistemology, the misperception by individuals and society of the characteristics of drugs and the consequences of drug use, and the promotion of one approach as being the most correct or acceptable, even if it is not empirically tenable. This can result in a number of serious misconceptions and problems in the use of drugs—as in the case of most psychoactive medications used for poorly defined mental illnesses, many chemotherapeutic agents designed for fatal diseases (e.g., AIDS, cancer), and some pharmaceuticals promoted for certain personal and social problems that have been medicalized. The instance of recent asthma mortality epidemics is also an example of clashing, and potentially incommensurate, views of a drug and its effects (Pearce, 1996).

Pharmaceutical scientists define or classify drugs based upon a physical, chemical, or physiological characteristic, such as structure, solubility, stability, or potency, and are interested in how drugs are isolated, synthesized, absorbed, distributed, metabolized, and excreted (Gilman et al., 1990). Most of the pharmaceutical sciences focus at a level that is not even connected consciously to a human being. Instead, for many of these researchers the drug itself is the all-important being. This is not an uncharacteristic approach. In fact, it is reflective of the dominant, biomedical approach to the study of drug taking which focuses on diseases and on the use of drugs to achieve normal functioning. The epidemiological approach is related, but focuses on the patterns, extent, and frequency of drug use at a population level (Anthony, 1983; Feinstein, 1985). The real emphasis is on identifying drug use problems.

Social scientific perspectives vary considerably, but mostly they look at drug-taking behaviors in individuals, groups, or societies; classify drugs based on social meanings and functions; and are interested in issues regarding the promotion, dispensing, control, and use of drugs (Young, 1971; Cooperstock, 1974; Svarstad, 1989). The media and society in general tend to focus on individual examples of good or bad drugs and their effects (Cohen, 1983; McCarthy and Montagne, 1992; Gabe and Bury, 1996). The emphasis often is on sensational cases of drug use, mostly in the course of selling a product (such as newspapers or airtime), presenting a political agenda, or encouraging a moral stance. The media can heighten public concern about certain types of drug use. They do this by providing opportunities for the expression

TABLE 1-1. Conceptual Foundation for Perceiving and Understanding Drugs and Drug Use

| | Pharmaceutical Sciences | Basic & Clinical Pharmacology | Medicine and Pharmacotherapeutics |
|---|---|---|---|
| Focus of Inquiry | Drug as object: its structure and properties | Drug's activity in living tissues and species | Drug's effects and responses in individuals and groups |
| Investigational Methods | Lab-based physical and chemical experimentation and analytical studies | Lab- or hospital-based biophysiological experimentation to assess activity | Clinical trials in humans to determine safety and efficacy; trial and error in clinical practice |
| Research Activity and Application | Working with chemical structures or compounds based on Structure-Activity Relationships and its physical properties | Screening or testing compounds for activity; tracking through the drug development process to market | Assessing clinically the best drugs for practice, in a variety of patients and conditions, noting adverse effect and specific problems |
| Major Issues | Understanding Structure-Activity Relationships, designing molecules that are optimally active with few adverse effects; getting drug to cellular site of action and drug stability | Testing drugs for effects to verify Structure-Activity Relationships and determining range of beneficial and toxic effects (dose-response) in "in vitro" tissues, animal models, and then humans | Healing with drugs in easiest, quickest, and simplest way in high-tech fashion, with tendency to use drug over nondrug alternatives; reducing adverse reactions and other problems |
| Metaphors | Lock and key; targeting; chemical structure terms: cradle, boat, rocking chair | Magic bullets; shooting or targeting drugs to the site of action in the body | Magic bullets; war on disease and illness; body as mechanistic and mind as computer; pharmakon meaning (remedy, poison, and magical charm) |
| Policy Implications | Attempts to generate and direct funding for drug development (with profit motive in capitalist systems and satisfaction of ego or knowledge pursuit for individual scientists/clinicians). Seeks to control nature and method of research process and perpetuation of certain ways (biologic) of assuring health and treating disease. Provides drugs to maintain mythic image of medicine and ability of Western health care to remedy human illness. | | |

*(Continued)*

TABLE 1-1. Conceptual Foundation for Perceiving and Understanding Drugs and Drug Use (*Continued*)

| | Epidemiology and Public Health | Social Sciences (Psychology, Sociology, Anthropology, Economics, History, Law) |
|---|---|---|
| Focus of Inquiry | Drug use problems at population level, and the limiting or preventing of them | Attitudes and behaviors regarding drugs and their use; drugs as commodities and characteristics, causes, and consequences of drug-taking behaviors in individuals, groups, and cultures |
| Investigational Methods | Population-based studies or interventions using a variety of methods | Method of primary discipline involved in study (experimental, survey, interview, observation, and cost analysis) |
| Research Activity and Application | Identifying risks of drug hazards in segments of the population, and testing prevention and intervention strategies | Conceptualizing and theorizing about drug use, its formation, causative factors and interrelationships; identfiying problematic attitudes and behaviors and attempting to change them |
| Major Issues | Reducing/preventing drug use problems; outbreak and spread of problem use; favor public health of society over individual rights | How and why people use drugs; social factors that influence drug effects and use; costs of drug use and its problems; differences in use cross-culturally and over time; influence of media and promotion; developing public policy from research |
| Metaphors | Drugs as tools/solutions for health problems. Drugs as contagions (epidemics) | War on drugs; a nonmechanistic view of drug action in the body (drug effects as semantic and hermeneutic) |
| Policy Implications | Seeks to link science to policy (formal social controls) with aim of limiting or preventing problems from any type of drug use (within confines of medical model) and at level of whole populations; attempts to direct funding to its goals; argues often for nondrug alternatives in health and wellness | Attempts to influence/create policy (formal and informal social controls) often for benefit of individuals/groups with diminished power/autonomy; seeks to validate/advance own theories and policies, often employing drug taking as representational of specific aspects of human endeavors and history and societal evolution; emphasizes drug use as human undertaking (as opposed to biological drive); influences policy often in opposition to (and less effectively than) medicine |

|  | *Media and Society* | *Individual Drug Users* |
|---|---|---|
| Focus of Inquiry | Drugs causing problems based on anecdotal accounts, often morally or politically based | Drugs as objects that heal (prevent, treat, or cure) illness and even solve other problems of life; and that create problems for people and society; what works best for specific conditions and problems |
| Investigational Methods | Investigative reporting and gathering information and quotes from sources of perceived importance/knowledge | Gather information from any source and from experiences of others that are part of social network/relations or society; influenced by media and promotional campaigns in capitalistic societies and folklore and personal knowledge in other cultures |
| Research Activity and Application | Investigating, making contacts and talking to people | Experimenting personally, seeking information from others to judge efficacy and safety of drugs for specific symptoms and conditions |
| Major Issues | High profile cases and problems that sell; also informing or protecting society from individual behavior | Optimal effects from drugs based upon perceived need, though many individuals using without clear need or reason; right of individual and privacy of action versus safety of society |
| Metaphors | War on drugs; drug is evil, demon, enemy; drug use as a plague; drugs as magic bullets | Magic bullets; great range of metaphors from patient and consumer perspectives (see Table 1-2 for some examples) |
| Policy Implications | Generates and controls policy through direct influence on both governmental systems and general society, mostly for political, economic, or ideological ends | Attempts to influence or control policy on drug development and use through voice (public forum), consumer power (market context), or individual action (often in disregard of professional standards, governmental policies, and social norms). Creates tension between individual right to drug use and societal need to control behavior, and in three functions of *pharmakon* |

of expert and lay viewpoints and by structuring the meanings of drug use into images and conceptions that are readily recognizable to the public at large (Gabe and Bury, 1996).

## The Nature and Meaning of Drug Effects

The impact of these different conceptions can be detected in a wide range of issues, problems, and conflicts concerned with the consumption of drugs. Their influence is particularly evident, however, in the way in which people perceive and describe drug effects. Drug effects are outcomes a user experiences after taking a drug. They include specific physiological and psychological changes, incidents of a more general behavioral or social kind.

The pharmacological theory of drug effects is now dominant. It controls not only health professionals' thinking about medicines but that of society at large (Basara and Montagne, 1994). This theory states that drug action results from the interaction, usually through a physicochemical bond, of a drug molecule with a cell, or constituent part of a cell, in the human body (Delgado and Remers, 1991). This notion has since evolved into the receptor concept which relates structural similarities in drug molecules with analogous biological mechanisms. The concepts of biochemical specificity, involving cellular receptors, and dose-response relationships have become the central tenets of this theory. These tenets have affected the ways in which drug effects are studied and measured, new drugs are developed and tested, clinical pharmacology is understood and taught, and drug therapy is prescribed and monitored (Montagne, 1995).

This theory has proved to be very effective in explaining how a wide range of drugs act in the body to produce effects, including antibiotics and chemotherapeutic agents, opiates and synthetic narcotics, and certain cardiovascular agents. But the theory does not explain or predict all aspects of the drug-taking experience. For example, the theory does not help account for the changes that often occur in the major indications for a drug over time. Nor is it effective in explaining many drug experiences such as placebo phenomena, anesthesia, most psychoactive drug effects, differences in main versus side effects, and descriptions of effects by drug user compared to those of an observer, like a researcher or clinician. Nor is it useful in making sense of effects that either are not detected in research studies or are not predicted from pharmacological information. For instance, recent research within this perspective has attempted to attribute the placebo phenomenon solely to the activity of endogenous neurotransmitters such as endorphins.

Sociological theories of drug effects are radically different in conception and description (Becker, 1967; Lennard, 1971; Orcutt, 1978; Montagne, 1995). From this perspective, drug effects are basically social in origin. The use of literary and other popular accounts of drug taking by users to construct a distinct social reality has led some social scientists to redefine the nature of drug effects in social terms, often in direct opposition to the chemicalistic fallacy (Dubos, 1964). This fallacy involves attaching specific effects to a particular drug and seeing them solely as a function of the biochemical properties of the drug. Sociological theories, on the other hand, do not assume that drug effects are a direct function of the pharmacological activity of the drug, but rather see them as being primarily shaped by social expectations and definitions.

Sociological theories have been helpful in explaining the effects of many types of drugs and in describing drug taking experiences that the user finds difficult to put into words (Montagne, 1995). These theories rest on the following tenets: 1. the user must perceive changes in body state or mood; 2. the user actively interprets these changes and defines them according to the social knowledge available; and 3. the defined effects must be attributed to the drug taken by the user, because only in this way can these effects become a part of that user's social knowledge about drugs. Within this theory the basis for perceiving, interpreting, and describing these drug effects is the metaphorical structuring of social knowledge.

## Metaphors for Drugs, Drug Giving, and Drug Taking

In this context, recent research has focused on the symbolic nature of drug giving and drug taking (Szasz, 1974; Burr, 1984; Rhodes, 1984; Montagne, 1988). Through studies of drug images and the meanings present in drug use, the functions that drugs serve in a society may be delineated more clearly. These images are created through the use of cultural metaphors. Such metaphors help shape the perception, interpretation, and description of drug experiences, as well as generating and structuring drug taking (Montagne, 1988; 1991).

Metaphor is important in language, epistemology and the generation of knowledge (Sacks, 1979; Lakoff and Johnson, 1980; Johnson; 1981). Symbols, images, and metaphors construct our social knowledge and assist us in giving meaning to our everyday life. In general, whatever we wish to explain and understand, be it a concept, object, entity, or experience, is defined through use of a metaphor or symbol, which in turn can be related to a concept or experience closer to personal experience. These symbols, images, and metaphors are preserved in our language and in the ritual of everyday life.

These images are influential in the development of patients' and health professionals' conceptions, attitudes and meanings about drugs and drug effects (Helman, 1981; Rhodes, 1984; Montagne, 1988; 1991). Such meanings are reflected in public debate and media accounts, and they can influence program planning, drug laws and regulations, and drug policy. Consumer advocacy groups and their associated networks, for example, work to create and disseminate alternative meanings around drugs (Mintzes and Hodgkin, 1996). For them the nature and meaning of health care must be defined from a consumer's perspective. Such a perspective can be influential during policy making. The more heterogeneous the various groups are in a consumer movement, however, the greater the range of possible metaphors, with both positive and negative connotations, each reflecting a different philosophical or political stance.

Metaphors exist for describing, understanding, and giving meaning to drug experiences, and they can be generated by different sources. Table 1-2 outlines a representative listing of predominant images and metaphors identified in medical and social research, the media, and public debate. The intended meaning and the reasons for the

TABLE 1-2.   Major Cultural Metaphors for Drugs and Drug Experiences

| Drug as [Is] | Drug Experience as [Is] |
|---|---|
| magic bullet/charm | panacea |
| cure/remedy/solution | life/death |
| poison/disease/killer | life change/lifestyle |
| pacifier/consoler/comforter | travel/trip/vacation/escape |
| helper/friend/missing mate | artificial paradise |
| hero/army/police | moral weakness |
| tool/vehicle/object | normal daily event |
| crutch/prop/support/security | military mobilization |
| lock/vice/prison | relaxing setting |
| ticket/passport | social image |
| money/barter | social control |
| food/fuel/tonic | barrier/imprisonment |
| devil/evil/plague/enemy | evil necessity |
| other drugs | other drug experiences |

creation of these metaphors can vary. It is therefore very important to note if the source is the patient, the healer (or health professional), the pharmaceutical manufacturer and promoter, the social researcher, or media commentators. In many instances it is difficult to know the original source of a metaphor. Often there is a complex intertwining of a metaphor coming from different sources (Montagne, 1988; 1991).

The presence and influence of metaphors in the use of pharmaceuticals are quite extensive. Metaphorical thinking in drug use becomes most apparent and important when the metaphors are applied in everyday interactions and take on very specific, local meanings. At this point a significant transformation takes place. As the metaphor and its meaning become fundamental to an individual or group, the analogue (indicated in Table 1-2 by "as") evolves into the related concept (indicated by "is"). In other words, the metaphor ceases to be an analogy. Instead, it becomes the related concept or entity, as signified in Table 1-2 by the semantic and conceptual transformation from "as" to "is" (Rhodes, 1984; Montagne, 1988; 1991). In consequence, these metaphors structure patients' and health professionals' knowledge, experiences, and behaviors at a very fundamental level of understanding. They are instrumental in the construction of social realities and cultural beliefs (Morgan, 1983; Conrad, 1985; McCarthy and Montagne, 1992). These metaphors influence cultural beliefs and perceptions to such a degree that social change is, or can be, brought about by a prevailing metaphorical structure.

## Balancing Public Concern and Private Interest

There is subtle ambiguity to the original meanings of *pharmakon*, but this has been lost in the technological advances of the pharmaceutical and biomedical sciences in the twentieth century. "Even though the word *drug* carries both positive and negative connotations in our own language, we have lost the powerful ambiguity of the original Greek word. Indeed, it is entirely absent in the word *medicine* which today (though not in the past) means only a beneficial drug" (Jonsen, 1988).

The metamorphosis of conceptions about drugs, while still rooted in the pharmakon phenomenon, is exhibited in the various epistemologies that influence drug taking in specific contexts. Throughout this chapter there has been an obvious tension between, on the one hand, the intellectual discussion of epistemologies about drugs and the policy applications of various cultural conceptions of drug use on the other. But how do epistemologies affect policy making and public debate, and how do they influence society's ability to use drugs rationally (that is, in safe, effective, and economical ways)? Moreover, in a world of culturally relative epistemologies, who defines "rational" and what are the implications of such relativity for drug policy?

Traditional beliefs about disease and treatment are used by many cultures in developing countries to reinterpret the function of many Western medicines. For example, the "hot" or "cold" classification of illness (Bledsoe and Goubaud, 1985). In a similar way, unique and innovative drugs can reshape dominant ideas and practices about health and illness. This is evident in the cases of oral contraceptives to prevent (control) pregnancy (Holmes et al., 1980), and human growth hormone for children who are just slightly short of average height (Benjamin et al., 1984).

In addition, with the dominance of biological models in medicine and health care, there are often attempts to define problematic human behaviors solely, or ultimately, in biological or biochemical terms. Medicalization, as this process is called, may have the effect of obscuring the diagnosis and treatment of certain conditions, especially those with poorly defined symptoms or diagnostic criteria (Lennard, 1971; Conrad, 1985; Pearce, 1996). There have been many examples of medications being promoted for "problems of life." These have included: the inability to cope with ordinary tension and emotional pressures, difficulties in personal relationships, stressful occupations, and even life in an urban setting.

Medicalization, however, can also involve "natural life processes." This is evidenced in the reconceptualization of mildly elevated blood pressure without apparent symptoms into the medical condition called hypertension (Kawachi and Conrad, 1996). This example is important because it differs from many other cases of medicalization in that elevated blood pressure can be measured, though the meaning of the measurement can be contested, yet does not involve a visible condition. In addition, it is not viewed as a disease itself, but as a risk factor for other medical conditions. With the development of antihypertensive drugs, "therapeutic empiricism, associated with the motto 'Control the hypertension and treat the disease,' replaced therapeutic rationalism as the dominant paradigm" (Kawachi and Conrad, 1996).

Though perhaps abstract in presentation, the cultural conceptions discussed in this chapter become most relevant in life when they serve to define and direct a society's authorized or approved uses of a drug, together with its channels of drug distribution and availability (Basara and Montagne, 1994). The distribution and use of drugs are either specified by codified law (formal social controls) or guided by ritual, custom, or social sanction (informal social controls). These controls can differ across cultures and within cultures, and they can vary over time (Zinberg, 1984).

In prescription drug use the role of health professionals is that of gatekeeper.

They provide access to drugs that are viewed as effective, but potentially unsafe. Thus prescribers exert greater influence and control over the drugs and are provided with professional conceptions that dominate drug taking decisions. The balance of power therefore shifts to the physician, the pharmacist, and the pharmaceutical manufacturer. In nonprescription (over-the-counter) drug use, however, consumers exert greater control through self-medication. While the symbolic paraphernalia of medical practice are less prominent in these circumstances (though they can be more important when health professional supervision is sought by the self-medicating patient) the distinction between prescription and nonprescription drug status is primarily legal in nature. It is adhered to more by the drug makers and drug givers than by the drug takers, and is ignored by those consumers who have gained power over drug taking decisions. These distinctions are being obscured or eliminated for many drug consumers with direct-to-consumer prescription drug advertising, prescription-to-nonprescription status switches, and prescription drug importation.

## Conclusion

It may be that the great strength of Western medicine, its intense technological development and the use of synthetic drug products, is also its major weakness. Has medicine become too reliant on the primary, or even universal, use of technology to solve problems (which in a majority of cases means therapeutic intervention with chemical substances)? Drug makers have tipped the balance of power in their favor through the evolution of the concept of the magic bullet this century. This mirrors very closely the growth and development of the pharmaceutical industry in western societies (Basara and Montagne, 1994). From the drug manufacturer's perspective the ideal drug would be inexpensive to make, protected by world wide patent, suitable for world wide promotion, create a mild psychological dependence in its users, give the appearance of answering some expressed medical need, and be free of unmanageable side effects (Melville and Johnson, 1982).

Drug regulators and policy makers attempt to maintain a balance, with the public interested in safe and effective drugs at as low a cost as possible and the drug industry focused on pursuing economic growth, profit, and autonomy. The potential perils in this balancing act are exemplified in Pearce's (1996) case study of two asthma mortality epidemics. This process is also problematic when the regulators and policy makers consist disproportionately of individuals sharing one particular view of the world. On some occasions attempts to protect one group of patients have arguably resulted in the premature removal of useful drug therapies—for example, Bendectin®, Halcion®—thus obstructing optimal care for another group of patients (Montagne and Bleidt, 1987). On other occasions—especially those involving diseases for which truly effective drug therapies have not been developed, such as AIDS, Alzheimer's disease, many cancers and psychiatric conditions—consumer activism sometimes has superseded the scientific research process, often to the detriment of the very patients whom these efforts are intended to assist.

In order to improve the therapeutic use of drugs there is a need for a better understanding of the social knowledge generated by different cultural conceptions. There also needs to be an appreciation of the conceptions about drugs which dominate research, practice, and policy. Scientists, educators, health professionals, and consumers all have their own cultural mind-sets about drugs and drug use. It is necessary to acknowledge them and to recognize—through symbols, images, and metaphors—the perceptions being portrayed in words and actions. Only then will society's ability to promote optimally safe and effective drug use be enhanced. There is a need to adopt approaches to the direction and monitoring of drug use that integrate the various conceptions and viewpoints, thus expanding our ability to identify and prevent, or limit, drug problems. There is also a need to focus more on behaviors, the how and why of drug taking, particularly those behaviors that put users at greater risk of developing problems.

In the end, an appropriate balance may be achieved through the proper management of health care technology. Does society possess the social maturity and ethical wisdom to control the power associated with drugs for human needs and for the public good, or will that power be used for exploitation and private gain? Some contemporary philosophers have argued that our industrialized world is evolving more rapidly than our moral and cultural development, leaving society poorly prepared to deploy technological advances, such as drugs, in a wise manner (Veatch, 1977). The processes of drug development and use have become institutionalized in western societies. It is therefore now necessary for those societies to address these institutions in a more conscious fashion, remedying imbalances in power when and where they occur.

# References

Anthony JC (1983) The regulation of dangerous psychoactive drugs. In: Morgan JP and Kagan DV (eds.) *Society and Medication: Conflicting Signals for Prescribers and Patients*. Lexington, MA: DC Heath Co., pp. 163–80.

Arluke A (1980) Judging drugs: patients' conceptions of therapeutic efficacy in the treatment of arthritis. *Human Organization* 39: 84–8.

Basara LR and Montagne M (1994) *Searching for Magic Bullets: Orphan Drugs, Consumer Activism, and Pharmaceutical Development*. New York: Haworth Press.

Becker HS (1967) History, culture, and subjective experience: an explanation of the social bases of drug-induced experiences. *Journal of Health and Social Behavior* 8: 163–86.

Benjamin M, Muyskens J and Saenger P (1984) Short children, anxious parents: is growth hormone the answer? *Hastings Center Report* 14: 5–9.

Berger P and Luckmann T (1966) *The Social Construction of Reality*. Garden City, NY: Doubleday.

Bledsoe CH and Goubaud MF (1985) The reinterpretation of Western pharmaceuticals among the Mende of Sierra Leone. *Social Science and Medicine* 21: 275–82.

Burr A (1984) The ideologies of despair: a symbolic interpretation of the punks' and skinheads' use of barbiturates. *Social Science and Medicine* 19: 929–38.

Cohen S (1983) Current attitudes about benzodiazepines: trial by media. *Journal of Psychoactive Drugs* 15: 109–13.

Conrad P (1985) The meaning of medications: another look at compliance. *Social Science and Medicine* 20:29–37.

Cooperstock R (ed.) (1974) *Social Aspects of the Medical Use of Psychotropic Drugs*. Toronto: Addiction Research Foundation.

Cooperstock R and Lennard HL (1979) Some social meanings of tranquilizer use. *Sociology of Health and Illness* 1: 331–47.

Delgado JN and Remers W (1991) *Wilson and Gisvold's Textbook of Organic Medicinal and Pharmaceutical Chemistry*, 9th ed. Philadelphia, PA: Lippincott.

DeRios MD (1976) *The Wilderness of Mind: Sacred Plants in Cross-Cultural Perspective*. Beverly Hills, CA: Sage.

DeRios MD and Smith DE (1977) The function of drug rituals in human society: continuities and changes. *Journal of Psychedelic Drugs* 9: 269–75.

De Toit BM (ed.) (1977) *Drugs, Rituals and Altered States of Consciousness*. Rotterdam: AA Balkema.

Dubos R (1964) On the present limitations of drug research. In: Talalay P (ed.) *Drugs In Our Society*. Baltimore: Johns Hopkins University Press, pp. 37–45.

Edwards G and Arif A (1980) *Drug Problems in the Sociocultural Context: A Basis for Policies and Programme Planning*. Public Health Paper #73. Geneva: World Health Organization.

Everett MW, Waddell JO and Heath DB (eds.) (1976) *Cross-Cultural Approaches to the Study of Alcohol*. The Hague: Mouton.

Feinstein AR (1985) *Clinical Epidemiology: The Architecture of Clinical Research*. Philadelphia, PA: Saunders.

Gabe J and Bury M (1996) Anxious times: The benzodiazepine controversy and the fracturing of expert authority. In: Davis PB (ed.) *Contested Ground: Public Purpose and Private Interest in the Regulation of Prescription Drugs*. New York: Oxford University Press, pp. 42–56.

Gilman AG et al. (eds.) (1990) *Goodman and Gilman's The Pharmacological Basis of Therapeutics*, 8th ed. New York: Macmillan.

Gusfield JR (1981) *The Culture of Public Problems: Drinking-Driving and the Symbolic Order*. Chicago: University of Chicago Press.

Habermas J (1984) *Theory of Communicative Action*, Vol. I. Boston, MA: Beacon Press.

Habermas J (1987) *Theory of Communicative Action*, Vol. II. Boston, MA: Beacon Press.

Helman CG (1981) "Tonic," "fuel," and "food": social and symbolic aspects of the long-term use of psychotropic drugs. *Social Science and Medicine* 15B: 521–33.

Hofmann A (1996) Planned research and chance discovery in pharmaceutical development. In: Bleidt B and Montagne M (eds.) *Clinical Research in Pharmaceutical Development*. New York: Marcel Dekker, in press.

Holmes HB, Hoskins BB and Gross M (eds.) (1980) *Birth Control and Controlling Birth: Women-Centered Perspectives*. Clifton, NJ: Humana Press.

Johnson M (ed.) (1981) *Philosophical Perspectives on Metaphor*. Minneapolis: University of Minnesota Press.

Jonsen AR (1988) Ethics of drug giving and drug taking. *Journal of Drug Issues* 18: 195–200.

Kawachi I and Conrad P (1996) Medicalization and the pharmacological treatment of blood pressure. In: Davis PB (ed.) *Contested Ground: Public Purpose and Private Interest in the Regulation of Prescription Drugs*. New York: Oxford University Press, pp. 26–41.

Kuhn TS (1970) *The Structure of Scientific Revolutions*, 2nd ed. Chicago: University of Chicago Press.

Lakoff G and Johnson M (1980) *Metaphors We Live By*. Chicago: University of Chicago Press.

Lennard HL (1971) *Mystification and Drug Misuse*. San Francisco: Jossey-Bass.

Mannheim K (1968) *Ideology and Utopia: An Introduction to the Sociology of Knowledge*. New York: Harcourt, Brace and World.

McCarthy RL and Montagne M (1992) Public perceptions and the therapeutic use of heroin. In: Trebach AS and Zeese KB (eds.) *Strategies for Change: New Directions In Drug Policy*. Washington, DC: Drug Policy Foundation, pp. 124–32.

Melville A and Johnson C (1982) *Cured to Death: The Effects of Prescription Drugs*. New York: Stein and Day.

Mintzes B and Hodgkin C (1996) The consumer movement: From single-issue campaigns to long-term reform. In: Davis PB (ed.) *Contested Ground: Public Purpose and Private Interest in the Regulation of Prescription Drugs*. New York: Oxford University Press, pp. 76–91.

Montagne M (1984) Social knowledge and experiences with legal highs. *Journal of Drug Issues* 14: 491–507.

Montagne M (1988) The metaphorical nature of drugs and drug taking. *Social Science and Medicine* 26: 417–24.

Montagne M (1991) The culture of long-term tranquilliser users: In: Gabe J (ed.) *Understanding Tranquilliser Use: The Role of the Social Sciences*. London: Tavistock/Routledge, pp. 48–68.

Montagne M (1992) The promotion of medications for personal and social problems. *Journal of Drug Issues* 22: 389–405.

Montagne M (1996) The nature and meaning of drug taking experiences: toward a social pharmacological theory of drug effects. *International Journal of the Addictions*, in press.

Montagne M and Bleidt BA (1987) Social forces in the premature removal of drug products from the marketplace. *Clinical Research Practices and Drug Regulatory Affairs* 5: 83–127.

Morgan JP (1983) Cultural and medical attitudes toward benzodiazepines: conflicting metaphors. *Journal of Psychoactive Drugs* 15: 115–20.

Orcutt JD (1978) Normative definitions of intoxicated states: a test of several sociological theories. *Social Problems* 25: 385–96.

Pearce N (1996) Adverse reactions, social responses: A tale of two asthma mortality epidemics. In: Davis PB (ed.) *Contested Ground: Public Purpose and Private Interest in the Regulation of Prescription Drugs*. New York: Oxford University Press, pp. 57–75.

Rhodes LA (1984) "This will clear your mind": the use of metaphors for medication in psychiatric settings. *Culture, Medicine and Psychiatry* 8: 49–70.

Rubin V (ed.) (1975) *Cannabis and Culture*. The Hague: Mouton.

Sacks S (ed.) (1979) *On Metaphor*. Chicago: University of Chicago Press.

Svarstad BL (1989) Sociology of drugs in health care. In: Wertheimer AL and Smith MC (eds.) *Pharmacy Practice: Social and Behavioral Aspects*, 3rd ed. Baltimore, MD: Williams and Wilkins, pp. 197–211.

Szasz T (1974) *Ceremonial Chemistry: The Ritual Persecution of Drugs, Addicts, and Pushers*. New York: Doubleday.

Veatch RM (1977) Value foundations for drug use. *Journal of Drug Issues* 7: 253–62.

Wallace AFC (1959) Cultural determinants of response to hallucinatory experience. *Archives of General Psychiatry* 1: 58–69.

Wuketits FM (ed.) *Concepts and Approaches in Evolutionary Epistemology*. Norwell, MA: Kluwer Academic.

Young J (1971) *The Drugtakers: The Social Meaning of Drug Use*. London: Paladin.

Zinberg NE (1984) *Drugs, Set and Setting*. New Haven, CT: Yale University Press.

# 2

# Medicalization and the Pharmacological Treatment of Blood Pressure

ICHIRO KAWACHI
PETER CONRAD

Blood pressure, like breathing, is a physiological property common to all animals born with a circulatory system. The existence of pressure in the arterial stream was first demonstrated in 1733 by Stephen Hales, an English clergyman. He stuck a goose quill in the carotid artery of a horse, fastened a long glass tube to the quill, and used this device to measure the resulting column of blood (about 9 feet). However, 143 years elapsed before an instrument was invented that could measure blood pressure in humans (Vertes et al., 1991). Even after the invention of the sphygmomanometer (blood pressure cuff), the meaning of elevated blood pressure was not appreciated. Well into the 1920s, physicians regularly measured blood pressure but considered an elevated level to be a harmless manifestation of the aging process (Farrar, 1991).

## The Medicalization Framework

This chapter examines how elevated blood pressure has become increasingly medicalized in the twentieth century. In general, *medicalization* is a process by which nonmedical problems become defined and treated as medical problems, usually in terms of illnesses and disorders (Zola, 1972; Conrad, 1992). While the medicalization of deviance has received much analytical attention (e.g., Conrad and Schneider, 1980a), there has also been considerable medicalization of what might be called "natural life processes." These include sexuality, childbirth, child development, menstrual discomfort (PMS), menopause, aging, and death (see Conrad, 1992). In all cases, new problems have been brought into medical jurisdiction, often leading to medical treatments.

Medicalization is a "process by which more and more of everyday life has come under medical dominion, influence and supervision" (Zola, 1983: 295). As Conrad (1975: 12) notes, it involves "defining behavior as a medical problem or illness and mandating the medical profession to provide some kind of treatment for it." It consists of "defining a problem in medical terms, using medical language to describe the problem, adopting a medical framework to understand the problem, or using a medical intervention to treat it" (Conrad, 1992: 211). In the case of elevated blood pressure, the issue is not defining behavior, but defining a naturally occurring attribute as a medical problem.

## Levels of Medicalization

Medicalization can occur on three distinct levels: the conceptual, the institutional, and the interactional (Conrad and Schneider, 1980b) (see Table 2-1). On the conceptual level, a medical vocabulary (or model) is used to order or define the problem at hand; few medical professionals need to be involved and medical treatments are not necessarily applied. On the institutional level, organizations may adapt a medical approach to treating a particular problem in which the organization specializes. Physicians may function as gatekeepers for benefits that are only legitimate in organizations that adopt a medical definition and approach to a problem, but where the everyday routine work is accomplished by nonmedical personnel. On the interac-

TABLE 2-1.   Levels of Medicalization

| *Level* | *Key Issue* | *Examples* |
|---|---|---|
| Conceptual | Medical vocabulary (or model) used to define the problem | Alcoholics Anonymous use of medical model; "battered child syndrome" for abuse of children; PMS; defining homosexuality as an illness |
| Institutional | Organizations adopt a medical approach; physicians function as gatekeepers to benefits | Alcoholism or substance abuse hospitals that adopt a medical approach but use primarily lay counselors; physicians certifying disability benefits |
| Interactional | Physicians define (diagnose) a problem as medical and/or provide a medical treatment | Medical diagnosis for behavioral (e.g., hyperactivity in children, chronic fatigue, or eating disorders) or body (e.g., obesity, menopause, or infertility) problems or providing medical treatment (e.g., drugs) without a specific medical diagnosis |

tional level, physicians are directly involved. Medicalization occurs as part of doctor-patient interaction, when a physician defines a problem as medical (e.g., gives a diagnosis) or treats a social problem with a medical form of treatment (e.g., prescribing tranquilizer drugs for an unhappy family life).

While this conceptualization is useful for showing the breadth of medicalization, it also illustrates that medicalization is not necessarily "medical imperialism," as some have argued (e.g., Illich, 1976), but rather that only a few physicians may be involved in medicalizing problems on the conceptual or institutional levels. Physicians surely have colonized certain problems such as childbirth, but just as often lay interests have championed the medicalization of human problems (see Conrad and Schneider, 1980a).

Pharmaceuticals and the pharmaceutical industry can affect medicalization on each of these levels. On the conceptual level, the promotion of a particular drug can help to define a problem as medical, even if the drug treatment is only rarely adopted. For example, the promotion of estrogen replacement therapy (ERT) for menopause has increased the medicalization of menopause as an illness, although at least one study shows the use of hormone treatments for symptoms is relatively low (Kaufert and Gilbert, 1986). On the institutional level, pharmaceuticals may be used for reasons that appear marginally medical. For example, the most common drugs prescribed in nursing homes are psychoactive medications, which are used more to control the behavior of patients than to treat an illness (Vladeck, 1980). On the interactional level, when physicians prescribe drugs like Valium for life problems, Prozac as a mood brightener, or prescribe diet pills for obesity, with or without medical diagnoses, medicalization has taken place.

## The Case of Blood Pressure

Using this conceptualization, we argue that blood pressure has been medicalized in the twentieth century. Of particular interest is how mildly elevated blood pressure without apparent symptoms has become a medical problem. We suggest that elevated blood pressure was first medicalized on the conceptual level as hypertension, and more recently in organizations through blood pressure screenings, and, most significantly, by physicians in their diagnosis of hypertension as a risk factor or illness and prescribing pharmaceutical treatment. Of particular interest are the contests around what constitutes hypertension (i.e., at what point measured blood pressure is defined as diseased) and the role of drug treatment in the expansion of the category of potential pathology.

In some respects, however, elevated blood pressure is different from other cases of medicalization. First, it is identified because it can be measured. Most elevated blood pressure is not noticeable unless it is measured by a sphygmomanometer. In medical terms, it is asymptomatic. It does not involve visible conditions like pregnancy, discomforts like PMS, or behavioral problems like alcoholism or hyperactivity. Second, not only is the ability to measure critical for blood pressure medicalization, but the meaning of the measurement, at least for some values, is contested. Thus there has been debate over what defines hypertension; where does one set the points of pathology and normality? Third, hypertension is not actually a disease in itself, but it is a risk factor for a variety of maladies. The problem is not that mildly or moderately elevated blood pressure directly affects functioning or behavior, but rather when it is uncontrolled it is deemed to increase the risk of other diseases (especially stroke and coronary heart disease). Finally, as with mental illness and hyperactivity, the pharmaceutical industry has been deeply involved in defining hypertension as a medical problem and promoting its treatment.

## Evolution of Hypertension as a Disease

### *"Judicious Neglect"*

The earliest recognition of the prognostic significance of elevated blood pressure came from insurance company data. In 1914, J. W. Fisher, of the Northwestern Mutual Life Insurance Company, was one of the first to demonstrate that a persistent increase of 15 mmHg in systolic blood pressure was associated with an unexpected rise in the mortality rate. Hence, he concluded that a deviation in systolic pressure of 15 mmHg or more above the age-specific norm should be regarded as pathological (Fisher, 1914). Subsequently, a large number of insurance company studies bearing similar conclusions were published throughout the 1920s, 1930s, and 1940s (Master et al., 1952). However, none of these studies made an impact on medical practice.

A general attitude of judicious neglect toward elevated blood pressure prevailed in the medical profession right up to the 1950s. Treatment was regarded as unwarranted except in the most severe and symptomatic forms of blood pressure elevation. In the early 1950s, a classification of elevated blood pressure was devised (Schroeder, 1953). Action was only called for in cases of "severe hypertension" (diastolic pressure between 120–160 mmHg), and "malignant hypertension" (diastolic pressure between 130–200 mmHg). Unfortunately, even when action was taken in cases of malignant hypertension, the results were not always clear-cut.

### *Effective Therapy*

The earliest effective therapeutic options for the treatment of malignant hypertension were rather draconian. The choices were between the extremely restrictive Kempner rice diet (1944), or surgical procedures such as surgical interruption of the sympathic nervous system (1951) or bilateral surgical removal of the adrenal glands (1952).

The introduction of ganglion blocker drugs for the treatment of hypertension in 1951 (Smirk and Alstad, 1951) is regarded as the beginning of the modern era of antihypertensive drug treatment. Although the effects of treatment were dramatic, it became apparent that the side effects of drug therapy were the limiting factor in broadening its general applicability. Patients who had previously been going blind or who had been disabled by heart failure were willing to tolerate the very significant discomforts induced by this form of treatment, but patients with less severe hypertension, particularly if asymptomatic, were understandably less compliant (Doyle, 1982).

A further breakthrough came with the discovery of thiazide diuretics in 1956. Here was the first class of drug that was effective at lowering blood pressure, could be administered by mouth instead of intravenously, and appeared to be well-tolerated. Other classes of drugs followed in quick succession. In hindsight, it is clear that the availability of these therapeutic regimens provided the impetus for the medicalization of blood pressure. Epidemiology has identified more than 240 risk factors for cardiovascular disease, including short stature, baldness, and being married to women in white collar jobs. Yet only a tiny fraction of risk factors has been medicalized so far, one reason being that there are no drugs available to treat the majority of identified risk factors.

## Preconditions for the Medicalization of Blood Pressure

### Treatment Moves out into the Community

The earliest antihypertensive drugs, such as the ganglion blockers, were associated with quite severe side effects. Consequently they were administered under close medical supervision in specialist clinics ("hypertension clinics"). The patient population at the time also reflected a more severe case mix. Most of the patients were symptomatic and felt ill (Dollery, 1982). Malignant hypertension was associated with a mortality rate of 90% in the first year after diagnosis. Emergency admission to the hospital was required for such patients, and the patient could quite legitimately adopt the sick role.

As the flood of new drug discoveries throughout the 1960s made treatment safer and easier to administer, the risk-benefit ratio of treatment shifted, and indications for the use of antihypertensive drugs were progressively widened. The definition of what constituted hypertension began to shift. Since the 1970s, most hypertensive patients have been cared for mainly by family physicians within the community, and the hypertension clinic only becomes involved when patients develop complications or fail to respond to conventional regimens. The development of effective, easily tolerated drugs thus opened the way for the mass medication of the population.

### Therapeutic Empiricism

Before 1950, the treatment of hypertension was never seriously considered because of a general belief that effective treatment of a disease was impossible without knowing the cause. The credo of this rationalistic approach to medicine was, "Find the cause and the treatment will become obvious." By contrast, once an array of effective, relatively safe drugs became available, the approach to the treatment of hypertension was reversed virtually overnight. Therapeutic empiricism, associated with the motto "Control the hypertension and treat the disease," replaced therapeutic rationalism as the dominant paradigm.

One of the consequences of therapeutic empiricism was the uncritical expansion of therapy to populations with mildly and moderately elevated blood pressure, even before rigorous proof of benefit was available in the form of randomized trials. This was assisted by the fact that the dividing line between normotension and hypertension is essentially arbitrary. Apart from the difference in pressure level itself, there is no identifiable biological property that marks the passage from health to disease. Even before the widespread use of effective drug therapy, the definition of hypertension fluctuated from year to year, and from one author to another (Table 2-2, adapted from Pickering, 1974).

The need for medicine to work within the framework of binary choices (either diseased or normal) has had enormous implications for the medical labeling of large sections of the general population. For example, according to Robinson and Brucer's definition of hypertension devised in 1939 (Table 2-2), nearly half of the U.S. population could be considered diseased. The authors defined it along the following lines: "Whatever the method of selecting any physiologic norm, the level cannot be interpreted medically as 'normal' *unless it is consistent with the longest possible life*" (emphasis added) (Robinson and Brucer, 1939: 442).

In the pursuit of the longest possible life, the labeling of large sections of the general population as abnormal is a characteristic shared by other common problems such as menopause, which is now defined as an estrogen-deficiency state (McCrea, 1983; Bell, 1987), and blue moods, increasingly viewed by some as a Prozac-deficiency syndrome!

### The Role of the Pharmaceutical Industry

The medicalization of blood pressure could not have been achieved without the massive investment of the pharmaceutical industry in developing a wide array of drugs. It seems remarkably prescient of the industry to have committed significant resources to develop new drugs during an era of therapeutic nihilism such as occurred before the 1950s.

In fact, there were several indications of the potential for antihypertensive drugs to become best sellers in the market: first, hypertension was (and continues to be) regarded as incurable, and hence drug treatment is lifelong. The discovery of hypertension in a patient is the starting point for decades of profitable drug therapy. Second, the infrastructure of the medical-industrial complex was already in place for

TABLE 2-2. Some Blood Pressure Levels
Suggested as Dividing Lines Between
Normotension and Hypertension

| Blood Pressure | Author |
| --- | --- |
| 140/80 | Ayman (1934) |
| 120/80 | Robinson and Brucer (1939) |
| 160/100 | Bechgaard (1946) |
| 180/100 | Burgess (1948) |
| 140/90 | Perera (1948) |
| 150/90 | Thomas (1952) |
| 180/100 | Evans (1956) |

the mass marketing of antihypertensive drugs to proceed. Mention has already been made of the devolution of treatment from specialists to generalists, and the shift in location of treatment away from hospitals into the community. The screening industry was similarly poised in the 1950s for a major campaign to detect hypertension in the general population. The non-invasive, portable nature of the sphygmomanometer meant that blood pressure screening could be carried out just as easily in "the corner drug store, street corner, or Atlantic City Boardwalk," as in the physician's office (Chasis, 1986: 936).

Third, owing to the arbitrary nature of the definition of hypertension, there was a high likelihood that need for treatment would be continually redefined by the medical profession to include increasing numbers of patients, a pattern that has also been evident in the case of blood cholesterol (Payer, 1992).

Fourth, the treatment of hypertension was congruent with a fee-for-service system of physician remuneration. By 1930, it was already apparent that hypertension was the most common diagnostic finding in office practice (Cabot, 1926). Therapeutic control of blood pressure with medication requires daily doses, and hence constant surveillance by physicians of both blood pressure levels and side effects of medication. The incentives for more aggressive screening and surveillance are greater under a fee-for-service system of physician remuneration.

The fifth reason for the successful diffusion of antihypertensive drugs was the fact that the timing of their introduction coincided with the rise of preventive medicine and epidemiology. Freis (1982a: 67) pointed out that before 1950, preventive medicine was not popular: "It failed to excite the imagination of either physicians or of the media." This attitude had changed by 1972, as is evident in an editorial written by the principal investigators of the Framingham Study (Gordon and Kannel, 1972: 565): "Prevention of cardiovascular disease may actually require the evolution of a new breed of physician and associated medical personnel concerned with adult preventive medicine."

Last, and perhaps most important, the twentieth century epidemic of coronary heart disease was approaching its peak in the 1950s (Stallones, 1980), and mass screening and treatment of hypertension came to be identified as one of the major planks of a national prevention policy. As will be apparent, the pharmaceutical industry remains a major player in the medicalization of hypertension.

## Recent Developments

### The Era of Therapeutic Enthusiasm

If the period before 1950 was the era of therapeutic nihilism, then the period from 1959 to 1985 could be characterized as the era of unbounded therapeutic enthusiasm.

In 1959, the Society of Actuaries published their Build and Blood Pressure Study, based on information gathered from 3.9 million policy holders between 1935 and 1954 (Society of Actuaries, 1959). The data were consistent with all the previous insurance studies that had been published up to that time, finding that mortality was smoothly and continuously related to successive elevations of blood pressure, with no discernible boundary between normal and abnormal. Whereas none of the previous insurance studies influenced clinical practice, in the era after the introduction of drugs, the new study was hailed as a landmark.

Nonetheless, the benefits of treating the less severe forms of hypertension continued to arouse controversy (Goldring and Chasis, 1966). Continuing uncertainty and debate provided the stimulus for the first randomized trial of treating mild-to-moderate hypertension, the Veterans Administration (VA) Cooperative Study on Antihypertensive Agents. The results, published in 1970 (VA Cooperative Study Group, 1970), suggesting a benefit of drug treatment even among individuals with mild elevations of blood pressure, sufficiently impressed the Secretary of Health, Education and Welfare, Elliot Richardson, that in July 1972 he launched the National High Blood Pressure Education Program (NHBPEP).

The NHBPEP developed two initiatives that had a lasting impact on antihypertensive therapy—namely, the formation of the Joint National Committee (JNC) on Detection, Evaluation, and Treatment of High Blood Pressure, which was to become the foremost body of U.S. experts on policies regarding hypertension control; and the initiation of the Hypertension Detection and Follow-up Program (HDFP), a multicenter randomized trial of treating mild-to-moderate hypertension in the community (HDFP Cooperative Group, 1979).

The lowering of the threshold for drug treatment of hypertension can be traced through the successive recommendations of the JNC. In its first report, the JNC advised that drug treatment was indicated for persons whose diastolic pressures exceeded 105 mmHg (JNC, 1977). In its next report, the JNC was much more demonstrative in recommending drug treatment for all patients with diastolic pressures above 90 mmHg (JNC, 1980). The difference between recommending drug treatment above 105 mmHg and above 90 mmHg diastolic is not trivial, since 85% of the total hypertensive population belong in this range, and hence qualified for treatment under the new definition of "disease."

Pharmaceutical advertisements in medical journals during this period reflect the emergent aggressive stance toward control of hypertension. In a full-page spread that appeared in a 1974 issue of the *American Journal of Cardiology*, drug therapy of apparently healthy persons with mild hypertension was already being advocated (years before the publication of the first JNC report). A 1977 advertisement for Catapres (clonidine, Boehringer Ingelheim), also appearing in the *American Journal of Cardiology*, implicitly claimed that lowering mild to moderate elevations of blood pressure can prevent heart attack—a claim that has still failed to be borne out by clinical trials 16 years after the advertisement appeared.

## Seeds of Discord

A virtual cascade of conferences, symposia, and editorials was unleashed during the decade of therapeutic enthusiasm, 1974 to 1985. However, not all the voices raised after the publication of the HDFP trial results were unanimously in favor of drug treatment. For example, Freis (1982b) and others (Peart and Miall, 1980) drew attention to serious methodological defects of the HDFP trial.

Further reservations about the mass treatment of hypertension appeared from an unexpected quarter—biomedical ethics. Guttmacher et al. (1981) and Brett (1984) drew attention to serious ethical dilemmas in the treatment of borderline hypertension. They questioned the wisdom of treating large numbers of asymptomatic people with drugs. The effects of the disease are probabilistic, as are drug benefits. On the other hand, taking any drug is associated with real risks of side effects.

These authors were also among the first to recognize that the overemphasis on pharmacological control of blood pressure had resulted in a neglect of social determinants, as shown by cross-cultural, social class, and racial differences in the prevalence of hypertension. They argued that adopting a purely medical approach was a way of dealing with the consequences of elevated blood pressure without addressing the underlying social order that increases risks for the disease.

### Therapeutic Retreat?

One of the crucial issues that remained unresolved by all the trials before 1985 was whether treating mild hypertension prevented coronary heart disease. With the publication of successive trials failing to demonstrate the efficacy of drugs at reversing coronary risk, commentators and experts nervously deferred their final verdict until the publication of the results of the largest clinical trial then in progress—the British Medical Research Council (MRC) trial on mild hypertension.

The MRC trial, started in 1977 and published in 1985, was by far the largest ($N = 17,354$) blinded, placebo-controlled trial of drug therapy for mild to moderate hypertension in history (MRC Working Party, 1985). If any trial was capable of definitively showing the effects of drug therapy on reversal of coronary risk, this was it. Consequently, the trial results caught everyone by surprise when it was announced that, "If 850 mildly hypertensive subjects are given active antihypertensive drugs for one year, about one stroke will be prevented. . . . Treatment did not appear to save lives or substantially alter the overall risk of coronary heart disease" (MRC Working Party, 1985: 104).

Fortunately for the medical care and pharmaceutical industries, the ultimate success of an innovation frequently has little to do with its intrinsic worth, but depends on the power of the interests that sponsor and maintain it (McKinlay, 1981). Even before the 1985 publication of the MRC trial results, the pharmaceutical industry had turned its attention to the next marketing strategy that would ensure the continued prescription of drugs to treat mild hypertension. That marketing strategy focused not so much on disease or prevention but emphasized quality of life.

### Reformulation of the Goals of Therapy

One of the major driving forces behind the concept of quality of life was consumer dissatisfaction with the biomedical model. Beginning in the 1970s, criticisms of medical care and skepticism of the value of health interventions emanated from major consumer groups, including women, minorities, and the holistic health movement (Illich, 1976; Ruzek, 1978).

Beginning in about 1984, the pharmaceutical industry seized upon the concept of quality of life and succeeded in appropriating it for use as a novel marketing tool. The advertisements of competing pharmaceutical manufacturers now make routine claims about the favorable impact of their products on aspects of quality of life, such as libido, mood, and general feelings of well-being. There has been a dramatic increase in the number of published studies that mention the expression "quality of life." The pharmaceutical industry has actively promoted the concept by producing journals with titles such as *Quality of Life and Cardiovascular Care* (Wenger, 1984), and financing numerous clinical trials.

In recent years, small clinical trials comparing the quality of life impacts of individual products have become a burgeoning cottage industry. Comparisons have been published for a stupefying combination of drugs. What is quite clear is that drug companies are financing such studies primarily for marketing purposes—to gain an edge on competitors. The rationale for antihypertensive therapy has been lost amidst the avalanche of these studies. Improving the quality of life has become a therapeutic goal in itself. By making drug treatment more acceptable in people's lives, the motive behind the industry's focus on quality of life appears to be to divert attention from the more fundamental question of whether such treatment is needed in the first place (Kawachi and Wilson, 1990). Quality of life is not the problem. Elevated blood pressure, and how we should go about preventing it and its consequences, is the problem.

## Antihypertensive Therapy—an Assessment

The virtual eradication of malignant and severe hypertension by drugs is justly regarded as a triumph of modern medicine. There is no question that the small fraction of people with severe and symptomatic elevations of blood pressure are at greatly increased risk of catastrophic disease, and consequently they demand urgent care.

On the other hand, treatment of hypertension is no longer a matter of putting symptomatic people on drugs. Modern antihypertensive therapy is about screening and identifying symptomless people in the general population considered to be at risk of developing disease, then starting them on drugs that in themselves impose real risks and are associated with uncertain benefits. The medicalization of mild and moderate blood pressure elevations has resulted in enormous numbers of people identified and treated with drugs. By 1984, antihypertensive medications were being taken on a daily basis by approximately 30% of U.S. adults aged 55 to 64 years, and over 40% of people aged 65 to 74 years (Havlik et al., 1989). They have become one of the best selling prescription drugs in the U.S. and elsewhere.

The most enduring legacy of adopting a biomedical approach to solve the problem of hypertension may turn out to be the neglect of sociocultural approaches to prevent it. It has long been known that elevated blood pressure is rarely seen in hunter-gatherer or pastoral subsistence societies. Cultural characteristics, such as a greater involvement in a money economy and more economic competition, have been found to correlate strongly with a rising prevalence of hypertension (Waldron et al., 1982). By extrapolation, the causes of elevated blood pressure are, to a significant extent, social. An established tradition of psychosocial research has demonstrated the relationship of blood pressure levels to acculturation (Dressler, 1984), status inconsistency (including "John Henryism" among U.S. black populations) (James, 1987), unemployment (Kasl and Cobb, 1970), social class and race (Williams, 1992), and job stress (Schnall et al., 1990; 1992). Yet with few exceptions, a sociocultural perspective has rarely informed policies dealing with America's "foremost public health problem." It is almost as though advances in technical solutions to control hypertension led to the simultaneous and progressive atrophy of interest in addressing its underlying social causes.

The alternative path is exemplified by the approach that Syme and colleagues have developed to deal with the problem of hypertension among San Francisco bus drivers (Syme, 1991). Previous studies had identified bus drivers to be at high risk of developing hypertension (Ragland et al., 1987). Whereas a conventional biomedical approach might have been to put the drivers on antihypertensive therapy, or to offer them individual counseling and relaxation, Syme and colleagues identified strategies that address the sources of stress in their social environment, such as changing the way schedules were arranged, or locating rest stops near city centers so that the normally socially isolated drivers would be more likely to meet other drivers (Syme, 1991).

Until now, such social interventions have not received the level of funding that drug trials have. Whether these approaches turn out to be as successful as drug therapy remains to be shown. But the crucial step before demonstrating the power of such approaches has to be to shift the concentration of resources away from drug therapy and toward primary prevention. Then the process of demedicalization would begin.

## The Legacy of Medicalization

What does the medicalization of blood pressure tell us about the process of medicalization? This is not a classic case of medical imperialism, since physicians already had jurisdiction over malignant hypertension and there were no contesting owners of the problem of blood pressure (Gusfield, 1981). Yet this is clearly an example of how the availability of a treatment (antihypertensive drugs) and an aggressive pharmaceutical industry can contribute to the expansion of the definition of hypertension and the promotion of widespread treatment of symptomless elevated blood pressure. The epidemiological paradigm that designated high blood pressure as a risk factor for heart disease and the various government reports that proposed screening and treatment certainly contributed to medicalizing elevated blood pressure.

The case of hypertension highlights several significant issues around medicalization. These can be termed the muddles of measurement, the social consequences of pharmaceutical intervention, and the dilemmas of the sick role.

### Muddles of Measurement

Compared to most other cases of medicalization, hypertension seems direct and straightforward. After all, blood pressure can be measured in consistent quantitative terms. For many other medicalized problems, diagnostic measurement is typically based on clinical observation of behaviors, and is usually inexact (e.g., hyperactivity, alcoholism). In other cases, clinical measurement is based on subjective experience (e.g., menopause, PMS) or experiential outcome (e.g., infertility, pregnancy). Obesity is one of the few medicalized conditions where a quantitative measure is significant: a certain percentage above ideal weight in terms of sex, height, and body type. But even with obesity, measurements are often subjective, based on appearance rather than rigid quantitative measurement. The question remains, however, not if there are measurable differences, but how are those differences characterized and with what consequences?

Mild and moderate hypertension is, of course, a function of the ability to measure blood pressure and attributing meaning to various measurements. Similar to many other examples of medicalized problems, there is nothing intrinsic in any level of blood pressure, except in rare instances of malignant hypertension, that designates it as illness or even a risk factor. It is the meanings medicine places on these measurements that makes them significant. In the case of hypertension, the meanings come largely from actuarial and epidemiological data, findings that suggest that elevated blood pressure is associated with the risk for certain cardiovascular diseases. It is interesting to note that the risk factor of high blood pressure has been designated a treatable illness, while the risk factors of cigarette smoking, or lack of physical activity, have not been medicalized in the same fashion. Is this an instance of available treatment increasing the likelihood of medicalization (Conrad, 1975)?

As we noted earlier, even with the ability for exact measurement (or perhaps because of it), there is still considerable debate over where to draw the line for illness and treatment. This measurement controversy has social consequences, in terms of the number of people identified and treated for hypertension. In the United States alone, if diastolic pressure of 90 mmHg or above is deemed hypertension, that would encompass approximately 58 million people; if it were 95 mmHg or above, 33 million people; or if it were 100 mmHg or above, 19 million people (Kaplan, 1990).

## Social Consequences of Pharmaceutical Intervention

In the annals of medicalization, we have several cases in which the advent of a pharmaceutical intervention has had a significant impact on the medicalization of a particular problem. These include stimulant medications and Hyperactivity-Attentional Deficit Disorder (Conrad, 1975), methadone and opiate addiction (Conrad and Schneider, 1980a), and estrogen replacement and menopause (McCrea, 1983; Bell, 1987). In the cases of hyperactivity and menopause, like hypertension, promotion and advertising by the pharmaceutical industry were important factors in medicalization. This of course has also been true for most psychiatric drugs, although the history of the medicalization of madness predates the pharmaceutical industry (Conrad and Schneider, 1980a). However, in all cases, the corporate strategy of expanding markets for one or another pharmaceutical product has significantly contributed to medicalizing human problems. Once there is a significant organizational investment supporting medicalization, demedicalization becomes much less likely (Roman, 1988).

Two other social issues emerge from extending pharmaceutical intervention. First, fusing medical and pharmaceutical intervention expands the range of medical surveillance (Foucault, 1977). When patients are medically treated with drugs that require regular visits to physicians, we can say they are subject to a form of medical surveillance. Their problems are considered medical ones and are monitored by medical personnel. In a society that values privacy and independence, this raises some discomforting issues.

Second, as noted earlier, medical and pharmaceutical intervention decontextualizes human problems and turns attention from the social environment to the individual. The "pill for every ill" approach to Western medicine has led to an inattention to social causes of problems and encouraged various types of technological fixes (Nelkin, 1973). When a pharmaceutical intervention "works" (i.e., modifies the designated problem), often the problem is considered solved and social changes and interventions are deemed secondary or irrelevant. This approach may skew our understanding of the situation and reduce our ability to intervene in other ways.

### Dilemmas of the Sick Role

One of the ramifications of medicalization is the extension of the sick role to human behaviors and conditions. The sick role legitimates certain conditions and reduces blame for related deviance so long as the individual seeks and cooperates with appropriate treatment (Parsons, 1951). By designating hypertension as an illness, an entire population of people who previously had not defined themselves as ill (since they had no symptoms) can at least theoretically take on the sick role. While this may be beneficial, at least not blaming them for their condition, it also has other consequences. For example, studies have shown that after individuals are diagnosed with high blood pressure they report more illness symptoms and have higher rates of absenteeism at work (MacDonald et al., 1984). Thus, labeling them hypertensive has an impact in itself; individuals begin to see themselves as more likely to be ill and reinterpret their bodily experiences as symptoms. Furthermore, labeling has been shown to have consequences for the chances of promotion at work as well as ability to obtain health insurance coverage. Thus, by medicalizing the blood pressure of larger segments of the population, we might be increasing the social incidence of illness and adoption of the sick role.

## Conclusion

The medicalization of elevated blood pressure is not complete, and indeed, in some quarters it remains contested. But to the extent that mild and moderate hypertension are medicalized, the social consequences of medicalization must be added to the clinical questions of diagnosis and treatment in any complete evaluation.

## References

Ayman D (1934) Heredity in arteriolar (essential) hypertension: a clinical study of the blood pressure of 1,524 members of 277 families. *Archives of Internal Medicine* 53: 792–802.

Bechgaard P (1946) Arterial hypertension: a follow-up of one thousand hypertonics. *Acta Medica Sandinavica* Supplement 172: 1–358.

Bell SE (1987) Changing ideas: the medicalization of menopause. *Social Science and Medicine* 24: 535–42.

Brett AS (1984) Ethical issues in risk factor intervention. *American Journal of Medicine* 76: 557–61.

Burgess AM (1948) Excessive hypertension of long duration. *New England Journal of Medicine* 239: 75–79.

Cabot R (1926) *Heart and Diseases*. New York: W.B. Saunders Co.

Chasis H (1986) A game of numbers: re-appraisal of antihypertensive drug therapy. *Journal of Chronic Disease* 39: 933–38.

Conrad P (1975) The discovery of hyperkinesis: notes on the medicalization of deviant behavior. *Social Problems* 23: 12–21.

Conrad P (1992) Medicalization and social control. *Annual Review of Sociology* 18: 209–32.

Conrad P and Schneider JW (1980a) *Deviance and Medicalization: From Badness to Sickness*. St. Louis: Mosby. [expanded ed., 1992, Philadelphia: Temple University Press.]

Conrad P and Schneider JW (1980b) Looking at levels of medicalization. *Social Science and Medicine* 14A: 75–79.

Dollery C (1982) A clinician looks at the future. *British Journal of Clinical Pharmacology* 13: 127–32.

Doyle AE (1982) The introduction of ganglion blocking drugs for the treatment of hypertension. *British Journal of Clinical Pharmacology* 13: 63–65.

Dressler WW (1984) Social and cultural influences in cardiovascular disease: a review. *Transcultural Psychiatric Research Review* 21: 5–42.

Evans W (1956) *Cardiology*, 2nd ed. London: Butterworth.

Farrar GE (1991) Therapy for hypertension. *Clinical Therapeutics* 13: 656–58.

Fisher JW (1914) The diagnostic value of the sphygmomanometer in examination for life insurance. *Journal of the American Medical Association* 63: 1752.

Foucault M (1977) *Discipline and Punish*. New York: Random House.

Freis ED (1982a) The Veterans Trial and sequelae. *British Journal of Clinical Pharmacology* 13: 67–72.

Freis ED (1982b) Should mild hypertension be treated? *New England Journal of Medicine* 307: 306–9.

Goldring W and Chasis H (1966) Antihypertensive drug therapy. In: Ingelfinger FJ, Relman AS and Finland M (eds.) *Controversy in Internal Medicine*. Philadelphia: WB Saunders Co., pp. 83–91.

Gordon T and Kannel WB (1972) Multiple contributors to coronary risk. Implications for screening and prevention. *Journal of Chronic Disease* 25: 561–65.

Gusfield J (1981) *The Culture of Public Problems*. Chicago: University of Chicago Press.

Guttmacher S, Teitelman M, Chapin G, Garbowski G, and Schnall P (1981) *Ethics and Preventive Medicine: The Case of Borderline Hypertension*. Hastings Center Report, February, pp. 12–20.

Havlik RJ, LaCroix AZ, Kleinman JC, Ingram DD, Harris T, and Cornoni-Huntley J (1989) Antihypertensive drug therapy and survival by treatment status in a national survey. *Hypertension* 13 (Supplement I): I28–32.

Hypertension Detection and Follow-up Program Cooperative Group (HDFP) (1979) Five year findings of the hypertension detection and follow-up program. I. Reduction in mortality of persons with high blood pressure, including mild hypertension. *Journal of the American Medical Association* 242: 2562–71.

Illich I (1976) *Medical Nemesis*. New York: Pantheon.

James SA (1987) Psychosocial precursors of hypertension: a review of the epidemiologic evidence. *Circulation* 76 (Supplement I): I-60–6.

Joint National Committee (JNC) on Detection, Evaluation, and Treatment of High Blood Pressure (1977) A cooperative study. *Journal of the American Medical Association* 237: 255–61.

Joint National Committee (JNC) on Detection, Evaluation, and Treatment of High Blood Pressure (1980) 1980 report. *Archives of Internal Medicine* 140: 1280–85.

Kaplan NM (1990) *Clinical Hypertension*, 5th ed. Baltimore: Williams & Wilkins.

Kasl SV and Cobb S (1970) Blood pressure changes in men undergoing job loss: a preliminary report. *Psychosomatic Medicine* 32: 19.

Kaufert DA and Gilbert P (1986) Women, menopause and medicalization. *Culture, Medicine and Psychiatry* 10: 7–21.

Kawachi I and Wilson NA (1990) The evolution of antihypertensive therapy. *Social Science and Medicine* 31: 1239–43.

MacDonald LA, Sackett DL, Haynes RB, and Taylor DW (1984) Labelling in hypertension: a review of behavioral and psychological consequences. *Journal of Chronic Disease* 37: 933–42.

Master AM, Garfield CI, and Walters MB (1952) *Normal Blood Pressure and Hypertension. New Definitions*. Philadelphia: Lea and Febiger.

McCrea FB (1983) The politics of menopause: the "discovery" of a deficiency disease. *Social Problems* 31: 111–23.

McKinlay JB (1981) From 'promising report' to 'standard procedure': seven stages in the career of a medical innovation. *Millbank Memorial Fund Quarterly* 59: 374–411.

Medical Research Council Working Party (1985) MRC trial of treatment of mild hypertension: principal results. *British Medical Journal* 291: 97–104.

Nelkin D (1973) *Methadone Maintenance: A Technological Fix*. New York: Braziller.

Parsons T (1951) *The Social System*. Glencoe, IL: The Free Press.

Payer L (1992) *Disease-Mongers*. New York: John Wiley & Sons Inc.

Peart WS and Miall WE (1980) The MRC mild hypertension trial. *Lancet* i: 104–5.

Perera GA (1948) Diagnosis and natural history of hypertensive vascular disease. *American Journal of Medicine* 4: 416–22.

Pickering G (1974) *Hypertension. Causes, Consequences and Management*. Edinburgh and London: Churchill Livingstone.

Ragland DR et al. (1987) Prevalence of hypertension in bus drivers. *International Journal of Epidemiology* 16: 208–13.

Robinson SC and Brucer M (1939) Range of normal blood pressure. A statistical and clinical study of 11,383 persons. *Archives of Internal Medicine* 64: 409–44.

Roman P (1988) The disease concept of alcoholism: sociocultural and organizational bases of support. *Drugs and Society* 2: 5–32.

Ruzek S (1978) *The Women's Health Movement*. New York: Greenwood Press.

Schnall PL, Pieper C, Schwartz JE, et al. (1990) The relationship between "job strain," workplace diastolic blood pressure, and left ventricular mass index. *Journal of the American Medical Association* 263: 1929–35.

Schnall PL, Schwartz JE, Landsbergis PA, Warren K, and Pickering TG (1992) Relation between job strain, alcohol, and ambulatory blood pressure. *Hypertension* 19: 488–94.

Schroeder HA (1953) *Hypertensive Diseases. Causes and Control*. Philadelphia: Lea and Febiger.

Smirk FH and Alstad KS (1951) Treatment of arterial hypertension by penta- and hexamethonium salts, based on 150 tests on hypertensives of various aetiology and 53 patients treated for periods of two to fourteen months. *British Medical Journal* 1: 1217–28.

Society of Actuaries (1959) *Build and Blood Pressure Study*, Vol. 1. Chicago: Society of Actuaries.

Stallones RA (1980) The rise and fall of ischemic heart disease. *Scientific American* 243: 53–59.

Syme SL (1991) Social epidemiology and the work environment. In: Johnson JV and Johansson G (eds.) *Psychosocial Work Enviroment: Work Organization, Democratization and Health. Essays in memory of Bertil Gardell.* Amityville, NY: Baywood Publishing Co., pp. 21–31.

Thomas CB (1952) The heritage of hypertension. *American Journal of the Medical Sciences* 224: 367–76.

Vertes V, Tobias L, and Galvin S (1991) Historical reflections on hypertension. *Primary Care* 18: 471–83.

Veterans Administration Cooperative Study Group on antihypertensive agents (1970) Effect of treatment on morbidity and mortality II. Results in patients with diastolic blood pressures averaging 90 through 114 mmHg. *Journal of the American Medical Association* 213: 1143.

Vladek B (1980) *Unloving Care.* New York: Basic Books.

Waldron I, Nowotarski M, Freimer M, Henry JP, Post N, and Witten C (1982) Cross-cultural variation in blood pressure: a quantitative analysis of the relationships of blood pressure to cultural characteristics, salt consumption and body weight. *Social Science and Medicine* 16: 419–30.

Wenger NK (ed.) (1984) *Quality of Life and Cardiovascular Care.* New York: Le Jacq.

Williams DR (1992) Black-white differences in blood pressure: the role of social factors. *Ethnicity and Disease* 2: 126–41.

Zola IK (1972) Medicine as an institution of social control. *Sociological Review* 20: 487–504.

Zola IK (1983) *Sociomedical Inquiries.* Philadelphia: Temple University Press.

# 3

# Anxious Times:
# The Benzodiazepine Controversy
# and the Fracturing
# of Expert Authority

JONATHAN GABE
MICHAEL BURY

On October 2, 1991 the Licensing Authority in Britain suspended the license for a leading benzodiazepine sleeping pill, Halcion (triazolam), produced by the American pharmaceutical company Upjohn. The branded drug and its generic form were both withdrawn overnight. The company appealed to the regulatory authority, the Committee on the Safety of Medicines (CSM), without success. Subsequent appeals to the CSM's Commission and to a special Committee of "persons appointed" led to recommendations that the drug should be allowed to return to the market with certain restrictions. This advice was, however, rejected by the British government, which revoked the drug's license in June 1993.

This unusual action is just the latest chapter in the controversial history of benzodiazepine tranquilizers and hypnotics. As we shall see, this particular group of drugs has had a checkered career. However, the debate surrounding their use also reflects what we believe to be the development of a more general crisis of legitimacy in the efficacy of medical treatments and trust in medical authority. As we hope to demonstrate, the controversy over benzodiazepines is illustrative of a fundamental shift in the social relations of health care.

Our argument will be developed as we chart the twists and turns in the history of benzodiazepines and how this history has been shaped by the activities of a range of collective agents ranging from medical experts and mental health consumer groups to the mass media and government regulatory agencies.

## Background and Origins of the Debate

Benzodiazepines are one of a long line of synthetic substances that have been produced to treat emotional distress and sleeplessness. The first of these drugs, bromide and chloral hydrate, were greeted enthusiastically by physicians in the middle of the nineteenth century as valuable sedatives and hypnotics that were believed not to have the addictive properties of the then-popular opium based preparations (Gabe, 1991). Evidence of their abuse by patients soon started to appear, however, and disillusionment set in, prior to a more judicious evaluation of their comparative worth.

### Recent History

This cyclical pattern of response has been repeated with each of the tranquilizers produced since that time (Cohen, 1983). For instance, the barbiturates, of which 50 compounds were marketed in the first half of the twentieth century (Lader, 1978), were initially welcomed as safer than bromide and chloral hydrate. Although cases of abuse and dependence on short-acting barbiturates were reported in the 1930s, it was only in the early 1950s that the risks involved were widely acknowledged and people became apprehensive (Hollister, 1983).

The barbiturates were in turn replaced by meprobamate (Miltown), again to wide acclaim. However, its reign was short-lived. In 1960 the first of the benzodiazepines, chlordiazepoxide (Librium), was introduced, followed in 1963 by diazepam (Valium), its more successful stablemate (Cohen, 1970). The product of an atmosphere of commercial competition (Smith, 1985), this group of drugs quickly made meprobamate obsolete, once it had become accepted that they were safer and more effective in alleviating anxiety (Lader, 1978).

This history of psychotropic drugs appears to follow McKinlay's analysis of the development of medical innovations, in each case moving from promising reports through professional and public acceptance to becoming a standard procedure (McKinlay, 1981). Critical evaluation may then have taken place, with the treatment being either confirmed or discarded. The benzodiazepine story contains elements of this model though, as we shall see, critical reactions have accompanied both the early development and the public acceptance of this class of drugs.

Between 1965 and 1970 prescriptions for benzodiazepine tranquilizers in England and Wales rose by 110%, compared with 9% for all psychotropic drugs (Parish, 1971); a similar pattern was found in the United States (Silverman and Lee, 1974). Over the same period barbiturate hypnotic prescriptions fell by 24%, while nonbarbiturate hypnotic scripts (mainly for the benzodiazepine Mogadon, and for Mandrax) increased by 145% (Parish, 1971). In other words, the "benzodiazepine era" had arrived (Hollister, 1983: 13).

During the early 1970s prescriptions for benzodiazepines continued to rise in Britain and elsewhere (Marks, 1983). However, growing concern about the number of prescriptions and their misuse as "pills for personal problems" (Trethowan, 1975) seemed to have some effect. Benzodiazepine prescriptions peaked in Britain in 1979 when 30.7 million scripts were dispensed (Taylor, 1987), and have fallen steadily each year ever since with 18 million prescriptions being recorded in 1990 (King, 1992). A roughly similar pattern has been noted in many other industrialized countries (Katschnig and Amering, 1990; Petursson, 1993).

## Elements of Controversy

Since the early 1980s there has been an increasing number of reports about the dependence potential of benzodiazepines at normal therapeutic dose. This shift in attention to the issue of dependence was always a developmental possibility, given the persistent concern about the harmful side effects of prescribed drugs (Smith, 1985). Early in the decade a number of studies were published that reported that patients withdrawing from long-term benzodiazepine use at therapeutic dose had experienced symptoms of physical dependence on withdrawal (such as intolerance of noise and light, bad headaches, and a dry mouth), and that these symptoms could last a year or more (Petursson and Lader, 1981; 1984; Tyrer et al., 1981; 1983; Rickels et al., 1983; Ashton, 1984). Furthermore, those studies that had used representative samples and control groups reported that between 27% and 45% of long-term users were dependent on their drugs (Tyrer et al., 1981; 1983; Rickels et al., 1983).

To these reports about unwanted side effects has been added evidence about the harm caused by particular short-acting benzodiazepines. For instance, it has been reported that Halcion has caused memory loss, agitation, and hallucinations in some patients (Bixler et al., 1987; 1991; Oswald, 1989) and "involuntary intoxication" from the drug has even been cited as a defense against murder in both the United States and Britain. Not surprisingly, these events had serious consequences for the prescribing of Halcion, with sales falling worldwide by 45% in 1992 to $131 million, and by a further 31% in the first quarter of 1993 (Anonymous, 1993). The banning of the drug in Britain has added to the company's problems.

In addition, attention has been directed recently to the use of certain benzodiazepines as drugs of abuse, being taken for purposes other than those for which they are legitimately prescribed (Woods et al., 1988). Survey evidence and case reports, however, indicate that the nonmedical use of these drugs is infrequent and generally restricted to multiple drug abusers who take benzodiazepines in conjunction with, but as secondary to, cocaine, heroin or alcohol (Dupont, 1988; Woods et al., 1988; American Psychiatric Association, 1990).

It is important to note that many of the claims concerning the benzodiazepines, especially those of a serious nature, have been the focus of intense controversy. The production of scientific knowledge in such circumstances constantly threatens perceptions of its reliability and trustworthiness, particularly when we look at the way such knowledge is represented in the public sphere. Therefore, in the next section we draw attention to the arguments concerning the benzodiazepines and the interests of those who have been participating in the debate. In so doing we examine the claims made about the drugs and the strategies developed to challenge or defend them.

## Making Claims About Benzodiazepines

The clinical and epidemiological evidence regarding benzodiazepines has provided a fertile terrain for the claims-making activities of interest groups ranging from medical experts and mental health consumer groups to the pharmaceutical industry. The potential gains, in terms of improved treatment of anxiety represented by these drugs, and the potential harm they might do because of dependence and serious side effects, indicate that there is much at stake in the controversies that have ensued.

### The Medical Authorities

The first point to note in this connection is the division of opinion among medical experts themselves. Hospital based medical experts, especially psychopharmacologists and psychiatrists, have played a central role in influencing the climate of opinion about benzodiazepines. Initially they warned of the overuse and misuse of the drug and the "total tranquillisation of society" (Tyrer, 1974). General practitioners (GPs) were singled out for particular opprobrium, being castigated for too often reaching out for the prescription pad instead of offering their patients talk (Trethowan, 1975), and then writing repeat prescriptions without seeing their patients personally (Parish, 1971). Patients were also criticized by some for conniving in the process by claiming that they could only manage the stresses of daily life with the help of the medical remedies their GPs could provide (Dunlop, 1970).

Subsequently, in the 1980s, these experts switched their attention to the dependence potential of these drugs and, on the basis of clinical and limited epidemiological evidence, claimed that they had identified a withdrawal syndrome among long-term benzodiazepine users. By this they meant intense physical disturbances when the administration of the drug is suspended.

While most experts have been careful to avoid treating benzodiazepine dependence as synonymous with addiction because of the lack of drug-seeking behavior, the absence of escalating dosage, minor use of the drug for nonmedical purposes, and the pejorative connotations attached to "addiction," there have been a few notable exceptions (Edwards et al., 1984; Lancet, 1984; Lader and Higgitt, 1986; Parish, 1992). Even such limited linking of benzodiazepines with addiction and, by implication, with illicit drugs about which there has been widespread public concern, has arguably further damaged the drug's reputation as a legitimate and safe medical treatment for anxiety and insomnia.

As during the earlier period, GPs have been singled out for particular criticism. They have been criticized for failing to establish the limits of therapeutic use, for writing repeat prescriptions without seeing the patient, and for subscribing to the belief that people troubled by family and occupational problems may legitimately seek help from the medical profession (Petursson and Lader, 1984; Lancet, 1985; Lader and Higgitt, 1986; Hallstrom, 1991). One expert has gone as far as to claim that behavior like this is souring the doctor-patient relationship (Lader, 1981) and has created a crisis of confidence among "the anxious members of our community" (Lader and Higgitt, 1986). Like other forms of psychotropic treatments (most notably the antidepressants), the wide availability and use of such drugs for emotional distress in everyday life cuts across their specific use in treating mental illnesses. The producers of these drugs and the doctors who prescribe them may be seen as little more than drug pushers in an era of "cosmetic pharmacology" (Kramer, 1993).

## The Lay Pressure Groups

Claims about physical dependence have not been restricted to medical experts. Various pressure groups on both sides of the Atlantic have used experts' claims about dependence to influence the recent debate. For instance, in the early 1980s Release, a British organization offering advice and referral on drug problems, argued on the basis of recent research concerning the physical withdrawal syndrome that tranx (benzodiazepines) are highly addictive to some users and that, in its experience, the degree of distress felt on withdrawal is often far more extreme than that which first led a user to seek help from a GP (Release, 1982).

Similar claims were made by DAWN (1984), the British feminist pressure group concerned with women drug users, and MIND, the British mental health pressure group. The latter invoked the U.S. Food and Drug Administration (FDA) which, it claimed, stated that "the danger of drugs in the benzodiazepine group are clear" and that "even very limited use may be ill advised" (MIND, 1984: 3).

In the United States equivalent claims have been made by the influential Washington-based Public Citizen Health Research Group. In 1982 it published a book for lay people entitled *Stopping Valium* that charged, among other things, that "Valium addiction is a major problem" in the United States and that many of the 1.5 million people who have taken benzodiazepines "continuously for over four months may be addicted" (Bargmann et al., 1982: 1,2). Quoting the results of epidemiological studies by certain British and American medical experts, alongside statistical evidence from the National Institute of Drug Abuse and the FDA, it concluded that there is "clear evidence that thousands of people are addicted to these dangerous drugs."

Its more recent publications, such as *Worst Pills, Best Pills*, aimed at older adults, warns that "a large fraction, probably the overwhelming majority of people who use any of the benzodiazepines at the recommended dose for more than one or two months will become addicted" (Wolfe et al., 1988: 151). Similar remarks have been expressed by the New York-based Center for Medical Consumers, in a report defending state legislation restricting prescriptions for benzodiazepines and requiring pharmacists to provide the state with a copy of every prescription filled (Center for Medical Consumers, 1989: 4).

It is noteworthy that these pressure groups have generally been less careful in their use of terminology than most of the medical experts whose work they have drawn on, and have used "addiction" and "dependence" interchangeably. At the same time they have shared with experts a willingness to attribute much of the blame for the problem of dependence to the GP, especially, again, in Britain. As previously,

GPs have been castigated for repeat prescribing and for failing to recognize that their patients might be dependent on benzodiazepines and in need of assistance in withdrawing from using them. In this way, pressure groups have also played a part in heightening public concern about the trust that can be placed in GPs' clinical judgments and medical treatments.

## The Pharmaceutical Companies

Against this background of divisions within medicine and increasingly vocal mental health pressure groups, pharmaceutical companies have made their own interventions in the debate. Three forms of action have been particularly apparent. First, they have funded a number of symposia in the United States, Britain, and elsewhere attended by experts of their own choosing who are considered largely sympathetic to their products. In each case the aim has been to try and develop a more balanced view of the risks and benefits involved in an attempt to challenge what the companies believe to be a "climate of confusion" on the part of many in the medical profession about their drugs' safety and efficacy.

For instance, in 1979, the Upjohn Company organized a symposium of experts in Boston to consider evidence about the benefits and risks of Halcion after the drug's suspension in The Netherlands. The symposium produced a favorable analysis of the evidence, derived from confidential data of clinical trials and postmarketing surveillance provided by the company, and reported its conclusions in the *Lancet* (Ayd et al., 1979).

Although at a later date the chair of the symposium accepted in a television interview that the experts had been misled about data provided by the company (BBC, 1991), at the time its results seemed to clear the air and helped Upjohn get Halcion approved by the FDA for the U.S. market. Indeed, the drug went on to become the most prescribed sleeping pill in the United States and the world during the 1980s (Medawar, 1992). More recent symposia and workshops (e.g., in Boston in 1988 and Leicester, England in 1989) have apparently been less successful in rehabilitating Upjohn's benzodiazepines.

Second, pharmaceutical companies have tried to influence the climate of opinion through academic research and critique. In some instances they have used their own staff to write academic reviews that question the credibility of their scientific critics. Most notably, Jonas (1992) has constructed a meta-analysis in which he attempts to cast doubt on the methodology employed by these critics; for example, the apparent publishing in several different articles of limited data from a single study to give the impression of a growing body of evidence.

More often the companies have financed independent researchers to undertake studies that might establish the benefits of benzodiazepines (Gabe and Williams, 1986). For instance, Upjohn funded a major cross-national randomized trial of the efficacy of Xanax (alprazolam) for patients with panic disorder with agoraphobia, and provided quality assurance (Marks et al., 1993a). However, when results appeared suggesting that behavior therapy was at least twice as effective as the drug, Upjohn reportedly withdrew their support abruptly and invited professionals to critique the study (Marks et al., 1993b). The publicizing of such a response has however backfired on the company and arguably reduced its credibility.

Finally, companies have resorted to litigation against those high-profile experts who have been perceived as undertaking a vendetta against one of their products. Such action was undertaken by Upjohn against Professor Ian Oswald in 1992. The company issued a writ in the British High Court claiming damages relating to Oswald's allegations about the safety of Halcion. In particular, they rejected his claim that the company had concealed data on the drug and stated publicly that his smear tactics were not fair either to their employees or to patients who had been "frightened and misled" and "deprived of a safe, effective and well tolerated sleep medicine" as a result of his "junk science" (Anonymous, 1992). The professor responded by filing a countersuit against Upjohn.

In May 1994 the High Court in London found in favor of Upjohn which was awarded £25,000 in damages, with a further £75,000 awarded to one of Upjohn's senior executives for being defamed by Oswald. However the company was criticized by the presiding judge for its behavior over admitted errors in the transcribing of drug trial data and Oswald was awarded £50,000 damages for allegations concerning his professional and academic integrity. Costs were awarded to Upjohn leaving the professor with a bill approaching £1 million which is reportedly being met by the Medical Defense Union (Frean, 1994).

Whatever the merits of this particular case it reveals, as do the other examples, how pharmaceutical companies have tried to influence the debate over benzodiaze-pines, in line with their own interests as profit-maximizing concerns. It also highlights a general process, now well under way in contemporary society, namely that expert knowledge is becoming "chronically contestable" both within expert systems and between them and lay publics (Giddens, 1990), thereby undermining a dominant source of authoritative interpretation. The fracturing of expert authority has in turn been compounded by the mass media, which have long taken a critical interest in benzodiazepines in both the United States (Cohen, 1983; Morgan, 1983; Smith, 1985) and the United Kingdom (Gabe and Bury, 1988; Bury and Gabe, 1990; Gabe et al., 1992). It is to the media's role as the potential amplifiers and legitimators of concern about these drugs that we now turn.

## Expressing Opinion Through the Mass Media—Especially Television

The importance of the media in heightening public concern about medical practice lies not only in its ability to provide opportunities for the expression of expert and lay views, but also in structuring meanings into recognizable images and narratives (Fiske, 1987). As regards benzodiazepines, our analysis of British mass media has revealed that they have played a central role in expressing and organizing critical expert and lay views and, in so doing, amplifying and legitimating concern.

We have examined all of the main television programs on this issue in Britain since the early 1980s (Gabe and Bury, 1988; Bury and Gabe, 1990). Perhaps the most important early coverage of problems with benzodiazepines was that of the British Broadcasting Corporation (BBC) magazine program *That's Life*, with an audience of around 10 million. It covered the issue of tranquilizer dependence in some depth on at least four occasions between 1983 and 1985. Others, such as Roger Cook's exposé program *The Cook Report*, transmitted in 1988 by Central Television to 6 million viewers, and BBC's current affairs program *Panorama*, broadcast in 1991, focused on one specific benzodiazepine, Ativan (lorazepam) and Halcion, respectively.

We see this coverage performing two broad functions. First, it has provided a key mechanism for literally mediating the massive explosion of information about benzodiazepine dependence and side effects. Information, and the claims of various groups, have been increasingly circulated, providing numerous opportunities for professional experts, individual patients, and consumer groups to enter and shape the debate.

As we have noted, many of these claims have focused on the role of GPs, and television has provided further opportunity for their expression. GPs thus have been severely criticized for allegedly prescribing tranquilizers to children (*That's Life*), for overprescribing these drugs to adult patients, for failing to warn these patients about the dangers of dependence and for not helping them to withdraw slowly (*That's Life*, *The Cook Report*). Some of these criticisms resulted in part from claims made by other medical experts. In turn, pharmaceutical companies have been severely criticized for their actions in the development and marketing of the benzodiazepines. Included here is the famous confrontation between Roger Cook (of *The Cook Report*) and the chairman of Wyeth while the latter was playing golf, and *Panorama*'s confrontation with Upjohn employees over the Halcion controversy. In all these ways television has played a major part in claims-making activity about benzodiazepines.

Second, we have tried to unravel the images and narratives that this television coverage has produced and disseminated in the process of covering the issue. At one level there is little doubt that the imagery employed can be seen as amplifying the reported effects of benzodiazepine dependence. For instance, these products frequently have been portrayed as drugs of addiction, with individual patients being described as hooked on them. This imagery has been reinforced in turn by pictures of the drugs themselves being manufactured in large quantities, emerging from the factory production line in their thousands and, in one instance (*The Cook Report*), showering down from the top of the screen in a colorful cascade. It is this imagery that leads to the countercharge by the defenders of the products that television exaggerates or sensationalizes the problems it tackles.

However, while there is undoubtedly an argument to be made here, our analysis has suggested that television coverage of health issues such as benzodiazepine dependence involves much more than sensationalism. Television frequently draws on a series of powerful narratives or stories (in this case often based on individual experiences) that touch on key elements in our cultural order (Silverstone, 1988). In the case of benzodiazepines, dependence and the problems of withdrawal are recast as moral tales about areas of behavior around which there is intense social ambiguity. In such tales the boundary between the consumption of licit and illicit drugs is frequently blurred and accounts develop by drawing on a series of oppositions such as innocence/guilt, good/evil, and hero/villain.

Similar arguments can be developed about television coverage of benzodiazepines in other countries. For example, U.S. television programs, such as the American Broadcasting Corporation's documentary news program *20/20* (ABC, 1989) and Columbia Broadcasting System's investigative news program *60 Minutes* (CBS, 1991), have both helped circulate the claims of experts and individual patients about the side effects of Halcion and criticized its makers for marketing it without due regard to its safety. They have also employed similar imagery and recast the story as a moral tale employing a narrative of innocence/guilt and good/evil to describe consumers and manufacturers of the drug.

In summary, the media, and especially television, provide the means for publicizing and legitimizing claims about the safety of benzodiazepines, but also create and recreate meanings around it. The images and narratives constituted by, and contained in, television programs present a picture that "imposes coherence and resolution upon a world that has neither" (Fiske, 1987). Those hoping to use the media, therefore, in order to advance their claims about benzodiazepines are confronted with the fact that they, in turn, become part of a more complex media agenda. At the same time, those at whom media messages are aimed, particularly state regulatory authorities, find themselves under scrutiny and may on occasion be forced to act despite themselves. The extent to which this has been so in the case of benzodiazepines is considered below.

## Policy Responses

Faced with the claims-making activities of professional and lay groups, and the amplification of concern by the media in the 1980s, one might have expected regulatory agencies on both sides of the Atlantic to respond robustly. In fact, this has not been the case in either the United States or United Kingdom, although the latter has finally bowed to pressure over one particular benzodiazepine, Halcion, as noted in the introduction. What actions have these bodies taken and for what reasons?

### The United Kingdom

In the United Kingdom the CSM, established in 1970 under the Medicines Act of 1968, is required to promote the collection and regulation of information relating to adverse drug reactions to advise on the safety, quality, and efficacy of medicines (Hallstrom, 1991). If one examines the actions of the CSM and other U.K. regulatory bodies on benzodiazepines it is clear that they have been extremely cautious, preferring to acknowledge side effects only when there is "pretty clear evidence of actual harm" (Medawar, 1992: 195) rather than acting earlier on evidence of risk. For instance, when the Committee on the Review of Medicines (CRM) published its guidelines in 1980, after a decade of concern among some medical experts, it took a conservative position. While casting doubt over the efficacy of long-term use, it stated that "on present available evidence the true addictive potential of benzodiazepines [is] low" (Committee on the Review of Medicines, 1980: 911). Even so its conclusions about efficacy and dependence were not incorporated in most data sheets for almost five years, apparently because of lack of cooperation by the drug companies (Medawar, 1992).

It was only eight years later that the first definitive statement was published by the CSM (1988). In it the committee reacted to the problem of dependence by advising doctors against long-term prescribing. It was suggested, following closely the recommendations of a Royal College of Psychiatrists (RCP) Working Party (RCP, 1988), that courses of treatment should be for no more than four weeks and only when anxiety or insomnia were disabling or severe. This advice was quickly incorporated into data sheets for doctors without the long delays that had occurred in 1980 (Medawar, 1992).

Even so, the CSM still refused to take action to revoke the license for any of the short-acting benzodiazepines that were causing particular concern among medical experts. As noted above, this only occurred in 1991 when it initially suspended the license for just one of the short-acting benzodiazepines, Halcion. Subsequently it revoked the license for this drug, despite appeals by its manufacturer, Upjohn, to the CSM's commission and to a committee of "persons appointed."

Though interpreting events as they unfold is difficult, this unusual decision may be explained in the following way. First, the CSM was no doubt mindful that its own actions in licensing benzodiazepines were likely to come under scrutiny from the courts as the litigation against the drug companies in the United Kingdom, involving 2,000 firms of solicitors and around 17,000 claimants, proceeded (Dyer, 1994). Second, the CSM may have acted as it did on this one occasion in order to defend itself from the intense gaze of the media, particularly the BBC's *Panorama* program, having already been savaged by the program on a previous occasion over the safety of Opren in 1983 (Brown, 1992). Third, the U.K. authorities, as defenders of national pharmaceutical interests alongside their responsibilities for promoting better prescribing (Stacey, 1988; Medawar, 1992), may have felt less compunction about revoking Halcion's license than would have been the case if the product had been made by a British rather than an American company. Fourth, it might have been influenced by the U.K. government's desire to have the proposed European Medicines Evaluation Agency (EMEA) located in the United Kingdom. In the event the decision was to locate the EMEA in London (Commission of the European Communities, 1993). At present no other benzodiazepine product license has been suspended or revoked in the United Kingdom.

## The United States

In the United States the machinery of drug control had been set up earlier, in 1962, when the FDA was required to obtain satisfactory evidence of drug efficacy as well as safety before a drug could be licensed for sale. One result of this was that U.S. doctors were first warned of the risks of benzodiazepine dependence in 1973, more than a decade before such warnings were issued in the United Kingdom (Medawar,

1992). Following evidence of symptoms after abrupt withdrawal, the U.S. authorities were persuaded that manufacturers should be required to warn doctors that the efficacy of benzodiazepines for anxiety was doubtful after four months of continuous use. As noted above, similar advice was only offered by the CSM in the United Kingdom in 1980.

Advice in the U.S. *Physician's Desk Reference* has continued to appear sooner and be more strongly worded than in the United Kingdom, reflecting the FDA's preference to act on evidence of risk rather than wait for clear evidence of harm. Yet it would be inaccurate to present the U.S. licensing authorities as any less cautious than their U.K. counterparts when it comes to the suspension of product licenses. For example, the FDA has shown itself to be reluctant to act against Halcion, despite the criticisms that have been levelled against the drug in the U.S. media (Ehrlich, 1988a; 1988b; ABC, 1989; PBS, 1989) and has consistently preferred to accept the word of the drug's manufacturer, Upjohn.

Thus, in 1988, when it was eventually forced to review adverse reaction reports showing that Halcion generated more reactions than other benzodiazepine sleeping tablets, its Psychopharmacological Drugs Advisory Committee continued to accept Upjohn's response that these reports were of limited scientific value. Part of the reason for this may lie in the FDA's reluctance to alter earlier decisions (especially regarding dosage) to avoid renewed scrutiny.

On this basis the FDA decided only to attach a stronger amnesia warning to the product, a recommendation that was subsequently heavily criticized by the U.S. consumer group, Public Citizen Health Research Group, for failing to draw attention to the drug's "possibly unique dangers" (Anonymous, 1990). Indeed it has remained cautious, despite the evidence of deficiencies in the drug trial data that led to Halcion getting a license in the United States and despite the United Kingdom's decision to suspend and subsequently revoke the license for Halcion. As a result, at the time of writing, Upjohn is still licensed to produce Halcion in the United States, as it is in most countries other than the United Kingdom.

## Conclusion

In this chapter we have presented a case study of one of the most controversial areas of medical treatment in recent times. To return to McKinlay's (1981) argument that medical innovations tend to pass from early recognition to become (usually unevaluated) standard procedures, the benzodiazepines offer an interesting variant. Criticism and disquiet about these drugs grew rapidly after their introduction, and only had a substantial impact on their use when the issue of dependence came to the fore. We have described the benzodiazepine issue as an instance of a general process, now well under way in contemporary society, in which expert knowledge is becoming chronically contestable both within expert systems and between them and lay publics (Giddens, 1990), thereby undermining a dominant source of authoritative interpretation. The fracturing of expert authority has in turn been compounded by the mass media.

While many medical experts today see themselves as beleaguered by external pressures, ranging from managerial imperatives to media attacks, our analysis has pointed to the role that medical experts have themselves played in the development of the controversy. Claims about the benzodiazepines have been fueled by the various positions taken up by medical researchers and practitioners. Consumer groups, though adding their particular concerns to the controversy, have often used evidence provided by medical critics.

We have also shown that, though the fear of the media's role may be overstated, there is little doubt in the case of the benzodiazepines that it has been important. It has permitted not only the rehearsal of many of the medical arguments, but it has also powerfully structured a range of meanings surrounding the use of psychotropic drugs—an area of social life that remains deeply ambiguous. It is for this reason that the media's coverage has been noteworthy, rather than any attempt on its part to influence policy in a direct or consistent way.

This also helps explain the mixed response by government drug regulatory agencies. Our analysis indicates that though these bodies have sometimes been under intense pressure to take action over the benzodiazepines, in reality they have been reluctant to do so. The case of the banning of Halcion in Britain stands out almost as an exception that proves the rule, indicating that many different pressures, including political and economic factors, may play a decisive role in the outcome of such processes.

Finally, our analysis of the benzodiazepines touches on more general trends in health care. There is now a persistent sense of ambiguity surrounding the development and use of modern medical treatments. The paradox here is that, as they become more effective, medical treatments also become more closely regulated. Moreover, the ever-wider accessibility and use of modern medicines leads simultaneously to the charge of the "medicalization of everyday life," and its challenge. The change in what we have called the social relations of health care is now potentially far-reaching. The story of the benzodiazepines indicates that, in the future, conflict and negotiation will color the relationships of medical experts, doctors, and their patients.

## References

ABC (1989) When sleep becomes a nightmare. *20/20*, American Broadcasting Co., 17 February.

American Psychiatric Association (1990) *Benzodiazepine Dependence, Toxicity and Abuse: A Task Force Report of the American Psychiatric Association*. Washington, DC: American Psychiatric Association.

Anonymous (1990) US FDA committee attacked on Halcion. *Scrip* 1662: 20.

Anonymous (1992) Warning against UK Halcion withdrawal. *Scrip* 1746: 18.

Anonymous (1993) Stop press. *Scrip* 1833: 24.

Ashton H (1984) Benzodiazepine withdrawal: an unfinished story. *British Medical Journal* 288: 1135–40.

Ayd F et al. (1979) Behavioural reactions and triazolam. *The Lancet* 1: 1018.

Bargmann E, Wolfe SM, and Levin J (1982) *Stopping Valium*. Washington, DC: Public Citizen Health Research Group.

BBC (1991) The Halcion nightmare. *Panorama*, British Broadcasting Corporation, 14 October.

Bixler EO, Kales A, Brubaker BH, and Kales JD (1987) Adverse reactions to benzodiazepine hypnotics: spontaneous reporting systems. *Pharmacology* 35: 286–300.

Bixler EO, Kales A, Manfredi RL, Vgontzas AN, Tyson KL, and Kales JD (1991) Next day memory impairment with triazolam use. *The Lancet* 337: 827–31.

Brown P (1992) Halcion and UK intransigence. *Scrip Magazine* 7: 3–4.

Bury M and Gabe J (1990) Hooked? Media responses to tranquilliser dependence. In: Abbott P and Payne G (eds.) *New Directions in the Sociology of Health*. Basingstoke, UK: Falmer Press, pp. 87–103.

CBS (1991) *60 Minutes*, Columbia Broadcasting System, 15 December.

Center for Medical Consumers (1989) *Triplicate Prescriptions for Benzodiazepines*. New York: Center for Medical Consumers.

Cohen I (1970) The benzodiazepines. In: Ayd FJ and Blackwell B (eds.) *Discoveries in Biological Psychiatry*. Philadelphia: J.B. Lippincott, pp. 130–41.

Cohen S (1983) Current attitudes about benzodazepines: trial by media. *Journal of Psychoactive Drugs* 15: 109–13.

Commission of the European Communities (1993) *The European Medicines Evaluation Agency*. London: Commission of the European Communities.

Committee on the Review of Medicines (1980) Systematic review of the benzodiazepines. *British Medical Journal* 280: 910–12.

Committee on Safety of Medicines (CSM) (1988) Benzodiazepines, dependence and withdrawal symptoms. *Current Problems* 21: 1–2.

DAWN (1984) *Women and Tranquillisers*. London: Drugs, Alcohol and Women Nationally.

Dunlop D (1970) The use and abuse of psychotropic drugs. *Proceedings of the Royal Society of Medicine* 63: 1279–82.

Dupont R (ed.) (1988) Abuse of benzodiazepines: the problems and the solutions. A Report of a Committee of the Institute for Behaviour and Health. *American Journal of Drugs and Alcohol Abuse* 14 (Suppl. 1): 1–69.

Dyer C (1994) Sad story of the happy pills. *The Guardian*, April 5, 21.

Edwards JG, Cantopher T, and Oliver S (1984) Dependence on psychotropic drugs: an overview. *Postgraduate Medical Journal* 60 (Suppl. 2): 29–40.

Ehrlich C (1988a) Halcion nightmare: the frightening truth about America's favorite sleeping pill. *California*, September.

Ehrlich C (1988b) Halcion: prescription for trouble. *California*, October.

Fiske J (1987) *Television Culture*. London: Methuen.

Frean P (1994) BBC faces £1.5 million legal bill for Panorama drug libel. *The Times*, 28 May, 2.

Gabe J (1991) Introduction. In: Gabe J (ed.) *Understanding Tranquilliser Use. The Role of the Social Sciences*. London: Routledge, pp. 1–12.

Gabe J and Bury M (1988) Tranquillisers as a social problem. *The Sociological Review* 36: 320–52.

Gabe J, Gustafsson U, and Bury M (1992) Mediating illness: newspaper coverage of tranquilliser dependence. *Sociology of Health and Illness* 13: 332–53.

Gabe J and Williams P (1986) Tranquilliser use. In: Gabe J and Williams P (eds.) *Tranquillisers: Social, Psychological and Clinical Perspectives*. London: Tavistock, pp. 3–24.

Giddens A (1990) *The Consequences of Modernity*. Cambridge: Polity Press in association with Blackwells.

Hallstrom C (1991) Benzodiazepine dependence: who is responsible? *Journal of Forensic Psychiatry* 2: 5–7.

Hollister LE (1983) The pre-benzodiazepine era. *Journal of Psychoactive Drugs* 15: 9–13.

Jonas JM (1992) Idiosyncratic side effects of short half-life benzodiazepine hypnotics: fact or fiction? *Human Psychopharmacology* 7: 205–16.

Katschnig H and Amering M (1990) Patterns of benzodiazepine use in Austria, Switzerland and the Federal Republic of Germany. In: Hindmarch I, Beaumont G, Brandon S, and Leonard BE (eds.) *Benzodiazepines: Current Concepts*. Chichester: John Wiley, pp. 169–80.

King M (1992) Is there still a role for benzodiazepines in general practice? *British Journal of General Practice* 42: 202–5.

Kramer PD (1993) *Listening to Prozac*. New York: Viking Press.

Lader M (1978) Benzodiazepines—opium of the masses? *Neuroscience* 3: 159–65.

Lader M (1981) Epidemic in the making: benzodiazepine dependence. In: Tognoni G, Bellantuono C, and Lader M (eds.) *Epidemiological Impact of Psychotropic Drugs*. Amsterdam: Elsevier/North Holland Biomedical Press, pp. 313–24.

Lader M and Higgitt A (1986) Management of benzodiazepine dependence—update. *British Journal of Addiction* 81: 7–10.

Lancet (1984) The benzodiazepine bind. *The Lancet* 2: 705–6.

Lancet (1985) Action on addiction to tranquillisers. *The Lancet* 1: 1521.

McKinlay JB (1981) From 'promising report' to 'standard procedure': seven stages in the career of medical innovation. *Milbank Memorial Fund Quarterly/Health and Society* 59: 374–411.

Marks IM, Swinson RP, Basoglu M, Kuch K, Noshirvani H, et al. (1993a) Alprazolam and exposure alone and combined in panic disorder with agoraphobia. A controlled study in London and Toronto. *British Journal of Psychiatry* 162: 776–87.

Marks IM, Swinson RP, Basoglu M, Noshirvani H, Kuch K, et al. (1993b) Reply to comment on the London/Toronto study. *British Journal of Psychiatry* 162: 790–4.

Marks J (1983) The benzodiazepines: an international perspective. *Journal of Psychoactive Drugs* 15: 137–49.

Medawar C (1992) *Power and Dependence. Social Audit on the Safety of Medicines*. London: Social Audit.

MIND (1984) *Tranquillisers: Hard Facts, Hard Choices*. London: National Association For Mental Health.

Morgan JP (1983) Cultural and medical attitudes towards benzodiazepines: conflicting metaphors. *Journal of Psychoactive Drugs* 15: 115–20.

Oswald I (1989) Triazolam syndrome ten years on. *The Lancet* 2: 451–52.

Parish J (1971) The prescribing of psychotropic drugs in general practice. *Journal of the Royal College of General Practitioners* 21 (Suppl. 4): 1–77.

Parish P (1992) *Medicines. A Guide for Everybody*. Harmondsworth: Penguin.

PBS (1989) Halcion. *MacNeil-Lehrer News Hour*, 1 September.

Petursson H (1993) An international perspective on benzodiazepine abuse. In: Hallstrom C (ed.) *Benzodiazepine Dependence*. Oxford: Oxford University Press, pp. 186–202.

Petursson H and Lader M (1981) Benzodiazepine dependence. *British Journal of Addiction* 76: 133–45.

Petursson H and Lader M (1984) *Dependence on Tranquillisers*. Oxford: Oxford University Press.

Release (1982) *Trouble with Tranquillisers*. London: Release Publications.

Rickels K, Case G, Downing RW, and Winokur A (1983) Long term diazepam therapy and clinical outcome. *Journal of the American Medical Association* 250: 767–71.

Royal College of Psychiatrists (1988) Benzodiazepines and dependence: a college statement. *Bulletin of the Royal College of Psychiatrists* 12: 107–9.

Silverman M and Lee PR (1974) *Pills, Profits and Politics*. Berkeley: University of California Press.

Silverstone R (1988) Television, myth and culture. In: Carey JW (ed.) *Media, Myths and Narratives: Television and the Press*. London: Sage, pp. 20–47.

Smith MC (1985) *Small Comfort. A History of the Minor Tranquillizers*. New York: Praeger.

Stacey M (1988) *The Sociology of Health and Healing*. London: Unwin Hyman.

Taylor D (1987) Current usage of benzodiazepines in Britain. In: Freeman H and Rue Y (eds.) *Benzodiazepines in Current Clinical Practice*. London: Royal Society of Medicine Services, pp. 13–17.

Trethowan WH (1975) Pills for personal problems. *British Medical Journal* 3: 749–51.

Tyrer P (1974) The benzodiazepine bonanza. *The Lancet* 2: 709–10.

Tyrer P, Owen R, and Dawling S (1983) Gradual withdrawal of diazepam after long-term therapy. *The Lancet* 1: 1402–6.

Tyrer P, Rutherford D, and Huggett T (1981) Benzodiazepine withdrawal symptoms and propranolol. *The Lancet* 1: 520–2.

Wolfe SM, Fugate L, Hulstrand EP, and Kamimoto LE (1988) *Worst Pills, Best Pills*. Washington, DC: Public Citizen Health Research Group.

Woods JH, Katz JL, and Winger G (1988) Use and abuse of benzodiazepines. Issues relevant to prescribing. *Journal of the American Medical Association* 260: 3476–80.

# 4

# Adverse Reactions, Social Responses: A Tale of Two Asthma Mortality Epidemics

NEIL PEARCE

Asthma has been known to occur for thousands of years, but very little is known about why it occurs. Even the definition of asthma has long been the subject of controversy, as has the form of treatment. One of the earliest documented examples of successful asthma treatment occurred in the sixteenth century, when Gerolamo Cardano came from Italy to Edinburgh to treat Archbishop John Hamilton. His treatment included diet, purging, regular exercise, sleep, and substitution of unspun silk for feathers in the Archbishop's mattress. This regimen succeeded in keeping Hamilton alive long enough to be hanged by the Scottish Reformers (Keeney, 1964).

Nowadays, asthma is considered to involve three main features: inflammation of the tissue lining the airways; bronchospasm, in which the muscles tighten around the airways; and mucus, which leads to obstruction of the airways. There has been considerable controversy in recent decades as to whether asthma treatment should concentrate on relieving bronchospasm (usually with beta-2 agonists) or reducing inflammation (usually with corticosteroids). Furthermore, there is increasing concern about the safety and efficacy of beta agonists and their possible role in asthma deaths.

This concern about the safety of asthma medications has arisen in parallel with other concerns about current approaches to the management of asthma. Asthma is a major cause of hospital admissions and accounts for a substantial proportion (10–20%) of pharmaceutical and health care expenditures in some Western countries; it is also an important cause of work and school absence and can severely affect the quality of life of individual sufferers and their families (Neville et al., 1993). Asthma has some parallels with diabetes, another major chronic disease that requires continual care and medication use, and that is life threatening in some instances; thus it is interesting to contrast the approaches that have been used in the management of these diseases in recent decades (Crane et al., 1991). Whereas patients with diabetes have been encouraged to learn self-management and to self-regulate their medication in response to changes in their disease, the management of asthma has been firmly in the hands of the physician. However, traditional approaches to asthma management have been questioned in recent years (Crane et al., 1991), and there is now increasing emphasis on self-management in asthma.

This chapter reviews the history of drug iatrogenesis and asthma treatment during this century. Above all, it is a story of two asthma drugs (isoprenaline forte and fenoterol), and of the two epidemics of asthma deaths that followed their introduction, why these epidemics occurred only in some countries while other countries (including the United States) were spared, and of the inadequate responses of physicians and the pharmaceutical industry to these epidemics.

## The First Epidemic—The International Evidence

Asthma death rates had been very low (Fig. 4-1) for more than a century (Speizer and Doll, 1968) until the 1960s, when asthma deaths increased suddenly in several countries, including the United Kingdom, Australia, and New Zealand (Fig. 4-2). One of the first published reports of the epidemic came in a letter to the *British*

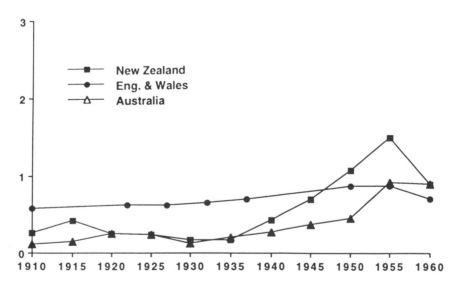

**Figure 4-1.** Asthma mortality in persons aged 5–34 years in New Zealand, Australia, and England and Wales, 1910–1960.
*Source*: Adapted from Beasley et al. (1990), Baumann and Lee (1990), Speizer and Doll (1968).

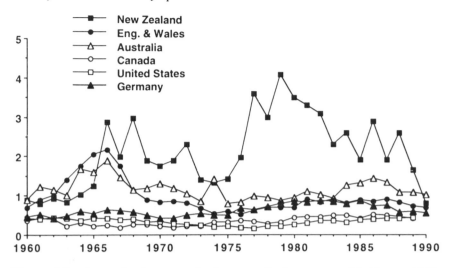

**Figure 4-2.**   International patterns of asthma mortality in persons aged 5–34 years, 1960–1990.
*Source*: Adapted from Jackson et al. (1988).

*Medical Journal* from two British researchers, Greenberg and Pines (1967). They warned that "patients with asthma may be killing themselves by the excessive use of sympathomimetic agents."

Speizer et al. (1968) subsequently studied time trends of deaths in the 5–34 age group (almost all studies of asthma deaths are confined to this age group because of problems of classification of deaths in other age groups). They concluded that the epidemic was real and was not due to changes in diagnostic criteria, certification, or coding practices. They also considered that it was unlikely to be due to a sudden increase in asthma prevalence, but was rather due to an increase in case fatality due to new methods of treatment. In particular, they found that the epidemic followed the introduction in 1961 of the pressurized beta agonist inhalers (including isoprenaline, known as isoproterenol in the United States), and the rise in asthma deaths paralleled the increase in sales.

This preliminary inhaler hypothesis echoed previous warnings that overuse of beta agonist inhalers could be causing asthma deaths. In response to these warnings, the Committee on Safety of Drugs distributed a pamphlet to all doctors in the United Kingdom in June 1967 warning of the possible dangers of overuse of inhalers, and these were removed from over-the-counter sale in December 1968. In addition, hospital admissions for asthma increased and there was also an increase in prescriptions of oral corticosteroids. The death rate fell following these moves.

## The Isoprenaline Forte Hypothesis

Despite the epidemiological evidence, and the presence of several plausible mechanisms (see next section), the inhaler hypothesis was regarded with skepticism by many respiratory physicians. This skepticism was partly justified by anomalies in the epidemiological data itself. In particular, there had been large sales of inhalers in the United States and several other countries that did not experience epidemics of deaths. This confusing situation was resolved by Paul Stolley, who was on sabbatical at Oxford, and became interested in this issue after attending a young man who had died after using isoprenaline in the village where he was living (Stolley, personal communication).

Stolley found that a high-dose version of isoprenaline (isoprenaline forte) had only been licensed in eight countries; six of these (England and Wales, Ireland, Scotland, Australia, New Zealand, and Norway) were the countries that had had mortality epidemics and these coincided with the introduction of the drug; in the other two countries (The Netherlands and Belgium) the preparation was introduced relatively late and sales volumes were low. Overall, there was a strong positive correlation internationally between the asthma death rate and isoprenaline forte sales in these eight countries (Fig. 4-3 shows data for England and Wales), whereas no mortality epidemics occurred in countries such as Canada and the United States in which isoprenaline forte was not licensed (Stolley, 1972). Stolley (personal communication) comments that:

> The company that made this drug cooperated with me when I first wrote to them, because I said that I was working on the problem [and that the theory that] these [beta agonist inhalers] were the cause of the epidemic was inconsistent with the American experience. So . . . they gave me lots of data. Then I sent them the manuscript when I finally finished and they told me they were going to sue me. I had to check with my university . . . and make sure the lawyers would defend me so I wouldn't go broke.

Stolley's paper was rejected by the *British Medical Journal* and the *Lancet*, but was finally published in the *American Review of Respiratory Diseases* in 1972 under the title "Why the United States was spared an epidemic of deaths due to asthma."

## Mechanisms

The asthma deaths during the epidemic were often sudden and unexplained, most occurred outside the hospital, direct information on drug usage was scanty, and the mechanism of death in individual patients was therefore unknown. However, the mechanism of death probably related to the fact that isoprenaline is a nonselective beta-receptor agonist. This means that isoprenaline also affects the beta-1 receptors (responsible for both an increase in inotropy and chronotropy) as much as the beta-2 receptors (responsible for smooth muscle relaxation). In particular, it increases the heart rate and blood pressure, and generally increases the workload of the heart. However, studies suggested that acute toxicity was unlikely to occur unless there had also been delays causing the patient's condition to deteriorate and hypoxemia (a shortage of oxygen) to occur. In this context, it was noted that the relief of symptoms could make it easier for a patient to tolerate worsening asthma, which might encourage delays in seeking medical help. This could be dangerous in itself, as well as increasing the chance of acute toxicity.

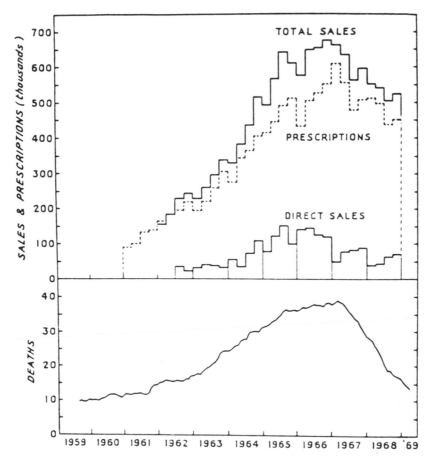

**Figure 4-3.**  Asthma deaths of persons aged 5–34 compared with sales and prescriptions of asthma preparations in England and Wales for 1959–1968.
*Source*: Inman and Adelstein (1969).

## History is Rewritten

By the early 1980s, the prevailing wisdom had changed, and the isoprenaline forte hypothesis was rejected in many medical texts and reviews (e.g., Olson, 1988). However, very little new evidence had appeared in the interim, and the process of reinterpretation of the 1960s epidemic was based on minor anomalies in the time trend data, which were emphasized, and to some extent exaggerated, in subsequent reviews (Stolley, 1993).

The tendency to discount the role of beta agonists received increasing emphasis as a result of the controversy following the decision of the U.S. Food and Drug Administration (FDA) in 1983 to license orciprenaline (a beta agonist drug that has cardiac side effects similar to those of isoprenaline) for nonprescription sale. The FDA decision was rescinded two months later, because of the concerns regarding the role of inhaled beta agonists in the 1960s mortality epidemic (Hendeles and Weinberger, 1983). Two reviews subsequently questioned the role of inhaled beta agonists in the 1960s mortality epidemic; one (Lanes and Walker, 1987) specifically acknowledged funding from the manufacturers of orciprenaline, Boehringer Ingelheim, whereas the other review (Esdaile et al., 1987) cited the FDA decision on orciprenaline as its justification. Both reviews dismissed the striking time trends in the six countries where isoprenaline forte was heavily sold, and instead emphasized the minor anomalies in the time trend data for other countries.

## The Second Epidemic—The New Zealand Case

In 1976, a second asthma mortality epidemic began in New Zealand, but not in other countries (see Fig. 4-2). It was first reported in 1981 by a Professor of Immunology at the Auckland Medical School, Doug Wilson, who noted an increase in young people dying suddenly from acute asthma in Auckland. Wilson speculated that the sudden nature of the deaths suggested a cardiac event, possibly due to overuse of beta agonists in combination with oral theophyllines. Jackson et al. (1982) subsequently studied the second New Zealand epidemic in depth, and concluded that it appeared to be real, and could not be explained by changes in the classification of asthma deaths, inaccuracies in death certification, or changes in diagnostic fashions. They concluded that it was very unlikely that the epidemic could be due to changes in the incidence or prevalence of asthma in New Zealand, and that the most likely explanation, as for the 1960s epidemics, appeared to be an increased case fatality rate related to changes in the treatment of asthma in New Zealand.

A national asthma mortality survey that was subsequently undertaken by the New Zealand Asthma Task Force (an ad hoc group funded by the former New Zealand Medical Research Council) included all of the 271 asthma deaths in persons under age 70 during 1981 through 1983 (Sears et al., 1985). However, the mortality survey did not include a control group, and (with one minor exception) the findings for individual asthma drugs were not reported. This reluctance to consider the possibility that the epidemic might be due to asthma drugs was surprising given the previous conclusions of Jackson et al. (1982). It may have been partly due to the difficulties of investigating this hypothesis, but it also reflected the prevailing sentiment among respiratory physicians that asthma drugs were not a major cause of asthma deaths.

### The Fenoterol Hypothesis

Thus, there was no tenable explanation for the second New Zealand asthma mortality epidemic until the fenoterol hypothesis was developed by the Wellington Asthma Research Group. This hypothesis stemmed initially from published reports of the greater cardiovascular side effects of fenoterol, and from incidental information in two previously published studies indicating that fenoterol was used by a relatively high proportion of asthmatics who died (Pearce et al., 1991). Fenoterol (a beta agonist that was marketed in a high dose preparation, like isoprenaline forte) was introduced to New Zealand in April 1976 and the epidemic of deaths began in the same year (Fig. 4-4). There was a rapid increase in the fenoterol market share to about 30%, and a similar rapid increase in the death rate, between 1976 and 1979. In contrast, the drug represented less than 5% of the market in most other countries and was not available in the United States. Although the market share in West Germany was 50%, use of inhaled beta agonists was relatively low in that country, and the per capita usage in New Zealand was greater than that of any other country and more than three times that in West Germany (Fig. 4-5). The reasons for the high sales of fenoterol in New Zealand are unclear but probably related to an effective marketing program. The company established good contacts with prominent New Zealand respiratory physicians through a series of annual asthma symposia in Rotorua, a major tourist resort.

Following these observations, our group conducted an experimental study that found that repeated use of fenoterol resulted in greater cardiac side effects than other commonly used beta agonists; these side effects were even greater than those of isoprenaline. The findings were similar to those in three previous studies that had tested fenoterol in relatively large doses, and also have been confirmed in subsequent studies conducted by our group and by others (Beasley et al., 1991).

Thus, by 1988 the epidemiological and experimental evidence strongly suggested that the high use of inhaled fenoterol could be the main cause of the second New Zealand asthma mortality epidemic. This evidence was comparable to that linking isoprenaline forte to the 1960s mortality epidemics. It had been generally agreed in discussions of the 1960s epidemic that the definitive method for testing such hypothe-

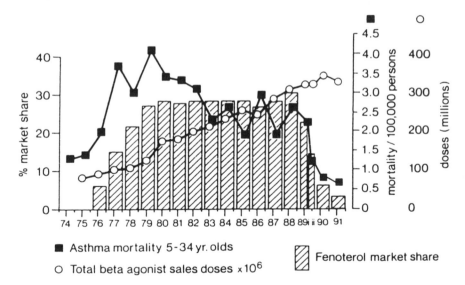

**Figure 4-4.** Fenoterol market share, total inhaled beta agonist sales, and asthma mortality in New Zealand 1974–1991.

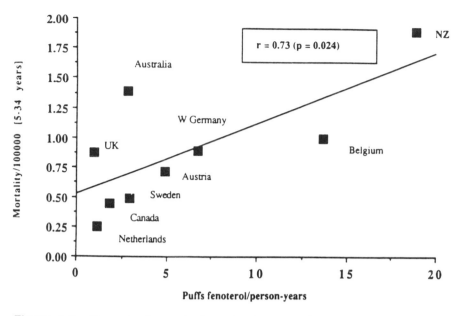

**Figure 4-5.** Per capita fenoterol sales and asthma mortality rates in 1985 in various countries.

ses was to conduct case-control studies of asthma deaths (Pearce and Crane, 1993). Because of the need to control for other risk factors for asthma death, such as chronic asthma severity, the ideal approach is to compare patients who died of asthma (cases) with a group of patients with nonfatal asthma of a similar chronic severity (controls). A suitable study design had been suggested in an internal Boehringer Ingelheim memorandum of October 1988:

> By comparing the exact drug medication of patients who died with hospital controls matched on the basis of severity (of past hospital admissions, of recent steroid use, and other factors) then any major disparity between the representation of [fenoterol], or other drugs, and the fact that they were compared with matched hospital controls, could be taken as positive evidence, and strong positive evidence, of a possible selective toxicity of the over-represented agent.

This approach was consistent with the findings of the only previously published case-control study of asthma deaths (Rea et al., 1986). Accordingly, our group conducted a case-control study (Crane et al., 1989) to investigate the possible role of fenoterol in the second New Zealand asthma mortality epidemic, using a design very similar to that outlined in the Boehringer Ingelheim memorandum. The study was partly based on drug data that had been collected for the previous New Zealand asthma mortality survey, but not previously reported; the cases (deaths) comprised all asthma deaths in New Zealand in the 5–45 year age group during 1981 through

1983, and for each case four controls were selected from records of hospital admissions for asthma during the same period (Table 4-1).

Information on prescribed drug therapy at the time of the last attack was documented for cases and controls. The only asthma drug found to be significantly associated with asthma deaths was fenoterol (Table 4-2); in patients with very severe asthma, the death rate in those prescribed fenoterol was more than ten times that in those prescribed other beta agonist inhalers (Crane et al., 1989).

## Problems With Publication

The case-control findings were very striking, and very consistent with the other epidemiological and experimental evidence. Nevertheless, we were aware that the findings of the case-control study were likely to come under attack, and this criticism began before the study had even been submitted for publication. The New Zealand Department of Health therefore convened an independent review panel to examine the research prior to its submission for publication. The review panel met with our research group and with members of the Asthma Task Force on December 20 and

TABLE 4-1. Studies of Fenoterol and Asthma Deaths

| | First New Zealand Study | Second New Zealand Study | Third New Zealand Study | Saskatchewan Study |
|---|---|---|---|---|
| Study period | 1981–1983 | 1977–1981 | 1981–1987 | 1980–1987 |
| Age group | 5–45 years | 5–45 years | 5–45 years | 5–54 years |
| Study base | All asthmatics | Patients with a hospital admission for asthma in previous year | Patients with a hospital admission for asthma in previous year | Patients with 10 different asthma prescriptions in 1978–1987 |
| Deaths (cases) | 117 | 58 | 112 | 44 |
| Controls | 468 | 227 | 427/448 | 233 |
| Matching for severity? | Yes (hospital admission controls) | Yes (hospital admission controls) | Yes (hospital admission controls) | Partial (matching for previous admission) |
| Information source Cases | Family doctor | Hospital records | Hospital records | Prescription records |
| Controls | Hospital records | Hospital records | Hospital records | Hospital records |
| Main exposure information | Prescribed medication* | Prescribed medication* | Prescribed medication* | Dispensed medication |
| Additional information | Nil | Nil | Nil | Number of units per month |
| Information on use? | No | No | No | No |

*Prescribed medication is synonymous with dispensed medication since prescribed beta agonists were free during the study period.

TABLE 4-2.  Findings from Studies of Fenoterol and Asthma Deaths

| | Relative Risk | | | |
|---|---|---|---|---|
| | First New Zealand Study | Second New Zealand Study | Third New Zealand Study[a] | Saskatchewan Study |
| Fenoterol | 1.6 | 2.0 | 2.1 | 5.3 |
| Salbutamol | 0.7 | 0.7 | 0.6 | 1.0 |

[a]Findings using control group A

21, 1988, and concluded that, although they had some criticisms, they would accept the study design as appropriate to the study and that "the findings of the study would be sufficient to justify public health action" (Leeder, 1988: 2).

The paper was submitted to the *Lancet* on February 3, 1989. The journal referred the paper to two independent referees who cleared it with very minor changes to the text, and it was accepted for publication on February 20, 1989. When the paper was submitted for publication, we gave a copy to the New Zealand Department of Health. We had repeatedly expressed our concern that there might be interference in the normal process of scientific peer review and publication if the manuscript were given to the manufacturer of fenoterol, Boehringer Ingelheim. However, we finally agreed for the then Director-General of Health to give a copy to the company on the written condition that the company would make no attempt to interfere with the paper's publication. Accordingly, on February 7, 1989 a copy of the manuscript was sent to the Medical Director of Boehringer Ingelheim (NZ), Doug Wilson (the former Professor of Immunology who had first raised the possibility that asthma drugs could have caused the second New Zealand epidemic). The first indication that all was not well came when an internal Boehringer Ingelheim report surfaced claiming that:

> There may be no formal protocol for the study. Information on this defect was provided by two Task Force members. . . . It appears that the protocol as such was developed during the course of the study as information came to hand.

This statement was incorrect, and was the first of many incorrect allegations from various sources to which we were subjected; the influence on reviewers of the study is a matter of speculation, although it is notable that at least one Boehringer Ingelheim reviewer subsequently referred to the possible lack of a formal protocol. Soon afterward, the first of many reviews commissioned by Boehringer Ingelheim began to arrive at the Department of Health. The first two reviews were written by the same groups that had previously disputed the role of isoprenaline forte in the 1960s epidemics, as a result of the FDA decision on the availability of orciprenaline, another Boehringer Ingelheim asthma drug. Although some reviews were relatively balanced, the overall weight of the Boehringer Ingelheim reviews was overwhelmingly negative, and quite emotional in defense of the drug. For example, Feinstein (1989: 3) argued that:

I shall be very surprised if the work is accepted by the Lancet. . . . If the work is accepted and published, the devastating criticism and subsequent embarrassment (for authors, editors, etc.) will occur afterward.

The approach of the Boehringer reviewers was predictable, given the history of similar epidemiological controversies. What was surprising in this instance was that some authorities apparently were influenced by these reviews, and even gave them equal weight with their own independent reviews. In particular, these reviews were sent to the *Lancet* by Boehringer Ingelheim, and on March 3, 1989 the *Lancet* wrote to our research group rescinding its previous unconditional acceptance of the manuscript.

In our reply of March 17, 1989, our research group stated that (Beasley et al., 1989: 1, 12):

We are concerned that our scientific paper, which was accepted unconditionally . . . could have this unconditional acceptance withdrawn following submissions made by a pharmaceutical company . . . we can counter convincingly the very critical comments . . . we look forward to seeing [the paper] in print.

The *Lancet* subsequently accepted these arguments, and the publication date was eventually set for April 29, 1989.

## The Department of Health Gets Lobbied

In the interim, the Boehringer lobbying was also operating in other spheres. On March 15, 1989, the New Zealand Director-General of Health wrote an internal memorandum stating that Boehringer Ingelheim was eager to work with the Department on contacts with the media. However, this joint approach apparently did not proceed, and just prior to the publication of the paper, the Department of Health and the company clashed over the Department's draft media release and its plan to send an abstract of the *Lancet* paper to all New Zealand doctors. Boehringer Ingelheim wrote to the Department that:

We are most concerned at your intended communication with doctors. . . . Enclosing a copy of the abstract suggests Departmental approval . . . unless the Department's approach is modified we are left with no option but to take every step available to us to protect ourselves.

The Department of Health's response to the company's lobbying was not helped by the fact that the Medicines Adverse Reactions Comittee (MARC) did not include an epidemiologist. However, the Department had commissioned its own review of the study by epidemiology Professors Mark Elwood and David Skegg. This, like the other independent reviews, was quite different in style and conclusions from the reviews commissioned by the company. It contained some criticisms of the study, but concluded (Elwood and Skegg, 1989: 35):

We recommend that action is taken on the basis that this study suggests there may be an increased risk of death from asthma in patients prescribed fenoterol by metered dose inhaler who have severe disease . . . This evidence, although far from conclusive, suggests that the current practice in the use of fenoterol should be modified.

## After Publication

The paper was finally published in the *Lancet* on April 29, 1989, and on that date the Health Department sent out a one-page letter advising doctors that "Fenoterol will not be withdrawn from the market, but doctors should review and perhaps modify the treatment of severe asthmatics."

However, this cautious advice was preempted by press releases from the company and the Asthma Task Force on April 28. The company's publicity package (the first of many over the ensuing two years) was sent by courier to most doctors, pharmacists, and health reporters in New Zealand, and was apparently also delivered to many respiratory physicians and pharmacoepidemiologists in other countries. It highlighted the conclusions of the New York meeting of Boehringer reviewers that the study had "serious flaws in design, execution and analysis which rendered its results uninterpretable." These conclusions received extensive coverage in the New Zealand media with headlines such as "Asthma study flawed say foreign experts."

## Further Investigations

### The Second Case-Control Study

Virtually all of the criticisms of the the first case-control study involved problems that were very unlikely to occur, were trivial, would tend to produce false negative results, or were simply incorrect. The most valid criticism was one that had been noted in the original report (Crane et al., 1989), and was also stressed in the review of Elwood and Skegg (1989), namely that the data for prescribed medicines was taken from different sources for the cases and controls. We therefore developed a new study design that enabled the information on prescribed drug therapy to be collected from the same sources for cases and controls. Using this design, we conducted a second New Zealand case-control study (Table 4-1) of asthma deaths in 5–45-year-olds during 1977 to 1981 (Pearce et al., 1990). This confirmed the findings of the first study that fenoterol was associated with asthma deaths (Table 4-2), and that in patients with very severe asthma the death rate in those prescribed fenoterol was much higher than in those prescribed other beta agonist inhalers.

### The Response

This second study was presented on June 29, 1989 at a Pharmacoepidemiology Symposium in Newcastle, Australia. The symposium, which included pharmacoepidemiologists and regulatory authorities from Australia, New Zealand, the United Kingdom, and the United States, concluded that the new study overcame the principal problems with the previous study, and that the evidence was now sufficiently strong that the drug should be withdrawn in New Zealand.

The Boehringer reviewers prepared their response at a meeting at the Beverly

Wilshire Hotel on July 28, 1989. Our group was excluded from the meeting, but the Director of the New Zealand Medical Research Council attended as an observer. His report was complimentary about some aspects of the proceedings, but noted that (Hodge, 1989: 4):

> [The participants] were under some pressure [during the preparation of the final report] from the PR representative . . . who clearly held partisan views in favour of Boehringer Ingelheim. . . . The company representatives prepared the ground for the meeting but stood back from the actual proceedings. . . . Nevertheless their presence could not be ignored and their hospitality was generous, to say the least.

The meeting concluded that "The second study avoids only one of the methodologic problems of the first study . . . but has retained others and introduced new methodologic problems" (Buist et al., 1989: 11).

The Department of Health also commissioned an independent review of the second study (Elwood, 1989: 7, 11) that reached the very different conclusion that:

> The balance of the available information is in favour of the causal rather than the confounding hypothesis . . . It is recommended that the drug regulatory authorities should take steps to ensure that the use of fenoterol is minimised.

The controversy in New Zealand was effectively resolved in December 1989 when it was announced that the drug was to be removed from the Drug Tariff. This action followed a recommendation from MARC (which by now included an epidemiologist) as a result of its examination of the Elwood review. Similar action was announced in Australia in March 1990, and the company subsequently halved the dose of the drug in the United Kingdom and other countries.

## Further Research in New Zealand

More recently, our group conducted a third national case-control study (funded by the Asthma Foundation) of deaths during 1981 to 1987 (Grainger et al., 1991); two control groups were used in order to address the remaining criticisms that had been made of the previous studies. Whichever control group was used, fenoterol was associated with an increased risk of asthma death, but the alternative control group suggested by Boehringer critics of the previous studies actually yielded stronger relative risks than the approach used previously.

The strongest evidence in support of the New Zealand findings has come from a Boehringer-funded study conducted in Canada by several members of the Boehringer consensus panels (Spitzer et al., 1992). This study examined 44 asthma deaths in the province of Saskatchewan during 1980 to 1987 and 233 controls (see Table 4-1). Nearly half of the deaths had been prescribed fenoterol compared with 16% of the controls; overall the death rate in those prescribed fenoterol was five times that in those prescribed other beta agonists (see Table 4-2). However, these results (which confirmed the New Zealand findings) were not mentioned in an abstract that was circulated widely prior to the publication of the paper (Bown, 1991). Instead, the abstract focused on the possibility of a general class effect of beta agonists. This abstract received extensive publicity in the *New York Times*, the *Lancet*, and the *New Scientist* (Bown, 1991) prior to the publication of the paper, thus leading to confusion about the safety of beta agonists in general, and obscuring the fact that the study had confirmed the New Zealand findings regarding fenoterol.

## Epilogue

Following the warnings about the use of fenoterol issued in mid-1989 (following the publication of our first case-control study), the asthma death rate immediately fell by half (Crane et al., 1992; Pearce et al, 1995). From 1983 to 1988 the New Zealand asthma death rate in the 5–34 age group had averaged 2.3 per 100,000, and the death rate was 2.2 in the first half of 1989. In the second half of 1989 (i.e., after warnings were issued about fenoterol), the death rate fell to 1.1, and fell further to about 0.8 during 1990–1992 (paralleling the fall in fenoterol market share). This sudden fall in asthma deaths coincided with warnings that fenoterol should not be used by severe asthmatics (and a corresponding decline in sales), just as the sudden increase in deaths coincided with the introduction of fenoterol in 1976 (see Fig. 4-4). On the other hand, the time trend data were inconsistent with the hypothesis (suggested by the authors of the Boehringer-funded study in Saskatchewan) that the epidemic may have been due to a class effect of beta agonists. The switch to regular use of beta agonists (and the sharp rise in overall beta-agonist sales) occurred in 1979, whereas the epidemic commenced in 1976. Furthermore, total sales of beta agonists actually increased slightly during 1989 and 1990, whereas fenoterol sales and asthma deaths both fell dramatically.

# Issues for the Future

The beta agonist story provides a rather extreme example of the problems of pharmaceutical safety. It is partly a story of epidemics in six countries (particularly New Zealand), but also of the avoidance of epidemics in other countries (including the United States). I do not intend to fully discuss all of the relevant issues here, but rather to raise some general issues, some of which are addressed elsewhere in this book. In doing so, I do not intend to imply that all of these issues relate specifically to the beta agonist story.

## The Company and Its Consultants

An article about the fenoterol controversy in the *Epidemiology Monitor* (Bernier, 1990) raised the issue of what limits should be set on a company's efforts to defend its products that have been implicated in serious side effects. Clearly a company has a right to argue against what it believes is weak data or incorrect conclusions, and it is not in the interests of society or the company to withdraw a drug that has been incorrectly implicated. However, a company's right to defend itself does not extend to interference with publication or impugning the integrity of the researchers concerned.

A common feature of controversies about drug safety is the use of hired consultants who review and criticize the research. A company clearly has a moral obligation to seek the truth of the matter when seeking advice from consultants, rather than just to prepare the "case for the defense." This is not to imply that deliberate corruption occurs; in fact, this appears to be very rare. However, a company that intends to prepare the "case for the defense" may seek out consulting firms or academics who (usually because of sincerely-held beliefs) have been very critical of similar studies in the past. Thus, the shaping of the "case for the defense" usually involves selection rather than coercion of experts, although subtle forms of influence may also occur.

The response of consultants may also depend heavily on what question is posed to them. One possible question would be "Is there any chance that the data are right?", to which the answer is invariably "yes." Most commonly, however, the question is "Is there any chance that the data are wrong?", to which the answer is also invariably "yes." This is perhaps the question that is most appropriate in the scientific context, where the emphasis is on scientific criticism and debate. However, in the context of public health decision making, the most appropriate question is "On balance, what conclusion is most likely true from the data?" Clearly, quite different reviews will eventuate depending on which question is asked.

A related issue is the attitude of the consultants toward the reviewing process. For example, several of the Boehringer Ingelheim reviews with regard to orciprenaline and fenoterol came from a group that has disputed most of the major epidemiological discoveries in the past 15 years, including such well-established associations as tobacco and lung cancer, oral contraceptives and stroke, diethylstilbestrol and vaginal cancer, estrogens and endometrial cancer, tampon use and toxic shock syndrome, and aspirin and Reye's syndrome (Savitz et al., 1990; Greenland, 1991). Although criticism is an important component of the scientific process, an overemphasis on it (sometimes justified by crude interpretations of the Popperian philosophy of science) can lead to almost any scientific study being dismissed as fatally flawed (Stolley, 1989).

This process can produce an apparent consensus that is quite different from the real consensus of independent scientists. This can be very influential since, although science is based on criticism and debate, public health policy is generally based on consensus. Thus, the selection by the company of a few scientists who are hypercritical of others' work can result in massive pressure on public health decision makers. This pressure is particularly effective since it apparently comes from independent scientists, whereas it would not be taken so seriously if it came directly from the company. In this sense, the company's reviewers have the privilege of acting as "lawyers for the defense" while presenting themselves as an independent jury.

This approach has become so widespread, in the United States in particular, that it has become accepted as part of normal epidemiological practice, and some industry consultants are now even arguing that there is no need to acknowledge industry funding of such reviews (Rothman, 1993).

## The Journal

This type of reviewing also poses problems for a journal that is considering for publication a paper implicating a particular drug in serious side effects. Ideally, a good journal should stand by its own reviewing process, and should not consider any unsolicited reviews. However, as the *Epidemiology Monitor* points out (Bernier, 1990: 4), if reviews commissioned by a company are sent to a journal, "the journal is placed in a difficult position because it may feel that it cannot prudently ignore the criticisms, yet they may not have been obtained during the normal process of peer review."

In the case of fenoterol, the *Lancet* has consistently denied that it suffered any undue pressure. For example, following the publication of our first paper, we submitted a letter for publication in the *Lancet*, stating that (Crane et al., 1989: 1):

> We would like to express our concern at the attempts by Boehringer Ingelheim to influence the normal process of publication of a scientific study, and to influence its subsequent assessment.
>
> . . . We are concerned at the precedent that Boehringer Ingelheim has set. . . . It is possible that a journal without the independence and integrity of the *Lancet* might have been influenced by these attempts.

Despite our attempts to let the *Lancet* off the hook, the journal resisted the notion that anything untoward had happened. In reply, the Deputy Editor of the *Lancet* claimed that (Sharp, 1989: 1):

> We were not put under pressure but merely asked if we would like to see copies of reports commissioned by the company. . . . I propose to put your letter on ice since I think you will be well advised to think again about it.

## The Researchers

Hostile reviews also pose a dilemma for researchers who have discovered evidence that a particular drug may have serious side effects. In theory, any evidence of hazard should be made immediately available to the scientific community, and should have some influence on public health decision making. In practice, researchers who have discovered evidence that a particular drug may be hazardous require very strong evidence, a fair amount of perseverance, a sense of humor, and a good lawyer. Even then, there is the danger that, despite the best of intentions, researchers may overreact to the resulting wave of criticism and may overstate the case against the drug, particularly if they consider that the company's criticisms are trivial, irrelevant, or incorrect. As Stolley (1989: 54) writes:

> The pharmacoepidemiologist must develop a thick skin; this is not a field for timid souls. More important, the pharmacoepidemiologist must have some historical and ideologic anchorage and perspective to be able to understand the nature of the attacks.

Ultimately, the best approach for researchers is to address any criticisms in further studies; certainly, this approach was the key factor that eventually led to the resolution of the fenoterol saga.

## The Future

There is an old saying that those who do not learn the lessons of history are condemned to repeat them. It is tempting to speculate whether the second New

Zealand mortality epidemic could have been avoided if knowledge gained from studies of the 1960s epidemics had been properly heeded. Certainly, the greater potency and greater cardiac side effects of fenoterol were known before its introduction and widespread use, as was the fact that fenoterol could cause death in baboons when infused in doses previously given to humans. Thus it is important that the lessons of the isoprenaline and fenoterol debates are not ignored again. More generally, it is important that new drugs are tested under the conditions and in the doses in which they are likely to be used, and that evidence of side effects is considered seriously. As Stolley (1991) noted in an FDA hearing on the safety of beta agonists:

> The United States has been spared two epidemics of asthma mortality, because . . . the FDA has not licensed either fenoterol or isoprenaline in its forte concentration. Now those people who believe that the FDA imposes an unnecessary burden on the industry because of their rigorous premarketing scrutiny of drugs, might rethink their position, because the epidemics occurred in those countries where drug regulatory agencies are unfortunately weaker than ours.

## Acknowledgments

Neil Pearce is funded by a Principal Research Fellowship of the Health Research Council of New Zealand.

# References

Baumann A and Lee S (1990) Trends in asthma mortality in Australia, 1911–1986. *Medical Journal of Australia* 153: 366 (letter).

Beasley R, Burgess C, Crane J, Jackson R, and Pearce N (1989) Unpublished letter to Deputy Editor, *The Lancet*. Wellington.

Beasley R, Pearce N, Crane J, Windom H, and Burgess C (1990) Asthma mortality and inhaled beta agonist therapy. *Australian and New Zealand Journal of Medicine* 21: 753–63.

Bernier R (1990) Asthma drug controversy climaxes with government decision to restrict use. *Epidemiology Monitor* 11(3): 1–5.

Bown W (1991) Warning letter links asthma deaths to drugs. *New Scientist* 27 July, p. 9.

Buist AS, Burney PGJ, Ernst P, et al. (1989) *Consensus Report: An Appraisal of a Manuscript by N. Pearce et al.* Unpublished report. Los Angeles: Boehringer Ingelheim.

Crane J, Pearce N, Burgess C, and Beasley R (1989) Unpublished letter to *The Lancet*. Wellington.

Crane J, Pearce N, Flatt A, et al. (1989) Prescribed fenoterol and death from asthma in New Zealand, 1981–1983: a case-control study. *Lancet* i: 917–22.

Crane J, Burgess C, Pearce NE, Beasley R, and Durham J (1991) Adult asthma management 1991: the patient takes the helm, health professionals chart the course. *Therapeutic Note* No 211. Wellington: Department of Health.

Crane J, Pearce NE, Burgess C, Beasley R, and Jackson R (1992) Asthma deaths in New Zealand. *British Medical Journal* 304: 1307 (letter).

Elwood JM and Skegg DCG (1989) *Review of Studies Relating Prescribed Fenoterol and Death from Asthma in New Zealand*. Wellington: Department of Health.

Elwood JM (1989) *Prescribed Fenoterol and Deaths from Asthma in New Zealand—Second Report*. Wellington: Department of Health.

Esdaile JM, Feinstein AR, and Horwitz RI (1987) A reappraisal of the United Kingdom epidemic of fatal asthma. *Archives of Internal Medicine* 147: 543–49.

Feinstein AR (1989) Unpublished letter to Medical Director, Boehringer Ingelheim (NZ) Ltd. New Haven, CN.

Grainger J, Woodman K, Pearce NE, et al. (1991) Prescribed fenoterol and death from asthma in New Zealand 1981–7: a further case-control study. *Thorax* 46: 105–11.

Greenberg MJ and Pines A (1967) Pressurized aerosols in asthma. *British Medical Journal* 1: 563 (letter).

Greenland S (1991) Science versus advocacy: the challenge of Dr Feinstein. *Epidemiology* 2: 64–71.

Hendeles L and Weinberger M (1983) Nonprescription sale of inhaled metaproterenol—deja vu. *New England Journal of Medicine* 310: 207–8.

Hodge JV (1989) *Fenoterol and Asthma Mortality: Report on Attendance at a Meeting in Los Angeles on 29 July 1989*. Auckland: Medical Research Council of New Zealand.

Inman WHW and Adelstein AM (1969) Rise and fall of asthma mortality in England and Wales in relation to use of pressurized aerosols. *Lancet* ii: 279–85.

Jackson R, Sears MR, Beaglehole R, et al. (1988) International trends in asthma mortality, 1970 to 1985. *Chest* 94: 914–18.

Jackson RT, Beaglehole R, Rea HH, et al. (1982) Mortality from asthma: a new epidemic in New Zealand. *British Medical Journal* 285: 771–74.

Keeney EL (1964) The history of asthma from Hippocrates to Meltzer. *Journal of Allergy* 35: 215–26.

Lanes SF and Walker AM (1987) Do pressurized bronchodilator aerosols cause death among asthmatics? *American Journal of Epidemiology* 125: 755–60.

Leeder SJ (1989) Unpublished minutes of a meeting of asthma investigators to discuss progress of a study of asthma deaths in New Zealand and their association with the use of inhaled fenoterol. Wellington.

Neville RG, Clark RC, Hoskins G, et al. (1993) National asthma attack audit 1991–2. *British Medical Journal* 306: 559–62.

Olson LG (1988) Acute severe asthma: what to do until the ambulance arrives. *New Ethicals* 105–16.

Pearce NE, Grainger J, Atkinson M, et al. (1990) Case-control study of prescribed fenoterol and death from asthma in New Zealand, 1977–1981. *Thorax* 45: 170–75.

Pearce NE, Crane J, Burgess C, et al. (1991) Beta agonists and asthma mortality: deja vu. *Clinical and Experimental Allergy* 21: 401–10.

Pearce NE and Crane J (1993) Epidemiological methods for studying the role of beta receptor agonist therapy in asthma mortality. In: Beasley R and Pearce NE (eds.) *The Role of Beta Agonist Therapy in Asthma Mortality*. New York: CRC Press, pp. 67–83.

Pearce NE, Beasley R, Crane J, Burgess C, Jackson R (1995) End of the New Zealand asthma mortality epidemic. *Lancet* 345:41–44.

Rea HH, Scragg R, Jackson R, et al. (1986) A case-control study of deaths from asthma. *Thorax* 41: 833–39.

Rothman KJ (1993) Conflict of interest: the new McCarthyism in science. *Journal of the American Medical Association* 269: 2782–84.

Savitz DA, Greenland S, Stolley PD, et al. (1990) Scientific standards of criticism: a reaction to "Scientific standards in epidemiologic studies of the menace of daily life." by A. R. Feinstein. *Epidemiology* 1: 78–83.

Sears MR, Rea HH, Beaglehole R, et al. (1985) Asthma mortality in New Zealand: a two year national study. *New Zealand Medical Journal* 98: 2715.

Sharp D (1989) Unpublished letter in reply to Crane J et al. London.

Speizer FE and Doll R (1968) A century of asthma deaths in young people. *British Medical Journal* 3: 245–46.

Speizer FE, Doll R, and Heaf P (1968) Observations on recent increase in mortality from asthma. *British Medical Journal* i: 335–39.

Spitzer WO, Suissa S, Ernst P, et al. (1992) The use of beta-agonists and the risk of death and near death from asthma. *New England Journal of Medicine* 326: 501–6.

Stolley PD (1972) Why the United States was spared an epidemic of deaths due to asthma. *American Review of Respiratory Diseases* 105: 883–90.

Stolley PD (1989) A public health perspective from academia. In: Strom BL (ed.) *Pharmacoepidemiology*. New York: Churchill Livingstone, pp. 51–55.

Stolley, PD (1991) *Testimony*. Pulmonary-Allergy Drugs Advisory Committee. December 12, 1991. Vol. I. Washington, DC: FDA, pp. 285–86.

Stolley, P (1993) The bellman always rings thrice. *Annals of Internal Medicine* 118: 158 (letter).

# 5

# The Consumer Movement:
# From Single-Issue
# Campaigns to
# Long-Term Reform

BARBARA MINTZES
CATHERINE HODGKIN

Until the 1960s there was little idea of patients' rights and no question of an organized consumer input into health policy. Although the Nuremberg Code, published in 1949, sought to prevent repetition of the atrocities carried out in concentration camps in the name of medicine, it was not until the publication of the Helsinki Declaration in 1964 that clear guidelines were adopted defining clinical investigation and treatment for the benefit of the patient (Medawar, 1992: 86).

Thirty years later, a widespread international consumer movement is concerned with the rights of users, safety, and access to independent information, and the elimination of double standards in international drug marketing. Increasingly, consumer groups have also focused on institutional reforms leading to effective consumer representation in all aspects of drug policy.

This chapter outlines the recent history of consumer involvement in drug policy, looking in more detail at how consumers have pushed for policies that reflect their needs and priorities through examples of specific campaigns. A final section assesses current gains and the major challenges presented by new developments in the regulation of pharmaceuticals.

## The Emergence of the Consumer Movement

Consumer involvement in the pharmaceutical arena can be attributed to the more general growth of the consumer movement worldwide, to a growing concern with the quality of goods and services, and to a more informed and demanding public. It also arose in response to specific tragedies that raised public awareness about the risks of drugs and caused anger about the apparent lack of caution contributing to drug-induced injuries.

### A Brief History

The use of organic arsenicals during World War I and Elixir of Sulfanilamide in the United States "drew attention to the fact that the new drug products could sometimes gravely injure or kill their users" (Dukes and Schwartz, 1988: 1). The U.S. Food and Drug Administration (FDA) was established after more than 70 people died from taking a sulfanilamide elixir containing ethylene glycol (Chetley, 1990: 22) and requirements for drug safety testing were introduced. However, it was not until early 1962 that regulations were tightened to require proof of efficacy. This followed the introduction of thalidomide in 1958 and its use during pregnancy, resulting in the birth of an estimated 8000 babies in 46 countries with severe birth defects (Braithwaite, 1984).

The 1970s saw the beginnings of an organized international consumer response to questions of drug safety. The work of the Swedish doctor Olle Hansson to ensure that those harmed by clioquinol were recognized and received compensation led to a prolonged conflict with Ciba Geigy and to a boycott of the company in some countries (Hansson, 1989). This campaign also brought together many of the groups that were to become part of the Health Action International (HAI) network, which was formed in 1981 to address drug issues from a user perspective.

While on one hand mistakes with drugs underlined the need for consumer protection, on the other hand consumer power in the industrialized world was growing and was increasingly acknowledged. The Consumers Union was formed in the United States in 1936, but was for many years the only organization of its kind (Sim, 1991: 1). By 1959 four additional consumer organizations had been founded in Europe: in the United Kingdom, Belgium, Holland, and France (Sim, 1991: 3), and, in 1960, 17 organizations from 14 countries joined to form the International Organization of Consumers' Unions (IOCU) (Sim, 1991: 26). The first consumer organizations in the developing world were established in the 1960s and many of these became members of IOCU.

### Defining Consumer Rights

Initially the national consumer associations were largely concerned with testing and the comparison of products, but this focus gradually changed to include advocacy, representation, and education.

In 1962 John F. Kennedy talked of consumers as "the largest economic group . . .

the only important group in the economy whose views are not heard." Kennedy defined four basic consumer rights: the right to safety, to be informed, to choose, and to be heard (Wells and Tiranti, 1985: 3). Consumer groups have since further defined and elaborated these basic principles, adding rights to access, equity, redress, and representation (National Consumer Council, 1993).

Consumer advocacy on health issues has addressed these principles at a number of levels. As mentioned above, safety and consumer representation remain key concerns. Questions of access and equity have been directed toward national governments providing health care services and toward international agencies. Well over half the population in developing countries still lacks access to essential drugs (Kanji et al., 1992). In this connection consumer groups have supported the introduction of national drug policies based on WHO's Model List of Essential Drugs as a means to increase access to needed drugs both in the public and private sectors.

The principle of choice cannot be applied to drugs and health services in the same way as to other consumer products. People do not generally choose to be ill and to need to use a medicine. A person is vulnerable when seriously ill or when caring for an ill child. In recognition of this vulnerability, consumer groups have argued for strong controls on drug promotion, better training for prescribers, guidelines governing health services and drug treatments, and access to full, independent information on which to base informed choices.

Redress for drug-induced injury remains inadequate. Injured users have addressed companies directly through litigation in individual and class action suits. Consumer groups have also argued for the need to introduce patient compensation schemes for injuries resulting from drug or medical treatment, such as Sweden's program (Dukes, 1990).

## A Broad and Diverse Movement

The consumer movement in the health and pharmaceuticals area is not homogeneous and consists of many types of groups and organizations. At the national level there are:

- national consumer groups whose primary focus is, in general, product testing and comparison. They increasingly also look at services and utilities and some of them produce publications on health issues, such as the magazine *Which Way to Health?* in the United Kingdom. Where consumer representation exists on government committees dealing with drug policy, it is usually through national consumer organizations.
- health rights groups, which focus on the quality of goods and services and on empowering users of drugs and health services. Examples include the Health Action Information Network in the Philippines, which has been influential in the development of a national drug policy, Social Audit in the United Kingdom, which has campaigned for greater transparency in medicines policy, and Public Citizen's Health Research Group in the United States.
- women's health groups, which have played a major role in breaking down traditional medical barriers. The publication of *Our Bodies Ourselves* in 1971 by the

Boston Women's Health Book Collective was an influential early example of information for the public that demystified medical procedures, pointed to existing discrimination, and advocated better medical care and increased consumer responsibility. The women's health movement has been primarily concerned with questions of equity and human rights and has brought broader concerns about women's position in society into the evaluation of health services and drug marketing.

- patient groups, which include organizations begun by people with specific health conditions as diverse as asthma, multiple sclerosis, endometriosis, AIDS, or physical and mental disabilities. They have mostly been formed by people suffering from chronic or serious conditions in order to provide information and emotional support to others in the same position and to lobby for better medical care. Some of these groups press for more access to new drugs or for more research funds for a particular illness.

- development-oriented groups in industrialized and developing countries, which aim to address inequalities in access to and quality of health care, such as BUKO in Germany (the federal Congress of Development Action Groups), the Association for Health and Environmental Development in Egypt, and the Voluntary Health Association of India. While working on national, international, and industry policies, they are centrally concerned with social justice, equity, and global disparities in wealth and power.

What the consumer organizations have in common is that they represent the special interests of people as users or potential users of pharmaceuticals and health care services. Their presence challenges the paternalistic model of medical care, redefining it from a user perspective with an increased emphasis on primary health care, prevention, and individual responsibility.

## An "International Antibody" to Marketing Excesses

At an international level, consumer interests on pharmaceutical questions have been raised through the HAI network and IOCU (one of its founding members). HAI was founded in Geneva shortly after the World Health Organization (WHO) passed an infant feeding code as the result of pressure from consumer groups in the International Baby Food Action Network, a loose coalition of nongovernmental organizations (NGOs) set up in 1979. HAI was to be an "'international antibody' to the worst effects of international pharmaceutical marketing" (Chetley, 1990: 71).

Initially the HAI network and its participants were dismissed by the pharmaceutical industry as extremists and attempts were made to discredit them as Moscow-funded communists (Chetley, 1990), but as more and more respected professionals allied themselves with the consumer critics and as their campaigns scored successes, it became impossible to ignore them.

In 1985 WHO organized the Nairobi Conference on the Rational Use of Drugs, which was intended to provide a new framework for the development of drug policy internationally. This meeting involved all the various interest groups including government, health professionals, the media, industry, and consumers. During the Nairobi Conference the role and responsibilities of consumers were clearly defined.

Since 1985, consumer representatives have been increasingly included in international policy discussions.

## Drug-Oriented Campaigns

Consumers have aimed to influence not only the pharmaceutical industry and regulatory authorities but also the general public, the medical profession, pharmacists, and medical insurance schemes. The brief sketches of consumer campaigns that follow have been chosen to show the variety of strategies consumers have used to make their voices heard and the range of levels at which they have worked. These sketches include campaigns focused on specific drugs at international and national levels. They also trace a growing demand for long-term structural changes leading to representation not only in solving existing problems, but also in policy development and access to the information on which regulatory decisions are based.

### Confronting International Double Standards

One of the key functions of the HAI network is to share information about national consumer campaigns and regulatory actions. Double standards almost always operate to the disadvantage of consumers in developing countries, where regulation is frequently very weak. Products that are banned or severely restricted in industrialized countries are often freely available in developing countries. Information given to consumers and prescribers, particularly on side effects, warnings, and contraindications, may be less complete. Greater claims are frequently made and a broader range of indications given (U.S. Congress, 1993; van Maaren et al., 1993). In confronting these problems consumer groups address not only national regulatory bodies, but also individual companies and industry associations.

### Pressuring Industry: The Example of Appetite Stimulants

In 1985, Social Audit, a U.K.-based organization, launched an international campaign against the promotion of appetite stimulants for children in developing countries. Internationally, the two leading drugs were cyproheptadine (Periactin), manufactured by Merck, Sharp and Dohme (MSD), and pizotifen (Mosegor), manufactured by Sandoz (Chetley, 1993: 106). These are both antihistamines that can increase appetite and promote weight gain as a side effect. The FDA judged that cyproheptadine was ineffective as an appetite stimulant in 1971, and MSD stopped promoting it for this indication in the United States (Chetley, 1993). In industrialized countries, cyproheptadine is used to treat allergic reactions and pizotifen is mainly used to treat migraines.

Appetite stimulants are popular in developing countries because loss of appetite is a common symptom of malnutrition and disease in children. However, they do nothing to combat the source of the problem—poverty and lack of adequate food—and lead to a waste of scarce resources.

Social Audit published an "antiadvertisement" on appetite stimulants in 1985, describing double standards in the promotion of these products. HAI Pakistan launched a national campaign against appetite stimulants during the same year. A U.S.-based organization, the Interfaith Center on Corporate Responsibility, made a complaint to MSD about their marketing of cyproheptadine in developing countries. In 1986, MSD declared that it would no longer promote cyproheptadine as an appetite stimulant. However, they stated, "the formal decision to discontinue promoting Periactin as an appetite stimulant . . . in no way reflects agreement with the implication of the Social Audit brochure. Appetite stimulation remains a medically valid, widely accepted use for Periactin" (Anonymous, 1986).

This was also the year in which HAI's first *Problem Drugs* pack was published; appetite stimulants were one of the categories of problem drugs highlighted (Chetley and Gilbert, 1986). In 1988, the Peruvian organization Tierra Nueva and national consumer organizations in India working within the All India Drugs Action Network also began public campaigns against the sale of drugs to stimulate appetite. MaLAM (Medical Lobby for Appropriate Marketing), an international network of health professionals that sends letters to industry questioning unethical marketing, also wrote to MSD in 1989 questioning their promotion of Periactin.

In 1993, HAI launched a revised edition of *Problem Drugs* that again drew attention to the continuing sale of Periactin as an appetite stimulant and criticized MSD for not acting to stop this (Chetley, 1993). During the launch of *Problem Drugs*, Australian HAI participants brought the sale of appetite stimulants to the attention of MSD Australia, which agreed to initiate a dialogue with MSD International. MSD announced in late 1993 that it would cease production of combination products containing cyproheptadine and vitamins and that it would delete the appetite stimulation indication for Periactin (Anonymous, 1993a). In early 1994, a Canadian generic manufacturer of cyproheptadine, Pharmascience, also agreed to withdraw the indication (Lexchin, 1994).

## Pressure For National Regulatory Action on Bromocriptine

In industrialized countries with a well-established regulatory system consumers are sometimes able to bring their complaints to the regulatory authority. A recent example is the U.S. group Public Citizen's work on bromocriptine as a lactation suppressant, a condition for which drug treatment is not needed.

In June 1989, the FDA Fertility and Maternal Health Advisory Committee recommended that the indication of postpartum breast engorgement (PPBE) be deleted for all drugs marketed for this condition, including bromocriptine. An expert review had concluded that these drugs were largely ineffective and unnecessarily risky. The FDA wrote to the companies asking that they voluntarily withdraw the indication of PPBE, and all complied except Sandoz (Anonymous, 1993a). The FDA did not press the issue, and bromocriptine continued to be prescribed to an estimated 300,000 women per year for this indication, with annual sales of $12.5 million (Wolfe and Moore, 1993).

In September 1993, Public Citizen's Health Research Group filed a citizen's petition with the FDA calling for the removal of the indication of PPBE for bromocriptine (Wolfe and Moore, 1993). They charged that the FDA had not followed up on recommendations of its advisory committee four years earlier. Their testimony criticized not only Sandoz's refusal to comply, but the FDA's inaction beyond a request for voluntary withdrawal of the indication. From 1989 to 1993, an additional 13 women had died from strokes and seizures after using bromocriptine and 14 had been permanently disabled.

The FDA announced in September 1993 that it would withdraw the PPBE indication for Parlodel, Sandoz's bromocriptine product, "within the next few months" (Anonymous, 1993a). Almost a year later, in August 1994, Public Citizen and the National Women's Health Network began a lawsuit against the FDA because of their "unreasonable delay" in acting to ban this indication. The FDA announced the next day, August 17, that it intended to withdraw approval of the indication. This was followed—again a day later—by an announcement by Sandoz that it was voluntarily withdrawing this indication for Parlodel. Sandoz also withdrew the indication in Canada, but maintained it in all other countries where Parlodel was sold. HAI passed the documentation from Public Citizen and the FDA to members of its international network, enabling them to pursue the issue. Within one month of the U.S. withdrawal of the indication, the issue had been raised in the press and with regulatory authorities and Sandoz in countries as diverse as Australia, Burkino Faso, Germany, Italy, Korea, Latvia, Mauritius, The Netherlands, Pakistan, Switzerland, Tanzania, Thailand, and Zimbabwe.

## DES: From Exposure to Expert Pressure

The campaigns on appetite stimulants and bromocriptine have been mainly directed at the pharmaceutical industry and national governments. They concern elimination of double standards in marketing and implementation of effective regulation to safeguard consumer health. The example of DES (diethylstilbestrol) illustrates how widespread exposure to a harmful drug has led to a campaign that broadened to include regulatory policy and standards of medical care, as well as the more immediate issues of safety and redress.

DES, developed in 1938, was used for a wide variety of indications, but became particularly commonly prescribed as a drug to prevent miscarriage and for other pregnancy problems. An estimated two to three million women in the United States took the drug during pregnancy (Orenberg, 1981).

A case-control study conducted by Herbst and his colleagues showed a strong association between prenatal DES exposure and clear-cell adenocarcinoma (Herbst et al., 1971). FDA regulatory action followed swiftly, banning use in pregnancy in 1971. Other national regulatory agencies in industrialized countries gradually followed suit, in some cases not until the early 1980s (Direcks et al., 1991). Although clear-cell cancer is relatively rare, reproductive tract abnormalities are common in women and men exposed prenatally to DES, leading to fertility and pregnancy problems (Kaufman et al., 1977; Leary et al., 1984).

There have been many successful lawsuits in the United States by women who were exposed to DES prenatally and developed cancer as a result. These cases have faced the barrier that women frequently cannot name the specific manufacturer of the DES their mothers took. DES was produced by many manufacturers because it was never patented. A ground-breaking case in New York in 1979 awarded Joyce Bichler compensation on the basis of market share liability (Orenberg, 1981), in which the companies selling DES were held liable for damages in proportion to the share of the market they held when it was prescribed. Other cases have successfully challenged state statutes of limitations that limit liability to no more than ten years after an injury has occurred. In October 1992, The Netherlands became the second country to pave the way for compensation for women with DES-associated cancer who could not name the manufacturer ('t Hoen, 1992).

Those involved in the various DES Action groups have gone much further than campaigning for compensation[1]. They want redress but also want to trace those affected by the drug, to get recognition of the scale of the problem, and to ensure that those affected have access to counseling, support, and appropriate medical care. This has included involvement in developing protocols for diagnosis and treatment of conditions associated with DES exposure and, in The Netherlands, pushing gynecologists to form a network of DES specialists (van den Berg, 1993). A survey of Dutch DES daughters found that women who had contact with DES Action experienced a better doctor relationship: "Doctors conduct better medical examinations and give more information and their patients are more assertive" (Zalmstra et al., 1989).

DES Action groups have also broadened their work to expand awareness of the potential dangers of using medicines during pregnancy and to call for higher standards for testing both the effectiveness and safety of new drugs and procedures such as infertility treatments and drugs prescribed to prevent breast cancer (DES Action Canada, 1993).

## From Drug-Oriented Campaigns to Long-Term Reforms

The work on specific drugs such as DES, appetite stimulants, and bromocriptine continues. However, these are classic examples of early consumer drug campaigns, which tended to target specific drugs or groups of drugs. Some consumer campaigns continue to be drug-oriented: examples include antidiarrheal drugs, which lead to especially acute problems in developing countries; and unnecessarily dangerous analgesics such as dipyrone, which is still commonly used in countries where regulation is weak. Increasingly, the groups involved have developed a broader perspective. It is not only a specific drug problem that is addressed but also the policies that allowed the problem to develop.

In a logical development from work on double standards in the marketing of specific drugs, European, North American, and Australian consumer groups have focused on drug export legislation. In France, Germany, and Australia the law has been changed to restrict the export of unapproved drugs as a result of consumer pressure. In the United States the consumer movement strongly opposed legislation enacted in 1986 that allowed companies to export unlicensed products to a limited number of countries. In 1993 the U.S. Office of Technology Assessment (OTA) published the report of a study of labeling in developing countries (U.S. Congress,

1993), which showed serious deficiencies in the information provided by U.S. companies in developing countries. This has led to renewed calls for control not only of the products exported but also the information provided with those products, as in a 1994 World Health Assembly resolution stating, "information for patients and prescribers which appears in leaflets of drugs in the manufacturing country should be supplied by the manufacturer to the countries to which the same drugs are exported" (World Health Organization, 1994).

## Drug Promotion: "The Truth, The Half Truth and Nothing Like The Truth"[2]

Standards of drug promotion and advertising are a consistent focus of international consumer advocacy. Since its inception in 1981, HAI has lobbied for strong controls on drug promotion. HAI continues to argue that industry self-regulation is inadequate and ineffective. The problem of unethical marketing, with negative consequences for public health, is particularly acute in developing countries (Chetley and Mintzes, 1992).

Recently, consumer advocacy at WHO has focused on obtaining a greater commitment to the implementation of a set of international ethical criteria for drug promotion that were developed as part of the Revised Drugs Strategy (WHO, 1988). The Ethical Criteria were developed by a joint committee with representation from WHO, national regulatory agencies, industry, consumer organizations, professional organizations, and the medical press.

HAI carried out a pilot survey of national implementation in 1992 and concluded "that the WHO Ethical Criteria have made minimal impact to the standards of promotional practice worldwide; that few countries have adequately addressed the call to 'monitor and enforce'; and that the standards in developing countries still lag greatly behind their more developed neighbours" (Harvey and Carandang, 1992: 3).

During the May 1994 World Health Assembly, HAI was again critical of the lack of initiatives by WHO to help national governments to implement or monitor controls on promotion, calling for concrete commitments from WHO and national delegates to take these criteria "off the shelf and into the legislatures" (HAI-Europe, 1994). Led by Norway and the other Nordic countries, over 50 countries sponsored a strong resolution to implement the Ethical Criteria, which was unanimously passed by the Assembly.

While arguing that strongly enforced national regulations are needed, HAI points out that promotional excesses are likely to continue as long as too many similar drugs compete for a limited market. A number of initiatives suggested by HAI in 1992 concern essential drugs policies and national formularies; the better regulation of advertising, postmarketing surveillance studies, and sponsorship of continuing medical education; anonymous hotlines to enable health workers and consumers to report inappropriate practices; and open access to information concerning malpractices and regulatory actions (Chetley and Mintzes, 1992).

## Secrecy – Anathema to Public Participation

Access to information on promotional malpractices forms one element of a larger consumer campaign for transparency and access to information:

> Secrecy in medicine is pervasive, largely unnecessary, and an obstacle to health. Lack of information limits freedom of choice, diminishes science and inhibits constructive participation. Secrecy tends also to hide evidence of inefficiency, incompetence, and inappropriate behaviour and therefore tends to reduce levels of public confidence and trust. [HAI-Europe, 1992]

HAI groups in Europe are advocating the rights of consumers to the information that forms the basis of regulatory decisions. The United Kingdom is one country where the issue has become important. In the United Kingdom, all information supplied to the Medicines Control Agency (MCA) is considered confidential. Secrecy is entrenched in Section 118 of the 1968 Medicines Act. Disclosure of safety data on which licensing decisions are based is prohibited. The advice of expert committees on issues of public safety, such as the withdrawal of a medicine from the market, is not available. A recent example is the sudden U.K. withdrawal of Halcion (triazolam), a widely-used sleeping pill, without adequate information to patients or prescribers. The information in media reports and the medical press ironically came from the United States (Anonymous, 1992), although the FDA did not decide to withdraw triazolam but only to restrict its use.

In December 1992, MP Giles Radice introduced a private member's bill, the Medicines Information Bill, with the sponsorship of three organizations: the Campaign for Freedom of Information, the National Consumer Council, and Social Audit. This bill would have restricted the scope of confidentiality to allow for protection only of genuine manufacturing secrets and sensitive information on products under development. The bill passed two readings and went to committee for discussion, but did not receive government support and never came to a vote. The Association of the British Pharmaceutical Industry opposed the bill, warning that if the bill became law its member companies would boycott the British licensing system (Webb, 1993).

The need for a transparent approach to medicines regulation has been reinforced by evidence of conflict of interest (National Consumer Council, 1993), inappropriate behavior by pharmaceutical executives, and particularly by the scandals emerging on an unprecedented scale during the investigation of Professor Duilio Poggiolini, head of the Italian drug regulatory agency and chair of the European Committee for Proprietary Medicinal Products (CPMP). The full extent of bribes received by Professor Poggiolini is as yet unknown; however, the value of the hoard found at his house was estimated at U.S. $188 million (Brown, 1993). Professor Poggiolini said, "the custom of exchanging costly gifts was widespread and tolerated if not condoned by everyone" (Anonymous, 1993b: 2). The trial revealed that these bribes affected not only pricing, but also product applications and licensing decisions that may have compromised the health of consumers.

## Australia – Exceptional but Limited National Consumer Representation

A transparent system for drug regulation can provide a degree of accountability to consumers. Consumer representation brings this accountability one step further, into the decision-making process. At the national level, consumer representation on drug committees is still the exception rather than the rule. Probably the most notable exception is Australia, where the Commonwealth (Federal) Department of Human Services and Health has made it a policy to seek consumer representation on a broad range of committees dealing with drug issues. One such committee is PHARM (Pharmaceutical Health and Rational Use of Medicines Committee), a multidisciplinary and cross-cultural group of consumer, industry, government, and health professional expertise brought together to develop "quality use of medicines."

> Consumers had not traditionally been involved in the decision making process . . . Ironically it was the consumers who were very instrumental in influencing thinking towards adoption of a formal policy. It is, of course, their safety and welfare which is paramount in the outcome of drug policy. [Hodge, 1993: 12]

In Australia, however, consumer representatives do not sit on the major regulatory committees. Recent reviews have recommended that consumer representatives be included on pharmaceutical manufacturers association committees that deal with complaints about the promotion of prescription and over-the-counter (OTC) drugs (Trade Practices Commission, 1992; 1994).

Accountability is an issue given that the constituency of consumers is ill defined. In Australia most consumer representatives are nominated by the Consumers' Health Forum of Australia, an organized coalition of consumer and public interest groups that receives some government funding. These representatives are almost always members of the public involved with a specific consumer health organization. Furthermore, committees usually have only one consumer representative, which makes it a challenging task for them to achieve a significant impact on the decisions reached.

## Shifting Sands and Solid Ground

What ground have consumers gained during the past two to three decades of campaigning? Can they claim to have achieved real change in medicines policy and increased consumer safety? What are the future directions for them to pursue?

Several of the drug-focused campaigns organized by consumers have led directly to regulatory action or industry withdrawals. These have been obvious and tangible gains for the organized consumer movement. However, consumer groups have become increasingly aware that the withdrawal of obsolete or dangerous drugs is hardly ever an aim in itself. All too often one problem drug is replaced by another. If real gains are to be made then policies need to be developed over the long term that take more account of consumer interests and rights.

## More Effective Regulation

While the regulatory system in industrialized countries offers some protection against ineffective or unsafe drugs, there are many areas in which consumers are pressing for stronger controls. Drug promotion is one such area. Consumer groups have also argued that only drugs that offer a comparative advantage over existing alternatives should be registered, advocating a model that was applied in Norway for many years in which "need" was one of the criteria for registration. Transparency, accountability, and public participation in the regulatory process are advocated, especially access to the information on safety and effectiveness on which regulatory decisions are based and continuing information from adverse reaction reports and postmarketing surveillance.

In developing countries there is frequently little or no control of the pharmaceutical market, and regulatory authorities are generally under-resourced and overburdened. Consumer and community based groups have been influential in pushing for better regulation. For example, the Philippines Drug Action Network, a broad-based coalition of many community and health organizations, was influential in campaigning for implementation of a comprehensive national drug policy (Tan, 1988). Consumer organizations also collaborate on many policy issues involving both industrialized and developing countries, such as exports, generics, quality assurance, pricing, promotion, and access to independent information. An underlying priority remains to limit the number of drugs marketed in both industrialized and developing countries.

## Representation

At an *international* level, consumer representatives have achieved considerable success in being recognized on committees concerned with drug policy. The Nairobi Conference on the Rational Use of Drugs provided a landmark in that the role and responsibilities of consumers were, for the first time, clearly defined and their legitimate place in policy debates acknowledged. At a *national* level, consumer representation in regulatory agencies exists in some countries, but generally at a level where effective impact on policy decisions remains minimal.

## A Better Doctor-Patient Relationship

Consumer organizations have promoted the idea that consumers have the right to expect both a high standard of care and information about their care. Prescribing is a fundamental but often unsatisfactory element of the doctor-patient relationship. Doctors frequently prescribe poorly (Garattini and Garattini, 1993) and consumers often do not comply with doctors' advice (Wright, 1993). Only about half of patients on long-term medication are thought to take their medicines in the way their doctors prescribed. "Too often a prescription signals the end of an interview rather than the start of an alliance" (Blackwell, 1973: 252). Better education is needed for prescribers, better drug and health information for consumers, and a change in the relationship between the two (de Vries, 1993).


## Dialogue with Industry

The pharmaceutical industry is heterogeneous and policy varies considerably from one company to another, and even within companies. In general the lesson learned by the industry over the last decade is that they should at least listen to critics: "ten years ago, claims by consumer or health defence organisations were frequently dismissed — not only by the industry — as extravagant. But today, as a result of some consistent demonstration of skill in making a case, health activist and consumer organisations have built for themselves a new level of credibility, which assures them of a respectful hearing in many serious forums" (O'Donnell, 1993).

There is some evidence that, where industry and consumers are brought into the processes of policy making, the possibilities for dialogue do improve: "the partnership so far developed between groups is fragile. But continued dialogue and experience in working jointly on projects show signs of significantly improving the understanding of each other's responsibilities and constraints" (Hodge, 1993: 13). In some cases, the national generics industry and consumer organizations have formed alliances, for example, opposition in Canada and India to new legislation introducing stronger patent protection.


## Strengthening the Consumer Voice

Increasing privatization and the deregulation of many prescription drugs has already led to changes in emphasis of the work of consumer organizations. In developing countries shrinking public health budgets due to the imposition of structural adjustment policies are seen as the biggest obstacle to tackle (Logie and Woodrofe, 1993), leading to a new focus for national and international advocacy. In industrialized countries, an increasing number of prescription drugs are being given OTC status. As a result, consumer organizations have begun to pay more attention to advertising standards for OTC products and the availability of independent information about these products.

In most developing countries the organized consumer movement is nonexistent or pitifully small. Even in industrialized countries consumer organizations often face difficulties of inadequate funding, lack of access to information, and reliance on volunteer labor. Consumer representation and community participation in health policy are increasingly accepted principles. However, further changes in the way policies are determined are a precondition for transforming these principles into effective practice.

## Conclusion

Consumers have been aiming to move from the "shifting sands" of drug campaigns to the "solid ground" of long-term reform by trying to achieve an adequate system of drug regulation and control, representation at international and national levels, transparency of decision making, an equal partnership with health care providers, a more responsive and responsible industry, and an independent and strong public interest and consumer movement. As this chapter shows, they have made some progress towards these goals—but much remains to be done.

## Notes

1. In 1985 DES Action International was formed by DES Action groups from eight countries and the DES Cancer network, an international support network for women with cancer associated with DES exposure.

2. Quote cited from Herxheimer (1993: 32).

## References

Anonymous (1986) Merck & Co stops promoting Periactin. *Scrip* (12 May), No. 1101, p. 7.

Anonymous (1992) Reasons for UK withdrawal of Halcion. *Scrip* (29 May), No. 1721, p. 25.

Anonymous (1993a) FDA to act on Sandoz' Parlodel. *Scrip* (14 September), No. 1855, p. 10.

Anonymous (1993b) Italian police raid Poggiolini home. *Scrip* (8 October), No. 1862, pp. 2–3.

Blackwell B (1973) Drug therapy: patient compliance. *New England Journal of Medicine* 289: 249–52.

Boston Women's Health Book Collective (1971) *Our Bodies Ourselves*. New York: Simon and Schuster.

Braithwaite J (1984) *Corporate Crime in the Pharmaceutical Industry*. London: Routledge and Kegan Paul.

Brown P (1993) No place for secrecy. *Scrip Magazine*, December, pp. 3–4.

Chetley A (1990) *A Healthy Business? World Health and the Pharmaceutical Industry*. London: Zed Books.

Chetley A (1993) *Problem Drugs*. 2nd edition. Amsterdam: Health Action International.

Chetley A and Mintzes B (eds.) (1992) *Promoting Health or Pushing Drugs?* Amsterdam: Health Action International.

Chetley A and Gilbert D (1986) *Problem Drugs*. Amsterdam: Health Action International.

DES Action Canada (1993) Alarming parallels between DES and new reproductive technologies, Press brief, 10 November. Ottawa: DES Action Canada.

de Vries T (1993) Presenting clinical pharmacology and therapeutics: a problem-based approach for choosing and prescribing drugs. *British Journal of Clinical Pharmacology* 35: 581–86.

Direcks A, Figueroa S, Mintzes B, and Banta D (1991) *DES European Study*. The Netherlands: DES Action.

Dukes MNG (1990) Drug-induced injury: the responsibility of the pharmaceutical industry. In: Mintzes B (ed.) *DES: A Drug with Consequence for Current Health Policy*. Utrecht, The Netherlands: DES Action, pp. 25–29.

Dukes MNG and Schwartz B (1988) *Responsibility for Drug-Induced Injury*. Amsterdam: Elsevier.

Garattini S and Garattini L (1993) Pharmaceutical prescriptions in four European countries. *Lancet* 342: 1191–92.

HAI-Europe (1994) WHO ethical criteria for medicinal drug promotion – off the shelf and into the legislatures. Briefing paper: drug policy at the 47th World Health Assembly, May.

HAI-Europe (1992) Resolution on secrecy in Medicines Control, 1 November. Unpublished.

Hansson, O (1989) *Inside Ciba-Geigy*. Penang, Malaysia: International Organization of Consumer Unions.

Harvey K and Carandang D (1992) The impact of WHO ethical criteria for medicinal drug promotion, unpublished survey, Health Action International.

Herbst AL, Ulferder H, and Poskanzer DC (1971) Adenocarcinoma of the vagina. Association of maternal stilbestrol therapy with tumor appearance in young women. *New England Journal of Medicine* 284: 878–81.

Herbst AL, Cole P, Colton T, et al. (1977) Age-incidence and risk of diethylstilbestrol-related clear cell adenocarcinoma of the vagina and cervix. *American Journal of Obstetrics and Gynecology* 128: 43–50.

Herxheimer A (1993) Independent drug information for prescribers and consumers. In: Chetley A (ed.) *Medicines and Independence: Towards Rational Drug Use in the Baltic States*. Amsterdam: HAI-Europe, pp. 31–36.

Hodge M (1993) Australia focuses on the quality use of medicines: policy and action. *Essential Drugs Monitor* 15: 12–13.

Kanji N, Hardon A, Harnmeijer JW, Mamdani M, and Walt G (1992) *Drugs Policy in Developing Countries*. London: Zed Books.

Kaufman RH, Binder GL, Gray PM, and Adam E (1977) Upper genital tract changes associated with exposure in utero to diethylstilbestrol. *American Journal of Obstetrics and Gynecology* 228: 51–59.

Leary FJ, Resseguie MJ, Kurland LT, et al. (1984) Males exposed in utero to diethylstilbestrol. *Journal of the American Medical Association* 252: 2984–49.

Lexchin J (1994) personal communication, March.

Logie DE and Woodroofe J (1993) Structural adjustment: the wrong prescription for Africa? *British Medical Journal* 307: 41–44.

Medawar C (1992) *Power and Dependence. Social Audit on the Safety of Medicines*. London: Social Audit.

National Consumer Council (1993) *Balancing Acts: Conflicts of Interest in the Regulation of Medicine*. London, PD 22/D4/93, September.

O'Donnell P (1993) Consuming passions. *Pharmaceutical Marketing*, October, p. 31.

Orenberg CL (1981) *DES: The Complete Story*. New York: St. Martin's Press.

Sim FG (1991) *IOCU on Record: A Documentary History of the International Organization of Consumers' Unions 1960–1990*. New York: Consumers' Union.

Tan ML (1988) *Dying for Drugs: Pill Power and Politics in the Philippines*. Quezon City, Philippines: HAIN.

't Hoen E (1992) Victory in DES lawsuit. *HAI Europe Update*, October.

Trade Practices Commission (1992) *Final Report by the Trade Practices Commission on the Self-Regulation of Promotion and Advertising of Therapeutic Goods*. Canberra ACT, Australia.

Trade Practices Commission (1994) *Determination: Application for Authorization under Sub-*

*section 88(1) of the Trade Practices Act, 1974 by the Proprietary Medicines Association of Australia Inc in Relation to its Code of Practice.* Canberra ACT, Australia.

U.S. Congress, Office of Technology Assessment (1993) *Drug Labeling in Developing Countries.* OTA-H-464. Washington, DC: U.S. Government Printing Office.

van den Berg A (1993) Patienten willen medisch handelen dat gebaseerd is op gedegen onderzoek: Ellen 't Hoen en Fons Dekkers in dialoog [Patients want medical care that is based on thorough research]. *Tijdschrift voor Gezondheid en Politiek*, November, pp. 12–15.

van Maaren PJM, van Mil JWF, Hardon AP, Haaijer-Ruskamp FM, and Dukes MNG (1993) *Nederlandse geneesmiddelen in ontwikkelingslanden; een farmacologische evaluatie* [Dutch drugs in developing countries; a pharmacological evaluation]. Groningen, The Netherlands: Noordelijk Centrum voor Gezondheidsvraagstukken (NCG)/WHO Collaborating Centre for Clinical Pharmacology and Drug Policy Science, Rijksuniversiteit Groningen.

Wells T and Tiranti D (1985) *IOCU: Giving a Voice to the World's Consumers.* The Hague: International Organization of Consumers' Unions.

Webb J (1993) Keep safety trials secret, say drugs companies. *New Scientist*, 9 January.

Wolfe S and Moore S (Public Citizen) (1993) Letter to David Kessler, Commissioner of Food and Drugs, US Food and Drug Administration, September 2.

World Health Organization (1988) *Ethical Criteria for Medicinal Drug Promotion.* Geneva: World Health Organization.

World Health Organization (1994) Forty-Seventh World Health Assembly, WHO Ethical criteria for medicinal drug promotion [WHA47.16], May.

Wright EC (1993) Non-compliance—or how many aunts has Matilda?, *Lancet*, 342: 909–13.

Zalmstra HAM, 't Hoen EFM, and Visser A (1989) DES Action: its influence on the awareness, experiences and doctor-patient relationships of DES daughters. *DES Action Voice* 39: 5.

# II

# THE PRODUCT CYCLE

# 6

# Market and
# Industrial Structure

## ROBERT H. BALLANCE[1]

The relationship between pharmaceutical companies and government regulators is a troubled one, but that was not always the case. During the 1950s and early 1960s the two groups maintained a relatively harmonious coexistence. The congenial atmosphere depended on regulators' acceptance of the argument that increases in prices and profits were essential if progress in research was to continue. That informal accord began to break down when the U.S. government launched a lengthy investigation of pricing strategies and monopolistic practices (see Comanor, 1986). In the years that followed economists have argued on both sides of issues concerning profit rates, pricing tactics, and research performance.

Behind this debate is an enduring conflict that pits the consumer's insistence on low-priced pharmaceuticals against society's desire for rapid development of new and more effective drugs. The conflict remains unresolved, although there has been a subtle change in the nature of the debate. Economists have convinced many public officials that policy recommendations that address current inequities without taking into account the longer-term repercussions will be costly.[2] To be effective, policy makers must weigh the present benefits for consumers against the long-term costs to society.

The shift in approach has introduced a more realistic element into the debate. Nevertheless, the industry poses exceptional challenges to the economist who seeks to provide guidance on critical issues of public policy. Difficulties stem from the unique combination of social, regulatory, and economic circumstances that surround the industry. Foremost among these is the number of different agents that are active participants in pharmaceutical markets. In the case of prescription drugs, the final consumer and the consumption decision maker (the prescribing physician) are not the same. The choice of a drug is further complicated by the thousands available in any industrialized country. As a result, neither of these groups is well informed about their alternatives. Nor is the cost of drug purchases borne solely by the final consumer. Third-party programs for reimbursement are operated by both governments and private insurers and their influence is growing. In the United States these groups accounted for 28% of all spending for prescription drugs in 1978, but by 1987 their share had risen to 44% (U.S. Office of Technology Assessment, 1993: 27). The result is a transaction process where the final consumer may neither choose which product is purchased, nor pay the full price associated with that decision.

In addition to the shared responsibilities for consumption decisions, the industry operates in a regulatory environment that is both complicated and unusual. Governments must intervene in the market to ensure that drugs are safe and efficient. Other forms of intervention follow from these objectives. For example, advertising is regulated, production processes are subject to inspection, price controls may be imposed and market access can be denied. These and other policies have created a powerful network of special interest groups that benefit from the existing regulatory system. Any changes in public policy, however desirable or efficient, will be opposed by at least some of these groups. In these circumstances it may not be enough that economists agree on which policies are efficient. To be successful, they may also need to devise a combination of policies and regulations that will be acceptable to a significant portion of the interest-group coalition.

The economist's role as a policy advisor is further complicated by the growing degree of internationalization within the industry. The interests of government regulators rarely extend beyond their country's borders. They have their own agenda and are unlikely to consider how their decisions might be coordinated or what impact they have on markets elsewhere in the world. Quite the opposite applies to the larger pharmaceutical firms. These companies aspire to sell in most, if not all, parts of the world and adopt a global perspective with regard to issues such as profitability and market presence.

The body of this chapter examines the pharmaceutical industry's performance from several different perspectives. The following section looks at the division of labor within the industry and makes some inferences about its internal priorities. In section two the degree of competition is analyzed, while in section three attention focuses on several of the industry's more important characteristics such as the pattern of ownership, the size of firms, and various forms of specialization. The concluding section of the chapter looks at some of the changes that may be in store for the industry, and then returns to consider the original conflict between the need for cheaply-priced drugs and the desire for rapid development of new medicines.

## Internal Structure of the Pharmaceutical Industry

Most industrial firms expect to devote the bulk of their resources to manufacturing operations. Pharmaceutical firms have a quite different set of spending priorities. At one end of the industry are large teams of chemists, biochemists, and pharmacologists who are concerned with research and development (R&D). At the other are huge networks for the distribution and promotion of products. Sandwiched between these two crucial parts of the industry is the manufacture of drugs.

The relative importance of each stage is evident from the data in Table 6-1. Integrated pharmaceutical companies (firms involved in all three phases of the industry) spend less than half their revenues on manufacturing operations. The share of manufacturing costs is not only small in comparison with other industries but has been falling since the 1970s. This decline has been offset by a rise in the portion of revenues devoted to marketing, R&D, and operating profits. The significance of the industry's manufacturing operations is further diminished by its modest impact on the competitive position of major firms. These companies employ very similar technologies, meaning that variations in production costs are modest so long as plant size and rates of capacity utilization are comparable. In contrast, the sums spent on research and marketing are rising and vary greatly across countries and between companies. The latter activities are more important sources of market power and competitive leadership.

Leading pharmaceutical firms assigned a high priority to research because they believed their competitive standing depended on access to marketable products. Given this orientation, they had little choice but to increase their outlays as more stringent regulatory requirements pushed up the costs of R&D. Spending for this purpose rose fourfold in the 1980s and industry sources put the worldwide total for 1993 at about $26.5 billion. The long-term increase in the share of R&D in total spending is evident from the data in Table 6-1. However, it is unclear that the industry can sustain this upward trend much longer. Fragmented data for the first few years of the 1990s provides a blurred picture. For example, a small survey conducted in 1991 indicates a continuation of the trends reported in Table 6-1, but a more recent study suggests the growth of research spending is slowing.[3]

Table 6-1 also shows a rise in marketing expenditures that did not become apparent until the mid-1980s. Firms had previously concentrated on only a few national markets whenever they launched a new product. Now, many seek to launch a new product in all major markets simultaneously to maximize the revenues earned. The new strategy requires a much bigger marketing force and heavy sales promotion. With additional resources at their disposal, large firms can accomplish a worldwide launch in only three years where they once required eight to ten years.

TABLE 6-1. The Changing Structure of Company Costs
in the Pharmaceutical Industry, 1973–1989[a]

|           | Manufacturing | Marketing | R&D | Operating Profit | Other |
|-----------|---------------|-----------|-----|------------------|-------|
| 1973      | 40.5          | 17.0      | 9.7 | 20.7             | 12.1  |
| 1975–1980 | 37.5          | 16.5      | 10.0| 25.0             | 11.0  |
| 1989      | 25.0          | 24.0      | 13.0| 28.0             | 10.0  |

*Sources*: Based on Cooper and Cuyler (1973); OECD (1975); and Ballance, Pogàny and Forstner (1992).

[a]All figures are based on data for leading research-oriented firms in Europe, Japan, and North America. However, the composition of firms and the size of each sample varies and may distort comparisons.

The consequence of all these trends is a unique division of labor between re-search, production, and marketing. New conditions are emerging, however, and it is inevitable that the industry will have to adapt. Several of the more important develop-ments are policy-induced changes. They include an expected squeeze on profits as governments tighten price controls and/or scale back on their reimbursement pro-grams, and renewed efforts to contain costs by encouraging the sale of generics and use of over-the-counter (OTC) medicines.[4] Many of the industry's operating princi-ples and practices will have to be altered as it comes to terms with these develop-ments.

Programs of cost containment will be pursued most vigorously in the field of research. Incremental adjustments such as greater reliance on parallel development (the practice of moving to the next research stage before completing the current one) and wider use of computerized systems to design new molecules and monitor clinical trials are being rapidly developed.[5] In addition to these innovations, firms are making fundamental changes in the way they manage research. Laboratories are already under pressure to set stricter research timetables and to ensure that every potential drug satisfies new, and much tougher, criteria. Projects that fall behind schedule or do not meet the new criteria will be scrapped more quickly than in the past.

There are two reasons why the industry is focusing so much attention on re-search. First, considerable savings can be realized by accelerating the pace of R&D. Firms presently need eight to ten years to convert a new discovery into a marketable drug (Scherer, 1993) and any reduction in this phase will increase the period of patent protection for the marketed drug. Second, the risks associated with any research bottleneck are greater than ever before. As the absolute size of the industry grows, the overall pace of innovation will quicken and the profitable lifetime of drugs is reduced. Millions of dollars could be lost if a successful product is preempted in even a few markets.

The marketing principles that have guided major firms until now are also being challenged. Integrated producers have long specialized in supplying prescription drugs but they are grudgingly beginning to move into markets for lower-priced medicines as well. Known within the industry as "dual production," this practice would not have been considered only a few years ago.[6] Producers feared that the move would threaten their profitability. In fact, there are several reasons why dual production could be attractive. First, the per-treatment price of generics and OTCs is low relative to the original drug but so, too, are the costs. Second, generics require little in the way of additional research expenditures: by definition, these costs were incurred when creating the patented version. Third, the per-unit costs of an elaborate market-ing apparatus should fall significantly as more generics are prescribed by doctors or when patented drugs are sold as OTCs. Finally, assumptions about the future profit margins of patent and nonpatent drugs appear to favor dual production. Govern-ments are likely to make a more concerted effort to reduce the prices and margins on patent-protected drugs than for off-patent products. If so, price differentials between the two groups should narrow, making off-patent products a more attractive proposi-tion.

The possibility that several large, research-oriented companies will eventually become dual producers could have widespread consequences. One change would be in the way these firms market their prescription drugs during the last few years of patent protection. In this crucial period, a company will want to build up consumer awareness so its product will have a reliable market base once it is off patent. Few of the larger companies have any experience with such a strategy, and even less in selling generic drugs.[7] Many will have to look for marketing assistance elsewhere within the industry, most often by establishing links with other firms that have specialized in this tactic.

Manufacturing operations will also see some changes, though not so drastic as in other parts of the industry. As margins fall, firms will come under pressure to abandon the dictum "one market, one factory." It is clear that a government's gratitude for local investment—expressed in the form of rapid product approval or the award of a favorable price—no longer offsets the penalties of an inefficient manufacturing operation. This issue may be of particular significance in Europe where production capacity does not conform to the region's demand patterns or market size. As a result, rates of use in some formulation plants are very low (50 to 60% of capacity). By the end of this decade the world's larger drug makers will need only about ten strategically located plants. No more than three to five should be in Europe, though all will probably be specialized in terms of chemistry and/or formulation type. Such a development would require a significant reorganization of the industry, particularly in Europe.

## Internationalization and Competition

Economists tend to gauge the degree and intensity of competition in general terms. They may focus on the market share of leading firms, their ability to set prices and squeeze distributors, the existence of barriers that inhibit the entry of new competitors, or similar characteristics. Aside from a lack of precision, the use of these indicators is complicated by the pharmaceutical industry's unique structure and the fragmented nature of its markets.

When markets for pharmaceuticals are pictured in global terms, a handful of research-based multinationals can be singled out. A group of about 25 companies accounts for around two-fifths of all the pharmaceutical preparations sold in world markets each year (*Scrip Pharmaceutical Company League Tables*, 1989; 1990; 1991; *Scrip Yearbook*, 1990). The composition of this group has changed very little over time, but there are frequent shifts in the relative standing of individual members. The leaders depend on a very small number of products for most of their pharmaceutical revenues: on average, about a fifth of each firm's earnings come from sales of a single drug (Ballance et al., 1992: 110 and Table 5.1). The launch of only one blockbuster drug can lead to a significant realignment of rankings and market shares among firms within this select group.[8]

Judged by these standards, the industry's leaders appear to be a powerful group but the picture changes remarkably when their shares in the world market are considered. The larger companies are far less prominent than in other industries such as aerospace, cars, computers, or telecommunications (Ballance et al., 1992: 110–

113). Even the very largest drug producers can claim no more than 3 to 4% of the world market in recent years.[9]

Estimates such as these have a drawback; they exaggerate the actual degree of competition if markets are highly fragmented. This is the case for pharmaceuticals. Unlike other consumer products, medicines are sold in many narrowly-defined and self-contained submarkets that reflect the diversity of diseases existing in any country. Around 20,000 different medicines are available in the United States and over 10,000 are found in many industrialized and developing countries. The degree of product differentiation is also extensive, depending not only on each medicine's characteristics but on methods of distribution, aspects of national policy, and the effectiveness of promotional campaigns. It follows that global estimates of market share understate the extent to which a few companies dominate each submarket.

A more detailed impression of the degree of competition is supplied in Table 6-2. The data shown there refers to the shares of the three best-selling brands in each of the three largest subclasses of selected countries. It is clear that a very small number of drugs accounts for a significant portion of sales in almost every therapeutic submarket.[10] The most obvious explanation for this dominance is that a few relatively efficient drugs are patent protected. However, there are many other instances in which the patents of leading brands have expired but the products still claim a significant portion of total sales.

Reasons for the success of off-patent drugs include the existence of brand-name loyalties, control over a key input, or policy decisions. The first of these explanations is the most common but also the most controversial. Aggressive promotion of branded drugs is part of the mechanism by which returns to innovation are realized. The success of advertising depends partly on the therapeutic novelty and efficacy of the drug. However, the hold of branded drugs on the market can be extremely powerful. Some analysts suggest that creation of brand loyalty may actually be a more effective method of guaranteeing high returns than the patent system itself (Lall, 1985).

Other reasons for market dominance without patent protection are less contentious. With control over a key input (for example, a medicinal chemical or active ingredient), the originating firm has a considerable degree of market power. It can sell the input to licensees or transfer the production technology. Alternatively, the originator may decide that it is more profitable to sell the drug itself, in which case the input will be denied to others.[11] A similar result can occur if policy makers decide to exclude certain drugs from their home market in the interest of greater efficiency or reduced costs. A few suppliers may dominate the national market but if government intervention (for example, price controls) is effective, the degree of market power should not be great.

The fact that the leading product may be an original that is no longer protected by patent is changing the nature of competition. Traditionally, the original market leader is expected to be replaced by a superior, research-based drug. That is still true in many markets, especially in those where demand is strong. But in markets that are rapidly maturing, the volume of research may be cut back and the overall pace of innovation will slow. Because the number of mature markets is greater than ever, a number of battles are being fought not between two patented drugs but between an

TABLE 6-2. Product Competition in Major Therapeutic Submarkets[a] of Latest Year[b] (by Product Class)

| Countries | Total No. of Products | Total Drug Sales[c] in Million US$ | Share of Largest-Selling Therapeutic Subclasses in Each National Market | | | Share of 3 Best-Selling Products in Each Subclass | | |
|---|---|---|---|---|---|---|---|---|
| | | | First Subclass | Second Subclass | Third Subclass | Largest Subclass | Second Largest | Third Largest |
| Austria | 2,700 | 1,046[d] | 3.8 | 2.5 | 2.4 | 35 | 31 | 65 |
| Belgium | 5,177 | 1,769[d] | 3.9 | 3.5 | 3.4 | 88 | 39 | 81 |
| Canada | 17,000 | 4,034 | 6.2 | 5.6 | 2.5 | 64 | 53 | 49 |
| Finland | 3,461 | 724 | 5.5 | 4.8 | 3.6 | 39 | 50 | 57 |
| France | 4,200 | 10,905[e] | 5.3 | 5.0 | 2.7 | 45 | 44 | 43 |
| West Germany | 8,429 | 13,131 | 3.2 | 1.8 | 1.7 | 59 | 35 | 43 |
| Italy | 4,210 | 11,865[d] | 4.7 | 4.7 | 3.0 | 52 | 62 | 64 |
| Japan | 13,589 | 30,355 | 8.4 | 5.4 | 2.3 | 29 | 44 | 59 |
| Netherlands | 7,990 | 1,484[d] | 8.2 | 3.2 | 1.8 | 75 | 97 | 70 |
| Spain | 5,400 | 4,325[f] | 6.0 | 4.7 | 3.8 | 19 | 37 | 63 |
| United Kingdom | 2,090 | 5,864[d] | 7.7 | 3.6 | 2.3 | 85 | 91 | 81 |
| United States | 19,000 | 44,260 | 6.5 | 5.2 | 5.0 | 77 | 49 | 67 |

*Source*: IMS (1992) and Farmindustria (1992).

[a] The major therapeutic subclasses differ from country to country. Systemic antibiotics, antacids/antiulcerants, and analgesics are most frequently represented among the largest-selling subclasses in the countries shown.

[b] Latest year is 1990 or 1992 except for Belgium (1989), Canada (1986), and the United Kingdom (1986).

[c] Unless otherwise indicated, figures refer to sales through retail pharmacies and hospitals.

[d] All outlets.

[e] Retail pharmacies only.

[f] Retail pharmacies and wholesalers only.

original and a copy. Factors like brand-name loyalty assume greater importance in these circumstances. This helps to explain why firms are now willing to spend more to maintain the marketability of older drugs.

In general, it appears that there is only a limited degree of competition. A small number of firms dominate the research end of the industry, accounting for an overwhelming portion of the new drugs brought to market. The same group wields less power in terms of world sales but their prominence reemerges when attention turns to individual markets in specific countries. A very few drugs claim the bulk of sales in a particular market. Rivals (which can be copies, molecular modifications, or originals) may compete and new products can enter. However, the markets themselves remain oligopolistic, marked only by changes in the leadership of firms.

## Nationality and Size

The nationality and size of drug companies are critical determinants of their behavior. The orientation and spending patterns of foreign-owned subsidiaries are quite different from those of domestically-owned firms. Research, for example, is a task seldom performed in overseas subsidiaries. It tends to be highly centralized and carried out in only a few locations, usually in the country where the firm has its headquarters and one or two of its major markets.[12] The only exception to this rule is the United States; in 1986, 26 foreign firms had research facilities in that country, and by 1992 the number had risen to 75 (OECD, 1993: 10). Such a locational pattern would be unusual in other industries, though several considerations make it appealing to drug producers. First, the difficult job of coordinating research becomes more complicated if facilities are widely dispersed. Second, firms are traditionally very secretive about their research programs and a highly centralized operation makes it easier to control information leaks. Finally, companies choose their research sites carefully to take advantage of research funding offered by host governments.

The modest research activities of most foreign subsidiaries are offset by a strong emphasis on marketing. Typically, the main function of subsidiaries is to provide a local managerial base for the distribution of drugs developed at research centers in the home country. There is also evidence that foreign-owned firms tend to spend proportionately more on marketing than their locally-owned counterparts (Ballance et al., 1992: 125). Should the number of foreign subsidiaries grow relative to the industry as a whole, the tendency to spend ever-greater amounts on marketing and distribution would be reinforced.

The contrasts between firms become even sharper when size rather than nationality is the focus of attention. Based on the data in Table 6-3, three broadly defined types of firms can be identified. Multinationals, which account for less than 7% of the total number, are represented by companies with annual sales of at least $200 million. This group can be distinguished by their research leadership and adherence to well-defined methods of operation with regard to patenting, licensing, and the acquisition of inputs from approved vendors. Surprisingly few of these multinationals are capable of competing vigorously in both research and marketing. The industry's rule of thumb is that about 2% of the world market for pharmaceuticals is necessary

TABLE 6-3.   Size Distribution of Pharmaceutical Firms in
Industrialized Countries, 1991

| Producer Category[a] | Annual Domestic Sales (in Million US$) | Number of Firms |
|---|---|---|
| Reproductive firms | 0–10 | 320 |
| | 10–25 | 381 |
| Innovative companies | 25–50 | 273 |
| | 50–75 | 303 |
| | 75–100 | 120 |
| | 100–200 | 230 |
| Research-oriented multinationals | 200–500 | 110 |
| | 500–1000[b] | 39 |
| | > 1000[b] | 15 |

*Source*: IMS (1992).

[a]For definitions of categories, see the text.

[b]All firms in these categories are in Japan and the United States.

if a company is to have the "critical mass" to succeed in both fields. Just 12 companies
were able to meet that standard in 1991 (Scrip, 1992).

Innovative companies have annual sales of $25–$500 million and make up more
than two-fifths of the industry. This group cannot afford the massive research programs of the multinationals but are still active in international markets. Some operate
foreign subsidiaries or participate in joint ventures with foreign partners. Many are
significant exporters, selling drugs directly through their own distribution channels or
via international trading houses on the open market. Reproductive firms make up the
remainder of the industry. These are generally small family-owned enterprises or
publicly-owned companies of modest size. Lacking any significant research capacity,
their products sell under brand names or as cheaply-priced generics.

It is unclear how these three groups will fare in the future. There is some
historical evidence to suggest that increased regulation had a particularly adverse
effect on small and medium-sized companies during the 1960s and early 1970s.[13] If
that finding were equally valid today, small and medium-sized firms would probably
face a difficult future as governments introduce more stringent price controls and
other regulations. The modern pharmaceutical industry, however, is quite different
from the one that existed 20 or 30 years ago and opportunities could vary accordingly. Some of these possibilities are considered in the closing section of this chapter.

## Conflict and Adjustment in the Future

Leading pharmaceutical suppliers devote a greater proportion of their revenues to
R&D than other research-intensive industries and spend as much on marketing as
most producers of consumer goods. Even more controversial is the industry's high
rate of profitability. In the United States the return on equity for pharmaceuticals
during the period 1960 through 1991 was 18.4% compared with 11.9% for all

industries.[14] These benchmarks are unlikely to be maintained as regulators and financially-pressed consumers struggle to bring down their health care costs.

Researchers should see the most dramatic changes. Spending cutbacks and other measures such as tighter managerial policies for R&D and new tools to bolster research productivity are already being implemented. Meanwhile, research-oriented firms will continue to press for favorable regulatory changes such as expedited review, accelerated approval of new drugs, and closer international alignment of testing requirements. These initiatives will help, but they probably will not be enough. Ultimately, the massive, independently-operated research programs conducted by some of the industry's leaders probably cannot be sustained. Big firms will come under increasing pressure to concede a portion of their research independence and penchant for secrecy.

Even the strongest supporters of the multinationals concede that little can be gained by building up even larger research operations. A more logical tactic may be to rely on small-scale research and large-scale development (for example, the performance of all the routine tests needed to satisfy regulatory requirements). The tighter controls that companies impose on their research programs will result in a large number of unfinished projects. Producers of varying sizes can then buy into research projects that fit their particular priorities and marketing strengths.[15] If such collaboration gains acceptance, some of the smaller innovative and reproductive firms would be drawn into the research sphere, albeit in a limited fashion.

Marketers in the industry can look forward to a less austere future. One reason is that these operations are subject to economies of scale while research is not.[16] Other explanations are the multinationals' conversion to dual production (brand-name prescription drugs and generics) and their newfound willingness to cooperate with drug firms that specialize in marketing operations. Such moves are logical but they can create problems of their own, since a measure of influence is ceded to wholesalers and others further down the distribution chain. These groups could eventually become powerful enough to wring significant price concessions from the industry without the help of government price controls.

Overshadowing this network of shifting alliances and changing priorities is the regulator's desire to create some form of managed competition. Many aspects of this new approach remain unclear, though drug prices and consumption decision makers appear to be the primary targets. As governments reorganize their health care systems, the influence of formulary committees in health maintenance organizations will grow at the expense of other decision makers. Advocates of managed competition see this as a desirable outcome. They believe that formulary committees are better able to weigh the costs and benefits of alternative drugs than individual physicians, whose choices can be undermined by insufficient information and the aggressive marketing tactics of drug firms. The principle on which this argument is based is that improved information and a more intelligent selection of drugs will lead to greater competition and eliminate some of the market imperfections that economists have noted.[17]

The impact of managed competition hinges on two critical issues. One is the extent to which research performance is affected by a decline in the rate of return on new products. If the two measures are closely linked, any fall in the rate of return would have serious repercussions for consumers. Economists have studied this point but have yet to assemble convincing evidence on the relationship between the two variables.[18]

A second issue concerns the way managed competition will alter the process of drug approval. A few governments have already begun to experiment with new criteria that are meant to reduce overall spending on drugs. In some countries, for example, it is no longer sufficient to show that a drug is safe and works; firms are also required to demonstrate that the drug is cost effective. Known as "pharmacoeconomics" within the industry, these studies are based on comparisons with existing treatments. They may concern the price of a drug, the impact on spending for other medical services, the time a patient spends in a hospital bed and, sometimes, the costs of social services.

The economic information to be compiled is relatively straightforward if the new product is only a marginal improvement on an existing one. However, the exercise becomes much more complicated and expensive when a highly priced breakthrough drug is submitted for approval. The drug company must then work hard to demonstrate conclusively that its product makes economic sense. It follows that the bulk of this additional work will be done by research-oriented companies and their development costs will increase accordingly. Moreover, these costs seem set to rise even more now that insurers, private clinics, health maintenance groups, and corporations are on the growing list of consumption decision makers. These groups will want to see such studies before entering into any price-setting negotiations with drug companies. They could soon be producing their own versions of pharmacoeconomic analysis as part of the preparations for these negotiations.

In conclusion, how will the pharmaceutical industry change in the future and what role will the economist play in its evolution? The demands on the industry's resources and areas of expertise are expanding at a pace that outstrips the capabilities of the richest firms. Very few firms will be able to excel at both research and marketing in the future. The industry faces a major transformation characterized by greater interfirm collaboration in both research and marketing, new types of marketing strategies, and lower (but probably still impressive) rates of profitability. These adjustments will strip the industry of some of its uniqueness, making it even more important to find sensible public policy choices that preserve the balance between consumer benefits and pharmaceutical innovation.

Those economists who have called for research to be treated as a public good— for example, Spence (1984)—will probably be disappointed with the changes to come. Governments cannot afford the huge amounts of public funds needed to divorce the financing of research from pricing decisions. Drug prices will continue to be set through a complex process of negotiation and argument rather than being dependent on demand and supply. But as the debate over prices and approval criteria enters uncharted territory, the role of economists may change. They are likely to become more deeply involved in matters of pharmacoeconomics and spend proportionately less time on matters relating to policy and industry performance.

The shift in focus carries its own dangers. Neither drug producers nor consumption decision makers in the private sector are unbiased. Left to their own devices, the pharmacoeconomic studies produced by either side will lack the credibility that impartial observers would demand. If economists do become actively involved in this field, they must first come up with credible and impartial methods of assessing the costs and benefits of any drug. Should they fail, it will be the consumer who suffers — either by paying unnecessarily high prices for drugs or by forgoing access to more effective products that could be developed if adequate financing were available.

## Notes

1. The views expressed in this chapter are those of the author and do not necessarily reflect the views of the Secretariat of the United Nations Industrial Development Organisation.

2. The economist argues this point in terms of static versus dynamic efficiency. There is a trade-off between short-term (static) and long-term (dynamic) concerns and an effective policy solution must take both sets of concerns into account.

3. The 1991 survey was commissioned by 17 large drug companies. On average, manufacturing accounted for only 20% of costs while marketing took 30%. An additional 30% was divided equally between R&D and operating profits and the remaining 20% was absorbed by other categories (cited in *The Economist*, 14 November 1992: 76). A different impression results from a survey of the 1993 spending pattern in 44 large pharmaceutical groups. Most of the companies included in this study reported only single-digit growth in this category and five actually reduced spending on R&D in both real and nominal terms. European companies with strong gains in sales volume (Astra, Glaxo, Wellcome and SmithKline Beecham) maintained their research budgets but overall results indicated a slowdown in the growth of expenditures for R&D (based on Pharmaceuticals: Research and Development, *Financial Times*, 23 March 1994).

4. The effects of these policies will be partially offset by extension of the effective patent life in industrialized countries and the wider acceptance of patent protection in world markets.

5. Parallel development accelerates the pace of research but also entails greater risks and higher costs. The wider use of computerized systems can reduce the attrition rate during the preclinical phase when thousands of molecules are tested in vitro and in animals (Scherer, 1993: 99). Despite these efforts, only 23% of the chemical entities put into human testing eventually receive approval and are marketed.

6. In addition to supplying the original, dual producers may produce a generic version or even an OTC.

7. Integrated firms are accustomed to selling their drugs through doctors or hospital administrators. To do so, they follow traditional marketing methods, known as "pushing" the product down the distribution chain. As suppliers of generics, these firms will have to handle multiple points of sale. Marketing methods must then be designed to "pull" products down the distribution chain by creating preferences among the end users or patients. Finally, price is very crucial in markets for generics and they must be sold in a manner quite different from on-patent drugs.

8. Glaxo, for example, was the 20th largest pharmaceutical company by sales in 1981 when it launched Zantac, the antacid for ulcers. After only five years, the drug's annual worldwide sales exceeded $1 billion and by 1988 Glaxo's revenues were the second largest of the major drug producers (*Scrip Pharmaceutical League Tables*, 1989; *Scrip Yearbook*, 1990; Ballance et al., 1992: 108–9).

9. The four firms with the largest pharmaceutical revenues in 1991 were Glaxo, Merck, Bristol-Myers Squibb and Hoechst. Their respective shares of the world pharmaceutical market ranged from 3.1 to 4.1% (OECD, 1993: 11; Table 5).

10. The sales volume in these therapeutic submarkets can be huge. In the United States, for example, the three leading brands in the largest therapeutic submarket reports combined sales of nearly $1.5 billion (Ballance et al., 1992: 136).

11. Such a situation can occur when the production technology is sophisticated and difficult to control. If competitors are unable to replicate the process exactly, their ability to compete with the original product is severely limited.

12. In fact, over 90% of the new drugs the industry has marketed since 1960 were discovered and developed in only 10 industrialized countries (Ballance et al., 1992: 10).

13. For example, the share of industry-wide R&D carried out by medium-sized innovative firms declined during this period (Thomas, 1987).

14. The pharmaceutical industry's profitability exceeded the median of the 500 industrials in the United States by 62% on average in the 1960s, by 39% during the 1970s, and by 53% in the 1980s (Scherer, 1993: 98).

15. The number of compounds under development is already beginning to fall. At Upjohn, the figure has been cut from 74 in 1991 to 34 in 1994 while at Bristol-Myers Squibb the total number in its research pipeline has been reduced by a third in recent years. One possibility is for small or medium-sized firms to purchase compounds relinquished by the multinationals because they judge the market to be too small. Other options are to buy the rights to complete testing on unfinished compounds discarded by larger companies, or to acquire drugs that have received government approval and then reformulate them to improve effectiveness.

16. Large research groups may consist of more than 200 scientists, all reporting to the same R&D director. The resultant confusion inhibits discoveries and the problem can only become worse as companies impose more stringent controls on drug development in the 1990s. These circumstances suggest that there is little to be gained by seeking economies of scale in research centers. In contrast, a cutback in marketing (where scale economies are already being exploited) would probably result in a rise in the unit costs of distribution.

17. Various types of market imperfections have been observed but pricing anomalies are the most relevant here. For example, suppliers of original products that are suddenly confronted with competition from generics may refuse to cut price, or to reduce it by only a negligible amount (see Frank and Salkever, 1992; Grabowski and Vernon, 1992). This practice prevails even when generic sellers offer prices 40 to 70% below that of the incumbent's drug (Caves et al., 1991). Such a strategy would not be practical if the competing products are roughly equivalent and consumption decision makers have good information on prices and product characteristics.

18. This issue is not the same as suggesting that a fall in expected profits prompts the research-oriented firm to reduce its investment in R&D. There is a broader question here that concerns the supply response of these firms when the rate of return on pharmaceutical innovation changes. If the supply of pharmaceutical innovation is particularly sensitive to the level of returns on innovation, any reduction (however small) would lead to a sharp decline in new products and be costly for society. The opposite applies if the supply of innovation is insensitive to the rate of return on innovation. For further discussion, see Comanor (1986: 1214).

# References

Ballance R, Pogany J, and Forstner H (1992) *The World's Pharmaceutical Industries, An International Perspective on Innovation, Competition and Policy*. London: Edward Elgar.

Caves R, Whinston M, and Hurwitz M (1991) Patent expiration, entry, and competition in the U.S. pharmaceutical industry. *Brookings Papers on Economic Activity*, Microeconomics: 1–48.

Comanor W (1986) The political economy of the pharmaceutical industry. *Journal of Economic Literature* 24: 1178–217.

Cooper M and Culyer A (1973) *The Pharmaceutical Industry*. London: Economist Advisory Group and Dun and Bradstreet Ltd.

*Economist* (1992) A modern smokestack industry. 14 November: 76.

Farmindustria (1992) *Indicatori Farmaceutici*. Rome: Farmindustria.

*Financial Times* (1994) Survival of the fastest. 23 March.

Frank R and Salkever D (1992) Pricing, patent loss and the market for pharmaceuticals. *Southern Economic Journal* 59: 165–79.

Grabowski H and Vernon J (1992) Branded loyalty, entry, and price competition in pharmaceuticals after the 1984 Drug Act. *Journal of Law and Economics* 35: 331–50.

IMS (International Medical Services) *World Drug Market Manual* (annual), Washington, DC.

Lall S (1985) Appropriate pharmaceutical policies in developing countries. *Managerial and Decision Economics* 6: 226–31.

Organization for Economic Cooperation and Development (OECD) (1975) *Transfer of Technology for Pharmaceutical Chemicals*. Paris: OECD.

Organization for Economic Cooperation and Development (OECD) (1993) *Globalisation of Industrial Activities: Sector Case Study of Globalisation in the Pharmaceutical Industry* (dsti/ind(93)4). Paris: OECD.

Scherer M (1993) Pricing, profits, and technological progress in the pharmaceutical industry. *Journal of Economic Perspectives* 7: 97–115.

Scrip, *Pharmaceutical Company League Tables* (annual). Richmond, UK: PJB Publications.

Scrip, *Yearbook*. Richmond, UK: PJB Publications.

Spence M (1984) Cost reduction, competition and industry performance. *Econometrica* 52: 101–21.

Thomas L (1987) Regulation and firm size: FDA impacts on innovation. *First Boston Working Paper Series*, FB-87-24. New York, NY: Columbia Graduate School of Business.

U.S. Office of Technology Assessment (1993) *Pharmaceutical R&D: Costs, Risks and Rewards*. Washington, DC: U.S. Government Printing Office.

# 7

# Pharmaceutical Innovation in a Changing Environment

## KENNETH I. KAITIN

## The Current Pharmaceutical Environment

Worldwide concern over the rising cost of health care has focused public and political attention on the role of the multinational pharmaceutical industry. In the United States, the research-based pharmaceutical industry has been the subject of unrelenting criticism, and even vilification, by public officials and the lay press. The industry's critics voice concern primarily that pharmaceutical products are too expensive and that drug firms focus too heavily on the development of so-called "me too" drugs, that is, drugs that offer little or no therapeutic advantage over available medications. This intense scrutiny of the pharmaceutical industry's activities has placed substantial pressure on drug firms to streamline their drug development process, reduce costs, and focus on medical therapies with demonstrable advantages over existing products.

Changing market conditions have also contributed to the pharmaceutical industry's burden. Over the past decade, several factors have profoundly transformed the pharmaceutical marketplace. One factor is the growth of generic competition. Spurred by concern over rising prices for prescription drugs, the U.S. Congress passed legislation in 1984 designed to reduce prescription drug prices by fostering competition in the pharmaceutical marketplace. The Drug Price Competition and Patent Term Restoration Act of 1984 (1984) revised and streamlined procedures under which the Food and Drug Administration (FDA) evaluates and approves generic drugs. The result has been the rapid approval of large numbers of generic versions of many top-selling brand-name products that have recently come off patent (Kaitin and Trimble, 1987). Moreover, the generics industry has emerged as a powerful new competitor in the pharmaceutical marketplace.

Another major factor that has altered the pharmaceutical environment has been the dilution of decision-making power regarding drug prescribing. Previously the exclusive domain of the physician, the decision about when to prescribe a drug and which drug to prescribe is now shared among several interested parties. These parties include managed care organizations, which showed explosive growth in the 1980s, insurers, employers, and the government (Boston Consulting Group, 1993). Economic considerations are now an integral part of the larger prescribing process. In efforts to limit health care expenditures, pharmaceuticals have been frequently targeted as an area for cost savings.

Various cost-containment measures have been used in an attempt to limit pharmaceutical spending. These include therapeutic substitution (i.e., dispensing of a less expensive therapeutic alternative to the prescribed drug) (Shulman et al., 1992), restrictive drug formularies (i.e., a preselected list of prescription drugs from which physicians are required to prescribe), Drug Utilization Review (i.e., a mechanism for health care providers to monitor the prescribing patterns of physicians), and Medicaid rebates (OBRA, 1992). These factors have transformed drug development and marketing strategies of pharmaceutical firms. Whereas in the past, companies emphasized product safety and efficacy, today firms must also demonstrate that their products are cost effective and represent value for the money.

Over the last few decades, the pharmaceutical industry has been remarkably successful in developing a broad range of therapeutically important and innovative new drugs. These drugs have had a major impact on morbidity and mortality rates associated with many infectious and chronic diseases (Brown and Luce, 1990). In light of the challenges posed by a rapidly changing marketplace, however, it is important to ask: Will the industry be able to sustain this level of contribution?

## Pharmaceutical Innovation and the Drug Industry

Pharmaceutical innovation, defined as the discovery and development of new medical therapies (Wardell and Scheck, 1984), is a time-consuming, risky, and expensive process. Following synthesis of a compound, animal studies are conducted to test for biological activity and toxicity. Those compounds that survive the high attrition rate of this preclinical development period then are subjected to clinical investigations in human subjects. In the United States, a firm must file an investigational new drug (IND) application with the FDA before human testing may commence.

The clinical development period is usually divided into three phases. Each phase progressively tests the safety and efficacy of the compound until enough evidence is obtained to file a new drug application (NDA) with the FDA. Only after the FDA approves the NDA may the drug be marketed in the United States.

The time required to bring a new drug from the start of clinical testing to NDA approval is considerable. Kaitin et al. (1994) recently showed that for new chemical entities (NCEs) approved by the FDA in 1990, 1991, and 1992, the mean length of the clinical phase (time from IND filing to NDA submission) was 6.1 years, while the mean length of the review phase (time from NDA submission to approval) was 2.6

years. Thus, it currently takes, on average, nearly nine years, excluding the preclinical testing period, to develop a new drug and approve it for marketing.

In addition to long development times, pharmaceutical innovation is associated with a high degree of risk. Although estimates vary widely, clearly the number of compounds synthesized per approved drug is formidable. For example, Wardell and Sheck (1984) estimated that 10,000 compounds are synthesized for each one that is approved. More recently, Halliday et al. (1992) determined that U.S. companies synthesize 6,200 compounds for every approved drug. Even for those drugs that enter the clinical testing phase, the likelihood of obtaining marketing approval is far from certain. Only 20 to 25% of the drugs that begin testing in human subjects are eventually approved for marketing by the FDA (DiMasi et al., 1991).

The substantial time and risk involved in bringing a new product from synthesis to market are reflected in the high cost of pharmaceutical research and development (R&D). DiMasi et al. (1991) calculated that the average cost to develop a new drug is $231 million, up from $101 million in 1976 (Hansen, 1979) (both figures in 1987 dollars). Converting to 1994 dollars, the current cost of drug development is $291 million.

Recently, the Office of Technology Assessment (1993), using data from DiMasi et al. (1991) but applying a higher rate at which these costs are discounted, put the cost of drug development at $359 million (in 1990 dollars per approved new drug). These figures include both out-of-pocket costs and time costs (investment income forgone from expending funds on R&D before any returns are realized). Moreover, the figures include the costs of failed projects.

## The Industry's Contribution to Medical Progress

Over the past 50 years, many factors have influenced medical progress. Certainly, the development of important new medical devices, such as magnetic resonance imaging and computed tomography, and major improvements in surgical techniques and procedures, have contributed greatly to the diagnosis and treatment of disease. Similarly, pharmaceutical innovation and the development of important new drug therapies have had a significant impact on the practice of medicine. Pharmaceutical products now provide therapeutic treatments for a broad range of previously untreatable, and sometimes fatal, diseases.

Although the importance of prescription drugs in medical practice is widely acknowledged, it is worth noting the degree to which the research-based pharmaceutical industry is responsible for developing these products and bringing them to market. To evaluate the relative contributions of the pharmaceutical industry, academia, and the government to the development of new drugs, Kaitin et al. (1993) recently examined the source of NCEs approved in the United States from 1981 through 1990. Of the 196 drugs approved during that ten-year period, the source of 181 (92.4%) was the pharmaceutical industry. Of the remaining 15 drugs, academia was the source of seven (3.6%) and government was the source of two (1%); the remainder were from miscellaneous sources.

To be sure, these findings in no way suggest that government and academia play an insignificant role in biomedical research and new drug development. The basic science contribution of academia and the National Institutes of Health (NIH) often provide the necessary foundation for drug discovery and development. Moreover, the pharmaceutical industry directly benefits from the government's investment in extramural and intramural research through its collaborations with academic research centers and through contacts and research agreements with the NIH and other government health research laboratories (Office of Technology Assessment, 1993). Nonetheless, the above findings clearly indicate that the research-based pharmaceutical industry is the primary source of prescription drugs marketed in the United States.

In light of these findings, it is worth noting that a recent Gallup Organization survey (1992) revealed a striking lack of appreciation by consumers of the role of the research-based pharmaceutical industry in the development of new drugs. For example, 70% of consumers surveyed did not know that the drug industry supports most pharmaceutical research and development. Moreover, consumers estimated that, on average, only 36% of all drug discoveries come from industry. It is worth emphasizing the critical implications of these findings. They suggest that the public is unaware of the degree to which the development and availability of new pharmaceutical products will be impeded by social policies that directly or indirectly lead to a decline in pharmaceutical innovation within the drug industry.

## Trends in Pharmaceutical Innovation

There is no single, simple measure of pharmaceutical innovation. Instead, various indices can be examined to create an overall picture of the drug development process. For example, trends in the level of clinical research activity by drug firms can be quantitatively measured by examining annual numbers of IND filings. Because firms must file an IND with the FDA before a new compound can be tested in human subjects, the rate of IND filings provides a gauge of the number of investigational compounds entering clinical trials in the United States during any given year.

At the other end of the drug development process, annual new drug approval rates can be used to measure the innovative output of the pharmaceutical industry. Trends in drug approval rates provide an estimate of the relative success of drug firms in bringing new products to market.

Other measures, such as clinical development and regulatory review times, allow one to assess the overall efficiency of pharmaceutical innovation. In addition, therapeutic ratings of new drugs and the time required to bring important new drugs to market provide a gauge of the quality of pharmaceutical innovation. In other words, what percentage of new products developed by drug firms represent important therapeutic advances, and how quickly are these products developed and approved for marketing?

In the following analyses, three aspects of pharmaceutical innovation will be explored. These are *quantity*, viewed in terms of input (IND filings) and output (NDA approvals) measures; *efficiency*, that is, the time required to bring new products to market; and *quality*, referring to the development of products that represent important therapeutic advances.

## Data Analyzed

The data used in the following analyses were obtained from confidential surveys of pharmaceutical firms and were cross-checked with data obtained through Freedom of Information (FOI) and from public source documents. These include FDA publications, as well as the Federal Register and FDC Reports (The Pink Sheet).

The analyses are based on NCEs either under investigation or approved for marketing in the United States. The Tufts Center for the Study of Drug Development (CSDD) defines an NCE as any new molecular entity not previously approved for use in the United States. Excluded are biologics, vaccines, diagnostic agents, and new salts, esters, and dosage forms of previously approved compounds. Note that, for simplicity, in the remainder of this chapter, NCEs will be referred to as "new drugs."

For investigational new drugs, data from the CSDD's triennial survey of a sample of major pharmaceutical firms with operations in the United States were used. These surveys ask firms both to update information provided in previous surveys and to provide new data on investigational new drugs that the firm either first tested in human subjects anywhere in the world or, as in the case of acquired new drugs, filed the first U.S. IND. The CSDD's database on investigational drugs currently contains information on more than 2,200 new drugs investigated during the period from 1963 to 1994.

For approved new drugs, data from the CSDD's annual survey of firms receiving an NDA approval during the year were used. In this survey, information is collected on each approved new drug's source, date of synthesis, clinical development, regulatory review, marketing (both in the United States and abroad), and relevant patent history. The CSDD's database on approved drugs contains data on every new drug approved by the FDA from 1963 through 1994.

## Trends in IND Filings and NDA Approvals

Figure 7-1 presents three-year moving averages of the annual numbers of IND filings and NDA approvals for 52 separate pharmaceutical divisions of 22 U.S.-owned firms and 14 U.S. subsidiaries of foreign-owned firms. These firms represent the majority of innovative pharmaceutical companies with operations in the United States. The upper line in the figure, which was recently presented in DiMasi et al. (1994), shows the annual number of INDs filed by these firms during the years 1963 through 1989. The lower line shows, for the same sample of firms, the annual number of NDAs approved from 1963 through 1993.

The average number of IND filings per year declined dramatically from the early 1960s to the mid 1970s. From a high of 111 in 1963–65, the annual filing rate decreased by 57%, to 48, in 1975–77. Although annual filings increased by 65% over the next seven years, to 79 in 1982–84, the number gradually declined through the remainder of the study period. Comparing mean IND filing rates for each of the three decades of the study period, there was a 34% decrease from the 1960s to the

**THE PRODUCT CYCLE**

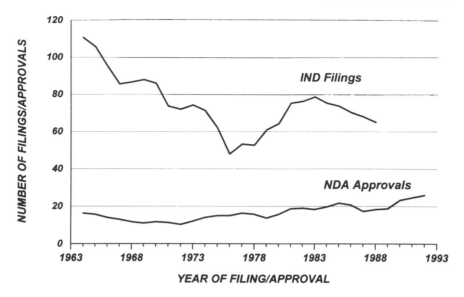

**Figure 7-1.** Annual number of investigational new drug (IND) application filings and new drug application (NDA) approvals for new chemical entities (NCEs), from 1963 to 1993. Data are from 36 major pharmaceutical firms with operations in the United States. Lines represent three-year moving averages.

1970s (from 97.9 to 64.7 filings per year, respectively). Average filings then increased by 10% in the 1980s (to 71.0 per year).

Because IND filings tell us the number of compounds that enter clinical investigation, one would expect that fluctuations in annual filing rates for a sample of firms would be roughly associated with corresponding changes in NDA approval rates for those same firms. Moreover, these changes in NDA approval rates would be expected to occur approximately five to nine years after the corresponding changes in IND filing rates, to account for the length of the clinical development and regulatory review phases. This was observed to some degree for the present sample of firms.

The lower line in Fig. 7-1 shows that the average annual number of NDA approvals for sample firms declined by 41% in the early years of the study period, from 13.6 in 1963–65 to 8.0 in 1971–73. This decline corresponds with the decline in IND filings during the 1960s. In the remaining 20 years of the study period, however, the average annual number of NDA approvals generally increased, to a high of 20.6 in 1991–93, an increase of 157%.

Interestingly, the gradual rise in NDA approvals began while IND filings were still decreasing. This paradoxical finding reflects, in part, changes in clinical success rates for new drugs during the 1960s and 1970s. That is, from the mid 1960s to the early 1970s, there was an increase in the percentage of new drugs with INDs filed that eventually obtained NDA approval (DiMasi et al., 1994). The rise in the rate of annual NDA approvals in the 1980s and early 1990s, however, in large part reflects the rapid rise in IND filings that occurred between 1976 and 1983.

The decline in the rate of IND filings in the mid to late 1980s suggests that the encouraging rise in annual NDA approvals through the 1980s and early 1990s will not continue indefinitely. Taking into consideration the average time from IND filing to NDA approval, one might expect that the annual rate of NDA approvals will decrease by the mid to late 1990s.

## Trends in Annual New Drug Approvals

Whereas Fig. 7-1 presents annual NDA approval rates for a sample of pharmaceutical firms, Fig. 7-2 displays the total number of new drugs approved each year between 1963 and 1993. There were 519 new drugs approved during this 31-year period. The trend over this time, depicted by the best-fit line superimposed on the annual approval bars in the figure, is upward, indicating a tendency toward increasing numbers of NDA approvals. Comparing approval rates by decade, there was a mean of 13.7 approvals per year in the 1960s, 13.8 in the 1970s, 18.8 in the 1980s (a 36% increase from the 1970s), and 24.3 in the 1990s (a 29% increase from the 1980s).

These findings suggest that pharmaceutical innovation in the United States has increased steadily over the last two decades. On the other hand, as noted above, a decline in the rate of IND filings may lead to an eventual reduction in NDA approval rates. The reduction in IND filings through most of the 1980s by major pharmaceutical firms operating in the United States (see Fig. 7-1), suggests that the rate of NDA approvals will begin to fall in the mid to late 1990s.

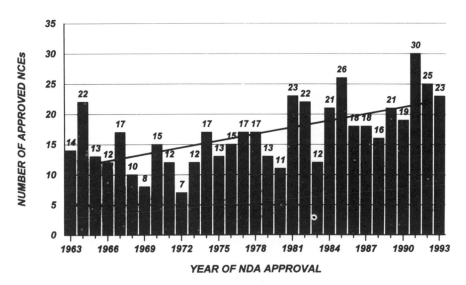

**Figure 7-2.** Annual number of new drugs (NCEs) approved from 1963 through 1993 (bars), and trend in approval rates represented by the best-fit line.

## Trends in Drug Development and Review

Whereas IND filing and NDA approval rates, respectively, are useful input and output measures of the quantity of pharmaceutical innovation, the lengths of the development and review times for new drugs measure the relative efficiency of the innovative process, that is, the speed at which new drug candidates are developed and approved for marketing.

Over the last three decades, there has been a substantial increase in the time required to bring a new drug to market. Figure 7-3 shows trends in clinical (IND filing to NDA submission) and review (NDA submission to approval) phases and total times (chemical synthesis or isolation to NDA approval) for new drugs approved in the United States from 1963 to 1993. The lines in the figure represent three-year moving averages.

The length of the clinical phase more than doubled during the study period, from 2.5 years in 1963–65 to six years in 1991–93. Most of this increase occurred in the 1970s; from 1970 to 1980, the clinical phase increased 60% (from 3.5 to 5.6 years, respectively). Although there were no clear trends through most of the 1980s, the clinical phase increased steadily from 1986–88 through the end of the study period.

NDA review times also increased over the study period, although not as dramatically as clinical development times. Between 1963–65 and 1991–93, the review

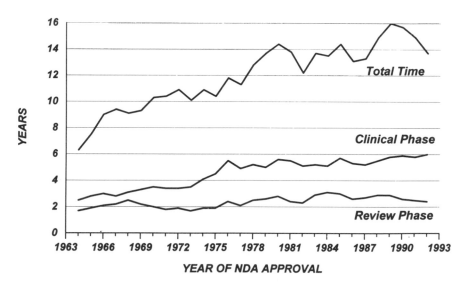

**Figure 7-3.** Length of the clinical development and regulatory review phases and total time for new drugs approved from 1963 through 1993. The clinical phase refers to the period from IND filing to NDA submission, the review phase refers to the period from NDA submission to approval, and the total time refers to the period from chemical synthesis or isolation to NDA approval. Lines represent three-year moving averages.

phase increased 41% (from 1.7 to 2.4 years, respectively). Over the last decade, however, the review phase generally decreased, from a high of 3.1 years in 1983–85 to 2.4 years in 1991–93.

There was a striking increase in total time over the study period. Total time refers to the period from chemical synthesis or isolation to NDA approval. This includes time spent in preclinical animal testing, clinical development, and regulatory review. Despite considerable variability in the 1980s and early 1990s, total time rose 156% over the study period, from a low of 6.3 years in 1963–65 to a high of 16.1 years in 1988–90. This increase was largely due to the trend toward longer clinical development times.

## New Drug Approvals by Therapeutic Rating

FDA-assigned therapeutic ratings allow one to assess the relative quality, in medical terms, of pharmaceutical innovation. Along these lines, development and review times for therapeutically important drugs offer a useful measure of how quickly new drugs that offer important therapeutic benefits are developed and approved for marketing.

The FDA's therapeutic rating system was implemented in 1976. To prioritize its application workload, the FDA began assigning therapeutic ratings to drugs filed with the agency, based on subjective assessments of the therapeutic value of these drugs (Food and Drug Administration, 1976). All commercially sponsored INDs and pending NDAs were classified by chemical type and therapeutic potential. Those new drugs considered to represent important therapeutic gains were rated 1A, those representing modest gains were rated 1B, and those representing little or no gain were rated 1C.

In 1986, the FDA added the classification 1AA for drugs intended for the treatment of AIDS and AIDS-related conditions. In 1992, at the recommendation of the President's Council on Competitiveness (1991), chaired by then-Vice President Dan Quayle, the FDA discontinued its A, B, C rating system and began designating applications as either "P" for priority review or "S" for standard review. Priority NDAs are earmarked for greater attention by agency reviewers and an expedited review process. Standard NDAs, in contrast, are given lower status and receive no special attention.

In the current analyses, new drugs rated 1P, 1A, 1AA, and 1B are grouped as "priority drugs" and those rated 1S and 1C are grouped as "standard drugs." Figure 7-4 shows mean clinical development and regulatory review phases for priority and standard new drugs approved in three six-year intervals (1976–1981, 1982–1987, and 1988–1993). Numbers of approved new drugs are also indicated. In each interval, priority drugs represented approximately 50% of total approvals.

Although the mean review time for priority drugs remained constant, at 2.1 years, over the 18-year period, in each interval priority drugs were reviewed more quickly than standard drugs. The difference was greatest in the 1988–1993 interval.

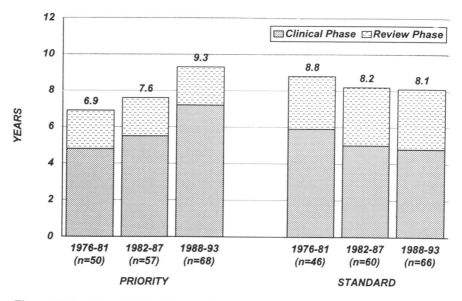

**Figure 7-4.** Mean clinical and review phases for priority and standard new drugs approved in three six-year intervals. *n* refers to the number of drugs approved in each interval.

During this period, priority drugs, on average, were reviewed 36% faster than standard drugs.

The constancy of the priority review time in each of the three intervals is discouraging in light of recent efforts by the FDA to accelerate the review of therapeutically important drugs. One explanation for the lack of change is that it is still too early for the full effects of these new initiatives to be felt. It is worth noting, however, that under a set of specific performance goals detailed in the recently enacted Prescription Drug User Fee Act of 1992 (1992), the FDA is committed to reduce review times for priority drugs to six months by October 1, 1997.

A particularly disturbing finding in the current analysis is the increase in the mean time spent in clinical development for priority drugs. From the earliest interval to the most recent interval, the length of the priority group's clinical phase increased by 50% (from 4.8 years to 7.2 years, respectively). In contrast, during the same period, the length of the clinical phase for standard drugs decreased by 19% (from 5.9 years to 4.8 years).

One result of these changes in clinical development times is that in the most recent interval, the total time from IND filing to NDA approval for priority drugs exceeded that for standard drugs by 1.2 years, a 15% difference. This finding supports the results of previous analyses (Kaitin et al., 1994; 1991; DiMasi et al., 1994) and suggests that despite the therapeutic importance of these drugs, the overall time taken for them to reach the market is greater than that for therapeutically less important drugs.

# Discussion

## Determinants of Pharmaceutical Innovation

No single factor can be considered the sole determinant of the quantity and quality of pharmaceutical innovation. Instead, various economic, regulatory, and scientific factors all contribute to the rate and efficiency of the new drug development process. From an economic perspective, current efforts to contain health care expenditures in general, and pharmaceutical spending in particular, have fundamentally changed the environment in which pharmaceutical firms operate (Boston Consulting Group, 1993). The spiraling increase in generic competition, the rapid growth of managed care organizations, and the proliferation of cost containment policies, such as therapeutic substitution, drug utilization review, price controls, mandatory rebates, and restrictive formularies, have substantially increased competitive pressures on pharmaceutical firms (Grabowski, 1994). If financial returns on drug development decline, some argue, firms may be less willing to invest in future research and development. The result may ultimately be a decline in drug innovation and pharmaceutical output.

Pharmaceutical innovation is also affected by the regulatory climate. Regulatory agencies, in their reviews of applications to market new drugs, must often balance two competing needs: ensuring that the public is protected from unsafe and ineffective drugs, and expediting the availability of effective new therapies. While stringent regulatory policies that demand extensive safety and efficacy data may reduce the likelihood of approving a drug that, with wider patient use, displays unacceptable toxicity, these policies may also delay the approval of valuable new medicines. Moreover, lengthy clinical development and review times serve as disincentives to pharmaceutical firms in their efforts to discover and develop new drugs.

Some have argued that in the United States, the stringency of the FDA's new drug approval requirements contribute to the high cost and excessive time required to bring new pharmaceutical products to market (Wardell, 1973; Cullen, 1983). One putative outcome of this regulatory stringency has been a delay in the availability of new drugs in the United States relative to other industrialized countries (Kaitin et al., 1994; 1989).

Scientific factors, such as the changing focus of drug discovery and development, also influence pharmaceutical innovation. Whereas in earlier decades, drug firms concentrated primarily on developing treatments for infection and other less complicated indications, firms are now targeting diseases of greater complexity and chronicity, such as Alzheimer's disease, AIDS, multiple sclerosis, and cancer. The drug development process for these persistent, degenerative, and life-threatening diseases is typically longer, more expensive, and more complicated. One result of this change in focus to more complex diseases may be a reduction in innovative output.

## Pharmaceutical Innovation in the United States

Based on the data presented here, there is some cause for concern about pharmaceutical innovation in the near term. The steady decline in IND filings through much of the 1980s suggests an imminent reduction in new drug approvals by the mid to late 1990s. This is further supported by the fact that the relatively large number of new drugs approved in recent years may be partially explained by the reduction in the FDA's formidable backlog of overdue NDAs (Food and Drug Administration, 1994). While the agency should be commended for its accomplishments in this area, elimination of the pool of backlogged applications will inevitably lead to a decline in the number of NDAs under review and available for approval. This in turn may contribute to a relative reduction in the annual rate of NDA approvals.

On a more optimistic note, however, two factors may offset the effects of the observed decline in IND filings. The first is the rapid rise in the number of INDs filed for biotechnology-derived products. Bienz-Tadmor et al. (1992) have recently shown that INDs filed for biotechnology products increased nearly tenfold between 1980 and 1988. If numbers of IND filings for biotechnology products and new drugs are combined, then the decline in filings described above disappears, and the rate of total INDs filed in the 1980s remains constant (DiMasi et al., 1994).

The second factor that may offset the effects of the observed decline in IND filings is the steady improvement in clinical success rates for new drugs (DiMasi et al., 1994). An improvement in clinical success rate indicates that a greater percentage of investigational drugs that enter the clinic eventually receive NDA approval. Thus, a decline in INDs filed may not necessarily result in a reduction in products approved. Over the next five to ten years, it will be important to monitor whether compensatory factors, such as higher clinical success rates and greater numbers of biotechnology product IND filings, can offset the effects of the observed decline in IND filings for new drugs.

In the current analysis, the length of the clinical phase increased markedly. This increase resulted in a striking rise in the time taken to bring a new drug from chemical synthesis to NDA approval, which was approximately 15 years for drugs approved in the 1990s.

The increase in clinical development times may be attributable to several factors. One factor is the change in focus within the pharmaceutical industry to developing drugs for more complex and chronic diseases. In many cases, these drugs require longer and more complicated clinical studies to assess efficacy and long-term toxicity. Another factor is increasing regulatory stringency by the FDA. Whereas the length of the clinical testing phase is, in theory, determined solely by the drug manufacturer, some have suggested that the FDA's continually increasing demand for more extensive safety and efficacy data has had a significant impact on the time required for firms to conduct the necessary clinical, as well as preclinical, studies (Smith, 1985).

The length of the regulatory review phase, in contrast, is directly related to the efficiency of the FDA review process (which, to be sure, involves drug sponsor response to the FDA's queries and criticisms). Over the past two decades, the FDA has been under growing pressure to accelerate its review procedures and hasten the availability of new drugs. In response, the agency has implemented several initiatives, such as prefiling conferences with drug sponsors and computer-assisted NDAs, to speed the drug approval process (Kaitin and Walsh, 1992). These initiatives have, no doubt, contributed to the gradual decline in the review phase observed during the last decade of the study period.

The current findings show that the average approval rate for therapeutically important new drugs as a percentage of total new drugs has remained relatively constant, at approximately 50% since 1976. These drugs represent important therapeutic breakthroughs and significant advances over current therapies. Given the therapeutic importance of these drugs, should one view the fact that they represent 50% of total new drugs as cause for optimism or concern? What percentage of new drug approvals can one reasonably expect will be therapeutic breakthroughs? There are no clear answers to these questions. It is worth noting, however, that medical progress generally occurs in small, incremental steps. Thus, one would not necessarily expect the number of therapeutically important drugs approved as a percentage of total drugs to be high.

On the other hand, the striking increase over the 18-year study period in clinical development times for these therapeutically important drugs is cause for serious concern. Current results show that in the most recent six-year period, the total time to bring priority drugs to market, from IND filing to NDA approval, exceeds by 15% the same time for drugs representing little or no therapeutic value. One possible explanation for this finding is that the longer development times for priority drugs reflect in part the novel nature of these drugs. In other words, more extensive and unusual clinical studies may be required to assess clinical safety and efficacy due to limited experience with that class of drugs. Nonetheless, these results suggest that current efforts to speed the availability of therapeutically important drugs must place greater emphasis on reducing the lengthy clinical development process, as well as on shortening the regulatory review phase.

It should be noted that several of the recent initiatives to facilitate new drug availability, such as the Treatment IND (1987), Expedited Approval (Subpart E) Regulations (1988), and Accelerated Approval Regulations (1992), focus exclusively on drugs to treat life threatening or severely debilitating diseases. These drugs represent a subgroup of the priority drug category. Interestingly, based on unpublished data from the CSDD, clinical and review times for these drugs were considerably shorter than those for other priority drugs. Thus, patients with life threatening and severely debilitating diseases have clearly benefited from the provisions of these regulations.

## Conclusion

Innovation in the pharmaceutical industry is responsible for a large majority of the therapeutic agents currently used in medical practice. These pharmaceutical products have had a substantial impact on the diagnosis and treatment of disease. Despite this progress, there are many areas that present either new or continuing medical challenges. AIDS, Alzheimer's disease, cardiovascular disease, and cancer are examples of diseases that exact a heavy toll in financial resources, human suffering, and death.

In the current study several measures were used to evaluate the quantity, efficiency, and quality of pharmaceutical innovation. The findings indicate that, whereas there has been a trend toward increasing numbers of new product approvals observed since the early 1960s, these numbers are likely to decline by the mid to late 1990s. On the other hand, evidence suggests that this decline may be offset by the rapid growth in biotechnology product development and improved clinical success rates for new drugs.

The findings also indicate that, while drugs for the treatment of life threatening and severely debilitating diseases enjoy relatively fast development and review times, there has been a growing delay in the time required to bring other therapeutically important drugs to market. Although the reasons for these trends are complex and difficult to define, they undoubtedly involve economic, political, regulatory, and scientific factors.

Social policies that lead to a decline in pharmaceutical innovation are certain to have dire public health consequences in terms of fewer new drugs and a reduction in R&D efforts toward the development of new treatments for diseases for which either no therapy exists or current treatments are inadequate. It will be imperative in coming years to continue to carefully monitor trends in new drug development and regulatory review and to critically assess the impact of the changing economic and political environment on pharmaceutical innovation.

## Acknowledgments

The author wishes to thank Mark Seibring, Information Systems Coordinator at the Tufts Center for the Study of Drug Development, for his technical assistance and helpful comments on the manuscript.

# References

Accelerated Approval Regulations (1992) Accelerated approval of new drugs for serious or life-threatening illnesses. 21 CFR 314.500.

Bienz-Tadmor B, DiCerbo PA, Tadmor G, and Lasagna L (1992) Biopharmaceuticals and conventional drugs: clinical success rates. *Bio/Technology* 10: 521–25.

Boston Consulting Group (1993) *The Changing Environment for U.S. Pharmaceuticals: The Role of Pharmaceutical Companies in a Systems Approach to Health Care.* Boston, MA: The Boston Consulting Group Inc.

Brown RE and Luce BR (1990) *The Value of Pharmaceuticals: A Study of Selected Conditions to Measure the Contribution of Pharmaceuticals to Health Status.* Washington, DC: Battelle Medical Technology and Policy Research Center.

Cullen R (1983) Pharmaceuticals inter-country diffusion. *Managerial and Decision Economics* 4: 73–82.

DiMasi JA, Hansen RW, Grabowski HG, and Lasagna L (1991) Cost of innovation in the pharmaceutical industry. *Journal of Health Economics* 10: 107–42.

DiMasi JA, Seibring MA, and Lasagna L (1994) New drug development in the United States from 1963 to 1992. *Journal of Clinical Pharmacology and Therapeutics* 55: 609–22.

Drug Price Competition and Patent Term Restoration Act of 1984 (1984) PL 98–417, 98 Stat. 1585, Section 505 (j)(7)(B).

Expedited Approval Regulations (1988) Drugs intended to treat life threatening and severely-debilitating illnesses. 21 CFR 312.80.

Food and Drug Administration (1976) Associate Director for New Drug Evaluation: Drug Classification. Staff Manual Guide. BD 4820.3. Washington, DC: Bureau of Drugs.

Food and Drug Administration (1994) Progress in Achieving the Performance Goals Refer-enced in the Prescription Drug User Fee Act of 1992: First Report to Congress for the

Period September 1, 1992 through September 1, 1993. Washington, DC: Public Health Service, Department of Health and Human Services, April 11.

Gallup Organization Inc. (1992) The Role of Pharmaceuticals in Medical Progress: A National Survey of Consumers and Experts. Washington, DC: Pharmaceutical Manufacturers Association Foundation, January.

Grabowski H (1994) Health reform and pharmaceutical innovation. *Seton Hall Law Review* 24: 1221–59.

Halliday RG, Walker SR, and Lumley CE (1992) R&D philosophy and management in the world's leading pharmaceutical companies. *Journal of Pharmaceutical Medicine* 2: 139–54.

Hansen RW (1979) The pharmaceutical development process: estimates of current development costs and times and the effects of regulatory changes. In: Chien RI (ed.) *Issues in Pharmaceutical Economics*. Lexington, MA: Lexington Books, pp. 151–87.

Kaitin KI and Trimble AG (1987) Implementation of the Drug Price Competition and Patent Term Restoration Act of 1984: a progress report. *Journal of Clinical Research and Drug Development* 1: 263–75.

Kaitin KI and Walsh HL (1992) Are initiatives to speed the new drug approval process working? *Drug Information Journal* 26: 341–49.

Kaitin KI, Bryant NR, and Lasagna L (1993) The role of the research-based pharmaceutical industry in medical progress in the United States. *Journal of Clinical Pharmacology* 33: 412–17.

Kaitin KI, DiCerbo PA, and Lasagna L (1991) The New Drug Approvals of 1987, 1988, and 1989: trends in drug development. *Journal of Clinical Pharmacology* 31: 116–22.

Kaitin KI, Manocchia M, Seibring M, and Lasagna L (1994) The New Drug Approvals of 1990, 1991, and 1992: trends in drug development. *Journal of Clinical Pharmacology* 34: 120–27.

Kaitin KI, Mattison N, Northington FK, and Lasagna L (1989) The drug lag: an update of new drug introductions in the United States and in the United Kingdom, 1977 through 1987. *Clinical Pharmacology and Therapeutics* 46: 121–38.

Office of Technology Assessment (1993) *Pharmaceutical R&D: Costs, Risks and Rewards*. OTA-H-522. Washington, DC: U.S. Government Printing Office.

Omnibus Budget Reconciliation Act of 1990 (1992) PL 101–158.

Prescription Drug User Fee Act of 1992 (1992) PL 102–571, 106 Stat. 4491.

President's Council on Competitiveness (1991) Improving the Nation's Drug Approval Process. Vice President Dan Quayle, chairman. Washington, DC: Author, November 13.

Shulman SR, DiCerbo PA, Ulcickas ME, and Lasagna L (1992) A survey of therapeutic substitution programs in ten Boston area hospitals. *Drug Information Journal* 26: 41–52.

Smith CG (1985) Past, current, and future safety and efficacy trends in the drug industry. *Regulatory Toxicology and Pharmacology* 5: 241–54.

Treatment IND Regulations (1987) Treatment use of an investigational new drug. 21 CFR 312.34, 312.35.

Wardell WM (1973) Introduction of new therapeutic drugs in the United States and Great Britain: an international comparison. *Clinical Pharmacology and Therapeutics* 14: 773–90.

Wardell WM and Sheck LE (1984) Is pharmaceutical innovation declining?: Interpreting measures of pharmaceutical innovation and regulatory impact in the USA, 1950–1980. In: Lindgren B (ed.) *Arne Ryde Symposium on Pharmaceutical Economics*. Swedish Institute for Health Economics and Liber Forlag, pp. 177–89.

# 8

# Prices for Prescription Drugs: The Roles of Market Forces and Government Regulation

DAVID J. GROSS, JOSEPH KILE,
JONATHAN RATNER, AND CELIA THOMAS[1]

Faced with urgent fiscal pressures, health care policy makers in many countries are considering whether new mixes of regulatory and market-oriented strategies might reduce health care costs. To predict how much a future shift in policy would restrain spending on pharmaceuticals, policy makers require more evidence and fewer assertions about the effect of today's regulatory and market factors on drug prices. Unfortunately, systematic evidence is in short supply. However, one source of information has been tapped too little—international data on drug prices. Analysis of these data can help illuminate the roles of various determinants of pharmaceutical prices.

Prescription drug prices differ between countries, even for identical products produced by the same manufacturer. To some extent, these differences reflect the different balances struck by each country's government between the desire to reduce drug costs to consumers and the conflicting desire to maintain incentives for pharmaceutical R&D. These choices are manifested in the differing degrees of price regulation, patent protection, and other policies in each country and, therefore, in average drug prices. But government regulation is not the only plausible determinant of a country's average prescription drug prices. Differences between countries in market factors, such as availability of therapeutic alternatives, can also create differences in drug prices.

This essay considers the two fundamental determinants of international price differentials: market forces and government actions. It is arranged in three parts. First, a conceptual model of the industry provides a framework for understanding why prices vary across international boundaries. In the second section, two case studies provide evidence on the determinants of differentials between the United States and Canada and between the United States and the United Kingdom. Finally, several observations conclude the essay.

## International Price Differentials—A Framework

This section develops a framework for understanding price differentials by addressing two questions. How can prices for identical products differ between countries? And what factors lead to average prices in one country exceeding average prices in another country? The focus is on the prices of patented, brand-name products that are sold in different markets. The focus has a dual rationale: to shed light on the pricing practices of research-based firms, and to ensure that drug prices are compared only for identical products.[2] For other purposes, such as international comparisons of the costs to consumers of products that are equivalent chemically but may differ in other respects, a wider focus that includes generics would be appropriate.

### How Can Prices for Identical Products Differ Between Countries?

The prescription drug industry operates in many markets, some defined for individual products or groups of products, some defined across international boundaries. Each country provides a separate market for each therapy. Therefore, a seller with market power supplying a product in more than one country would be expected—absent regulatory restraints—to set prices in each according to the characteristics of demand and the seller's costs.

When cost conditions in the two countries are the same, for example, when the costs of supplying additional units of a drug do not vary across units or countries, sellers may still charge different prices in different markets, or "price discriminate."[3] Two conditions allow this. First, each manufacturer has market power based on patent protection and on brand loyalty. Second, arbitrage is limited because it is generally illegal or impractical to buy pharmaceutical products in inexpensive markets and resell them in more expensive markets.[4]

When the conditions for price discrimination obtain, and production and distribution costs are relatively low, profit-seeking firms can supply some markets at correspondingly low prices. For example, in price-sensitive markets or in low-income markets, pharmaceutical firms can profitably sell their product at a price that covers only their marginal costs of production and distribution while charging higher prices in less price-sensitive or wealthier markets.

## What Factors Lead Prices in One Country to Exceed Prices in Another?

International differences in average drug prices depend, of course, on the extent to which price differentials exist for individual products. Underlying these differentials are disparities between countries in market and regulatory factors – some that are common to most, if not all, products within a country, and others that differ among individual products. We focus first on several broad factors: international differences in the general price responsiveness of prescription drug consumers, the extent of market organization among buyers, and the extent of government intervention in the marketplace. We then provide a discussion of drug-specific factors, such as the availability of substitutes, that lead to average price differences and variation in price differences across drugs.

### Broad Factors

In the absence of price controls, prices that a company sets in different countries depend, in part, on the average elasticity of demand, or price responsiveness, of consumers in the respective countries. Where consumers' prescription drug buying patterns are generally more insensitive to price changes – relatively less price elastic – pharmaceutical firms would be expected, other factors equal, to charge higher prices. The extent and type of third-party payment for prescription drugs could, for example, influence the price responsiveness of consumers. For example, the German method of subsidizing drug purchases, in which consumers pay flat fees for prescriptions, might be expected to decrease price sensitivity more than a system in which the insurer pays a certain percentage of a prescription's cost. In addition, a common conjecture is that consumers in a country with relatively high average income have more inelastic demand, compared to consumers in less affluent countries and could, others factors equal, be charged higher prices.

International price differentials are also likely to depend on the nature and extent of organization among buyers. Buyers who act together gain strong positions from which to negotiate for low prices. Traditionally, most drugs in the United States have been sold through retail pharmacies that had little power to negotiate with large drug manufacturers.[5] In many other countries, however, the government takes a more active role in organizing buyers and creating buying power. This gives public and quasi-public payers a form of buying power – the buyer is too big for the seller to ignore. In Canada and the United Kingdom, for example, this is accomplished with a single payer for those citizens covered under a prescription drug benefit program. In France and Germany, buying power is achieved through government regulations on reimbursements that apply to quasi-public insurers.

The average price of drugs in any country, and hence international price differentials, also depends on the extent and type of government regulation.[6] In many countries, the government intervenes directly or indirectly in the marketplace for prescription drugs. In addition to indirect intervention in the form of government-sponsored purchasing groups as described above, governments may directly control prices or corporate profits on prescription drugs, or choose not to enforce patent laws. France, for example, until 1994 directly regulated the prices of prescription drugs. Germany, Sweden, and The Netherlands set maximum reimbursement rates for some drugs. In the United Kingdom, the government regulates the rate of return for pharmaceutical firms, though it does not control directly the introductory or launch price of newly marketed drugs. (Gross et al., 1994).[7] Also, several developing countries do not enforce patent laws for prescription drugs; access to drugs is seen as too important to be limited by high prices (see, e.g., Redwood, 1994).

## Drug-Specific Factors

Drug price differentials are affected by factors that can vary not only across countries but also across individual drugs, some of which are similar to the influences affecting all drugs in a country. For example, differences in the elasticity of demand between products or types of products and differences in the effects of regulation on drugs within the same country can lead to price differentials. In addition, differences in costs of supplying a product in one country vis-à-vis another could lead to price differences.

The presence of therapeutic substitutes can affect the relative elasticities of demand for different products and, thus, the price differential for those individual products. Two examples illustrate this effect. First, the emergence of a generic alternative to a brand-name drug can lead to an *increase* in the price of the brand-name drug—an effect that is counterintuitive. For example, one study demonstrated that the price of cephalexin, which is sold under the brand name Keflex, increased with the entry of generic alternatives, even though generic alternatives were launched at prices below the price of Keflex (and subsequently declined).[8] Some consumers or their physicians value the reputation of a brand-name product more than they value low price while others value low price more than their preference for the brand name. Producers of the brand-name product recognize that even if they maintain prices that significantly exceed the generic price, some physicians will continue to prescribe the brand-name product. The drug company willingly cedes the price-sensitive segment of the market to the generic product in order to charge a higher price to those people who are most loyal to the brand-name product. Thus, the availability of generic drugs in some countries but not in others may affect price differentials. For a more complete discussion of this effect, see Comanor (1986).

Second, a similar phenomenon may also occur with the entry of a new drug that is therapeutically similar to an existing drug. A well known example of this is found in the U.S. market for ulcer medication. Tagamet revolutionized the treatment of certain types of ulcers when it was introduced in 1977. Several years later, Zantac came on the market as a therapeutically similar treatment. Although the two drugs were slightly different in their effectiveness and their side effects, neither was uniformly preferred to the other. Recognizing that each drug had advantages for certain patients, each manufacturer was able to charge a price higher than the original Tagamet price in supplying consumers who preferred its product.[9]

Price differentials may also be related to differences in how government regulations affect particular drugs. For example, in some countries, pricing regulations are not applied uniformly across all drugs: Canada's federal pricing regulations apply only to drugs under patent, while Germany's limits on drug reimbursement prices apply only to drugs with generic or nongeneric therapeutic substitutes. Also, regulations that exercise tighter controls over drug price increases than on introductory prices are likely to have a more stringent effect on older products while the converse is true for regulations that exercise tighter controls on introductory prices than on price increases.

The effect of regulation may be unrelated to product characteristics or it may vary with each product's determinants of demand elasticity, such as therapeutic category. For example, if the government mandated a reduction in the prevailing market prices of all drugs by a fixed percentage, the regulatory effect would be independent of each product's characteristics. In contrast, however, a regulatory authority may seek to control more tightly the prices of products for which the demand is insensitive to price. In this case, the effect of regulation would vary with the market characteristics of each drug. These alternative schemes for effecting price restraint illustrate the importance of the goal and the sophistication of the regulatory authorities: Do they set price or profit constraints in a vacuum, or do they take into account the differences between drugs' market characteristics? When government regulators follow this latter approach, price differentials between any two countries may vary substantially from product to product.

## Two Case Studies of International Price Differentials

With this conceptual framework in mind, we turn to two case studies of international price differentials. This section explores the differences in manufacturers' prices for identical drug products sold in the United States and two other markets, Canada and the United Kingdom. It is broken into two sub-sections: the first spells out significant differences in the institutional arrangements in each country while the second presents an empirical analysis of price differentials.

### Institutional Differences in the Pharmaceutical Markets

The regulatory institutions and market organization factors that can influence pharmaceutical prices vary widely among the United States, Canada, and the United Kingdom. The United States is almost alone among Western industrialized countries in its absence of drug pricing regulations (Redwood, 1993). While some managed care organizations are able to negotiate discounts, and state Medicaid programs receive rebates from manufacturers, discounts are not typically available to the wholesalers and other buyers that serve cash paying retail customers.

By contrast, both Canada and the United Kingdom have national policies for restraining prescription drug prices. These policies are, however, quite different in the way that they operate. In Canada, where pharmaceutical products are paid for by a variety of public and private third-party payers, manufacturers' drug pricing is reviewed by a national board whose jurisdiction is limited to drugs that are under patent. (Drugs not under patent are exempt from national price regulation.) This federal price-monitoring body, known as the Patented Medicine Prices Review Board

(PMPRB), establishes guidelines for defining excessive drug prices. The introductory price of a drug is not to exceed the daily dosage price of therapeutically comparable medicines; in some cases, the board takes as its benchmark the median of prices for the new drug in seven industrialized countries. Increases in drug price are to be limited to the three-year cumulative increase in the consumer price index. Unlike a conventional price control body, the PMPRB can neither set prices nor keep products with excessive prices from being sold on the market. Instead, the board relied until recently on the threat of public hearings (a form of "jawboning") and of removal of market exclusivity for some of a firm's patented products.[10]

In contrast to the Canadian system, the United Kingdom's health insurance system, administered by the National Health System (NHS) is virtually a single payer for pharmaceuticals. As a result, its policies influence prices for the whole country. Products sold to the NHS are subject to a national regulatory framework known as the Pharmaceutical Price Regulation Scheme (PPRS). In fact, this scheme controls not the price of each separate product but the profits of the company. Each individual firm is allowed to set the introductory prices on its new drug products at any level, provided the firm's profits do not exceed a rate negotiated with the government.[11] However, price increases on existing products are generally prohibited without prior permission of the government; they are usually restricted to companies that have not reached their profit limit.[12]

Drug prices in Canada are also subject to the market leverage exercised by large third-party payers—specifically, the Canadian provincial governments. Each provincial government, through its participation in Canada's national health insurance system, has its own health benefit plan that buys drugs for some or all of the population.[13] While these governments do not regulate drug prices, each typically issues a drug formulary that lists the amount it will pay for each drug.[14] The potential for the formulary prices to be lower than the prevailing prices stems from the concentrated buying power of the provincial benefit plans. Furthermore, the public availability of information on the prices paid by these provincial plans assists private third-party payers in their negotiations with pharmaceutical manufacturers. Indeed, factory prices for drugs listed in the Ontario formulary, covering Canada's most populous province, tend to set factory prices throughout Canada.

## Empirical Analysis

Drawing on the preceding discussions of institutional factors and factors affecting consumers' price responsiveness for specific drugs, this section develops empirical approaches that yield evidence about the determinants of product-by-product price differentials. After describing the data for each case study, we present results on these market and regulatory determinants. The character and level of detail of our findings differ between the case studies. For the U.S.-Canadian comparison, we estimated a regression model that relates price differentials to a set of explanatory factors. The multivariate approach permits (but does not guarantee) the estimation of each determinant's effect, free of the influences of other determinants. For the U.S.-U.K. comparison, a similar multivariate analysis was not possible (or more accurately, would not have been meaningful). Whereas regulatory variables could be constructed for the Canadian data—because Canadian regulation applies to some products but not others—U.K. regulatory variables could not be constructed because U.K. regulations apply to all prescription drugs uniformly. With the multivariate approach ruled out, we present the results of bivariate analyses of the U.S.-U.K. data. Because these analyses cannot control for confounding influences, the U.S.-U.K. results are only suggestive and qualitative, though broadly consistent with our findings from the U.S.-Canadian multivariate analysis.

## Datasets for the Analysis

The empirical analysis exploits two datasets compiled by the U.S. General Accounting Office (GAO, 1992; 1994). They contain information on drug prices, the types of regulations applied to drug prices, the degree of organization among buyers, and characteristics of each drug that might affect the demand for it in any given market. The U.S.-U.K. dataset also includes for each product the quantity sold in the United States. These country-by-country and product-by-product differences permit an analysis of drug price differentials in the two cases we examine. This empirical analysis assumes similar marginal costs of supplying drugs across the countries. Moreover, these drug-specific data do not enable us to identify the separate effects of factors that might vary by country but not by drug.

   In these datasets, the price measure is the factory price charged by a drug manufacturer for sales to buyers serving the cash-paying retail market. The price of each specific drug product pertains to a single, commonly used U.S. dosage form and dosage strength.[15] For each case study, the sample was drawn from *American Druggist*'s annual list of the 200 most frequently dispensed drugs in the United States,[16] and includes only those drugs that could be matched by identical dosage form, dosage strength, and drug manufacturer (or licensee). In making accurate product-by-product price comparisons, these criteria for matching are important: they eliminate price differences due to disparities between the two countries in the drug itself.[17] The dataset on U.S. and Canadian drug prices, which represent the prices charged on May 1, 1991, has 121 observations. The U.S.-U.K. dataset, which has prices charged on May 1, 1992, has 77 observations.[18] Because the datasets measure prices at different times, the U.S.-Canadian comparison is based on *American Druggist*'s 1991 list, and the U.S.-U.K. comparison is based on the 1992 version of the same list.[19]

## Analysis of Differences in U.S.-Canadian Drug Prices

Factory prices of most drugs in the sample are, on average, higher in the United States than in Canada; however, individual price differentials display significant dispersion. U.S. factory prices of the 121 drugs in that dataset ranged from being 44% lower to 967% higher than the corresponding Canadian prices. The variation in price differentials between the United States and Canada is shown in Fig. 8-1. Lack of data on quantities sold prevents the calculation of the appropriate, quantity-weighted average price differential; nonetheless, the figure makes apparent that factory prices

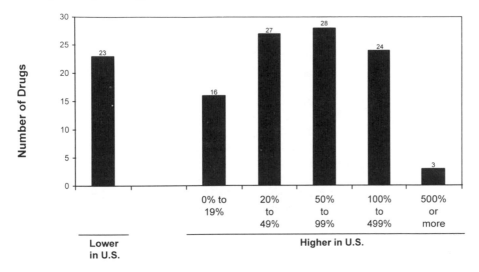

**Figure 8-1.** The range of U.S.–Canadian drug price differentials.

were generally higher in the United States than in Canada.[20] In fact, almost half of the 121 drugs cost 50% more in the United States than in Canada, and almost a quarter were more than twice as costly in the United States.

Table 8-1 describes in detail each independent variable used to analyze U.S.-Canadian drug price differences and also presents the average value of the variable. The dependent variable, LFRAC, is the log of the U.S. price relative to the Canadian price. Four independent variables measure the effect of government intervention on price differentials. Three variables capture distinct effects of the federal PMPRB while the remaining variable measures the effect of the provincial Ontario Drug Benefit (ODB).[21]

Several variables represent factors affecting the relative elasticity of demand for a drug in the United States and Canada. First, three dummy variables reflect the availability of generic substitutes, with those drugs with generic products in neither country constituting the reference group:

- GENERIC-US indicates that a brand name drug has generic substitutes available only in the United States. If brand name drug manufacturers react to generic competition by, for example, raising their U.S. prices, thereby widening the U.S.-Canadian drug price differential, then the coefficient on GENERIC-US should be positive.
- Similarly, GENERIC-CAN indicates generic substitutes are available only in Canada. If drug manufacturers react to this generic competition by raising Canadian prices, then this would result in lower relative prices in the U.S., and the coefficient on GENERIC-CAN would be negative. Alternatively, the coefficient would be positive if manufacturers reacted by lowering Canadian prices of brand-name drugs.
- GENERIC-BOTH indicates generic substitutes are present in both countries. A positive coefficient would imply that manufacturers facing generic competition can

TABLE 8-1. Definitions of Variables Used in Multiple Regression Model

| Variable | Definition | Mean[a] |
|---|---|---|
| LFRAC | Natural logarithm of the ratio between the price per package (in U.S. dollars) of a prescription drug in the United States and Canada | 0.406[b] |
| PRE-C22[c] | Dummy variable: 1 for patented drugs subject to PMPRB review of price increases but not introductory prices (i.e., drugs introduced before 1988), 0 otherwise | 0.331 |
| D88/89[c] | Dummy variable: 1 for patented drugs subject to PMPRB review of price increases and retroactive review of introductory price (i.e., drugs introduced during 1988 or 1989), 0 otherwise | 0.066 |
| POST89[c] | Dummy variable: 1 for patented drugs subject only to PMPRB review of introductory prices (i.e., introduced after 1989), 0 otherwise | 0.058 |
| ODBDATE | Interaction term between time that drug is on the Canadian market (truncated at 15 years) and a dummy variable that is equal to 1 if the drug is on the Ontario Drug Benefit formulary and 0 otherwise | 9.52 |
| GENERIC-US | Dummy variable: 1 if generic substitutes for the drug are available in the United States, 0 otherwise | 0.479 |
| GENERIC-CAN | Dummy variable: 1 if generic substitutes for the drug are available in Canada, 0 otherwise | 0.562 |
| GENERIC-BOTH | Dummy variable: 1 if generic substitutes for the drug are available in both countries, 0 otherwise | 0.372 |
| ANTI-INFLAM | Dummy variable: 1 for anti-inflammatory drugs, 0 otherwise | 0.174 |
| CARDIO | Dummy variable: 1 for cardiovascular drugs, 0 otherwise | 0.190 |
| NERVSYS | Dummy variable: 1 for central nervous system drugs, 0 otherwise | 0.207 |
| HORMONES | Dummy variable: 1 for hormones or synthetic substitutes, 0 otherwise | 0.107 |
| SKIN | Dummy variable: 1 for skin and mucous membrane agents, 0 otherwise | 0.066 |
| GASTRO | Dummy variable: 1 for gastrointestinal medicines, 0 otherwise | 0.049 |
| ENT | Dummy variable: 1 for ear, nose, and throat medicines, 0 otherwise | 0.049 |
| RANK | Drug's rank among 200 most frequently dispensed drugs in the United States | 90.16 |

[a]With the exception of LFRAC, ODBDATE, and RANK, all mean values denote the percentage of total observations in each category. For instance, 33.3% of the observations are PRE-C22 drugs.

[b]The standard deviation for LFRAC is 0.52, for ODBDATE is 5.60, and for RANK is 59.78.

[c]The excluded group is unpatented drugs that are not subject to PMPRB regulations.

raise prices on brand name drugs relatively more in the United States than they can in Canada.[22]

Quantifying the effects of other plausible determinants of the relative elasticity of demand for individual drugs between countries is particularly difficult. Many of these factors, such as differences in medical practices and in availability of alternative drug and nondrug therapies, are difficult to measure with available data. Proxies can, to some extent, capture the effects of several of these factors. In particular, a drug's therapeutic category may represent characteristics unique to certain classes of drugs, such as the number and nature of nongeneric therapeutic substitutes available. For example, compared to anti-inflammatory drugs, central nervous system drugs tend to be less substitutable for each other, decreasing price sensitivity. The model includes seven dummy variables intended to capture drug characteristics associated with therapeutic categories—ANTI-INFLAM, CARDIO, HORMONES, NERVSYS, SKIN, GASTRO, and ENT. Drugs not in one of these therapeutic categories constitute the reference set.

One other variable, RANK, measures each drug's ranking in *American Druggist's* 200 most widely dispensed drugs. It is a proxy for volume, testing whether there is a relationship between the drug's sales volume in the U.S. and the magnitude of the price differential.

The regression results are presented in Table 8-2. Coefficients on six of the

TABLE 8-2. Estimate of the U.S.–Canadian Regression Equation Dependent Variable: LFRAC

| Variable | Coefficient | t-statistic |
|---|---|---|
| Intercept | −0.386[b] | −2.17 |
| PRE-C22 | 0.244[a] | 2.43 |
| D88/89 | 0.336[a] | 1.73 |
| POST89 | 0.484[a] | 2.24 |
| ODBDATE | 0.039[a] | 4.06 |
| GENERIC-US | 0.247 | 1.61 |
| GENERIC-CAN | 0.067 | 0.51 |
| GENERIC-BOTH | −0.017 | −0.09 |
| ANTI-INFLAM | −0.006 | −0.04 |
| CARDIO | 0.078 | 0.54 |
| NERVSYS | 0.376[b] | 2.67 |
| HORMONES | 0.410[b] | 2.49 |
| SKIN | 0.180 | 0.90 |
| GASTRO | 0.391 | 1.82 |
| ENT | 0.051 | 0.24 |
| RANK | −0.0003 | −0.45 |

[a]Significant at the .05 level (one-tailed test).

[b]Significant at the .05 level (two-tailed test).

R-squared = 0.3664; Adjusted R-squared = 0.2750; Observations = 120; F-Statistic = 4.010.

explanatory variables have the predicted sign and are statistically significant at the .05 level. The coefficients on the four regulatory variables are individually and jointly significant at the .05 level. These results are consistent with the following hypotheses:

- The federal PMPRB price regulations were effective at restraining Canadian drug prices. All three PMPRB coefficients had the predicted positive sign and were significant.
- The market power exercised by the provincial ODB reduced the prices paid by Canadian private purchasers, relative to what they would have been in the absence of the ODB.
- Price differentials vary with factors associated with particular therapeutic categories. Differentials are higher, relative to drugs in the excluded therapeutic categories, for central nervous system drugs (NERVSYS) and hormones and synthetic substitutes (HORMONES). The estimated effects of the other included therapeutic categories are not statistically significant at the .05 level.

The regression provides weak statistical evidence, at best, for the hypothesis that drugs with generic substitutes have larger price differentials. The coefficient on GENERIC-US has the expected positive sign but a marginal significance level (two-tailed test) of roughly 0.11.

A richer regression model could be developed if better data were available. In particular, future research should explore whether there might be differences in supply costs across countries and products.[23]

## *Sources of Differences in U.S.-U.K. Drug Prices*

Analysis of the U.S.-U.K. price differentials shows they have an even wider dispersion than do the U.S.-Canadian differentials. For the 77 drugs in the U.S.-U.K. dataset, U.S. factory prices ranged from being 62% lower to 1,712% higher than the corresponding prices in the United Kingdom. Eleven drugs (14%) were priced lower in the United States than in the United Kingdom, while over 60% were priced more than twice as high in the United States than in the United Kingdom. The quantity-weighted average price in the United States was 60% higher than in the United Kingdom.[24] Figure 8-2 shows the dispersion of drug price differentials.

As mentioned earlier, the lack of variation in types of drug regulation among products prevented a multivariate analysis of the causes of drug price differentials. However, bivariate analyses are consistent with the qualitative conclusions that follow from the multivariate analysis of the U.S-Canada data: that both pricing regulation and market factors affect the size of the price differential for particular drugs.

Figure 8-3 shows that the price differentials for the drugs in our data set are, on average, greater for older drugs than for newer products. A volume-weighted market basket of the 39 drugs introduced in the United Kingdom before 1980 would cost (at factory prices) 121% more in the United States than in the United Kingdom. In contrast, the market basket of 22 drugs introduced between 1980 and 1985 would cost 59% more in the United States; the market basket of the 16 drugs introduced after 1985 would cost only 17% more in the United States. This is consistent with

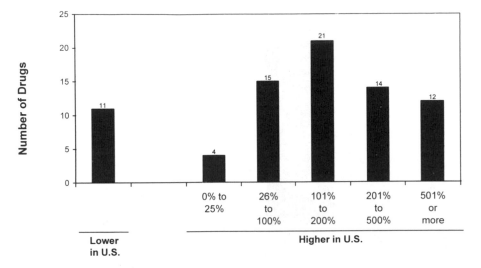

**Figure 8-2.** The range of U.S.–U.K. drug price differentials.

the hypothesis that the United Kingdom's price regulations contribute to the price differentials, since restrictions on price increases could lead to wider differentials (lower U.K. prices) for drugs on the market longer. However, this evidence is not conclusive, since it does not take into consideration the introductory pricing strategy of manufacturers.

The data shown in Fig. 8-4 suggest that manufacturers' pricing behavior also reflects differences in the demand for particular products. Figure 8-4 shows that U.S. prices exceed U.K. prices more, on average, for drugs with generic substitutes than for single-source drugs. A market basket of brand name drugs with generic substitutes

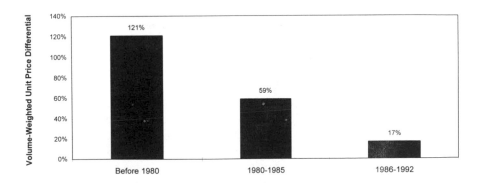

**Figure 8-3.** More recently introduced drugs have smaller U.S.–U.K. price differentials.

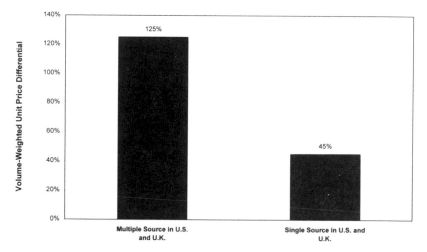

**Figure 8-4.** Drugs with multiple sources in the United States and United Kingdom have larger U.S.–U.K. price differentials.

in both countries would cost 125% more in the United States than in the United Kingdom, while a market basket of drugs that are single source in both countries would cost 45% more in the United States. These results support the contention that in the unregulated U.S. market, manufacturers can raise prices on brand-name products even when generic substitutes are available. Because the U.S.-U.K. dataset is smaller than the U.S.-Canadian dataset, there are too few observations to warrant examining how the price differentials vary among drugs in different therapeutic categories.

## Conclusions and Observations

This essay explores the reasons that manufacturers' prices of prescription drugs differ from country to country from the standpoints of theory and evidence. Economic theory suggests that drug price differentials occur because individual manufacturers possess market power for their products and because arbitrage is either impossible or unprofitable. The size of price differentials, both on average and for individual products, is expected to depend on differences in market factors and government intervention in the marketplace. Empirical analyses of drug price differences between the United States and two other countries, Canada and the United Kingdom, indicate that price differentials are due, in part, to the drug price regulations present in Canada and the United Kingdom, but absent in the United States. However, differences in market demand and organization among buyers also affect prices and, hence, price differentials. These market-induced price differences could persist even if regulatory intervention were absent in all countries.

We end on a cautionary note about drawing normative and policy implications from, first, our findings about determinants of price differentials, and second, the findings of substantial U.S.-foreign price differentials themselves.

## Policy Options for Reducing Drug Prices

When a government determines that existing drug prices are not in the short-term or long-term interest of its citizens, what alternative policies can it consider? Debate in the United States has centered on variants of drug price regulation, such as Canadian-style price review. Our analysis shows that drug price regulations can be effective tools for restraining pharmaceutical prices. But our analysis also points to other policy instruments that are discussed less frequently. By developing evidence that differences in the elasticity of demand across countries contribute to differences in drug prices, this research suggests that drug prices can be reduced through the use of tools that make buyers and prescribing physicians more price sensitive. In particular, encouraging greater organization among buyers may give these buyers the leverage to use market forces, such as competition between alternative innovative products, or between innovative and generic products, to obtain lower prices for the drugs that they purchase. Encouraging price sensitivity among both buyers and providers, and providing them with information about competing products, may increase the elasticity of demand for products they buy or prescribe, thereby eventually leading to price reductions.

## Normative Evaluation of International Price Differentials

Some policy makers and consumers may disapprove of international price differentials because they view such differentials as evidence that pricing practices are unfair, especially to those consumers who pay higher prices. However, international differences in market prices should not be considered surprising or necessarily undesirable. While price differentials often signal the exercise of market power, international price differentials for prescription drugs may be desirable for two reasons:

- First, because high prices in wealthy countries may in effect subsidize consumption in relatively poor countries, more consumers worldwide may have greater access to drugs than if price differentials were narrowed by lowering wealthy countries' prices or, in the extreme, if prices were identical in all countries.
- Second, profit opportunities linked to such differentials encourage drug companies, at least to some extent, to engage in research activities that may provide new drug therapies. In principle, the desirable extent of price differentials can be separated from the desirable level of the average world price of pharmaceuticals. In practice, the two are intertwined. Decisions by large countries, such as the United States, or a group of countries, such as the European Community, about their own average drug prices significantly alter the average global price as well.

These efficiency-based defenses of price differentials notwithstanding, charging different prices to similar consumers for an identical product still may offend policy makers' and public concepts of fair play and horizontal equity. Such conflicts between efficiency and equity cannot be resolved by analysts, but are faced in the policy arena.

## Notes

1. Seniority of authorship is shared equally. The opinions expressed in this essay are those of the authors and are not necessarily the opinions of Barents Group of KPMG or the U.S. General Accounting Office.

2. The focus on research-based companies and identical products requires the exclusion of generic drugs, which typically are produced by different, unaffiliated companies.

3. Price discrimination is a standard, nonpejorative term that refers to the practice of charging different prices to different consumers of the same product, when those differences are not attributable to differences in manufacturers' costs.

4. In the European Community, it is legal for a distributor to buy in a relatively inexpensive country (e.g., Greece), and resell in a relatively more expensive country (e.g., the United Kingdom). Although this practice, known as parallel importing, does occur, transport costs and differences in language on labels have limited the practicality or cost effectiveness of this practice to some extent. However, reimbursement systems in some countries (e.g., the United Kingdom, Germany, and The Netherlands) encourage the practice of parallel importing.

5. During recent years in the United States, there has been an increasing trend for HMOs and large purchasing cooperatives to concentrate their buying power and negotiate lower prices with drug makers. The U.S. Medicaid program, which pays for health benefits for low-income individuals, has also enacted policies to reduce prices it pays for prescription drugs. These factors have lowered the price of drugs to some American consumers and has increased the dispersion of prices within the United States.

6. Even without the enactment of price regulation, the anticipation of such regulation can affect manufacturers' pricing decisions. In a political climate that the manufacturer with market power views as dangerous, it may choose a price below the monopoly price to reduce the likelihood of price controls being implemented. The firm's ability to engage in such price restraint may depend on its own financial condition, stockholder pressure for short-term income, and the firm's ability to send and receive signals to others in the industry about its pricing strategy, without drawing the attention of antitrust authorities. (This channel for policy is interesting for other applications, such as explaining U.S. drug prices in 1991–94, though not for the empirical analysis presented below.)

7. Price regulations can also include price freezes or price reductions. Such approaches have been used in recent years in France, Germany, and the United Kingdom (Gross et al., 1994).

8. For more details, see Griliches and Cockburn (1993).

9. For a discussion of issues relating to therapeutic substitution, see Shulman and Gouveia (1993).

10. For more details on the PMPRB and the sanctions available to it, see GAO (1993); Schulman (1994).

11. This profit rate is generally 17 to 21% of the capital invested in the United Kingdom for the purpose of sales to the National Health Service. The particular rate is negotiated between the NHS and each firm.

12. See GAO (1994) for a more detailed description of drug price regulations in the United Kingdom.

13. Most provincial drug programs provide benefits for the elderly, the disabled, and poor persons. Only three provinces provide universal drug coverage.

14. See GAO (1992) for a more detailed description of these federal and provincial policies.

15. Of the three countries examined, the United States is the only one where a significant share of the market can obtain factory prices less than those charged to buyers serving the cash-paying retail market. Some U.S. third-party payers, such as some managed care organizations, are able to negotiate discounts with drug manufacturers. GAO found, however, that inclusion of the prices paid by this segment of the market did not change the conclusion that manufacturers' U.S. prices for brand-name drugs substantially exceed equivalent U.K. prices. See GAO (1994). Data on discounted U.S. prices were not publicly available for the U.S.-Canadian comparison.

16. These top 200 drugs represent more than 50% of all prescriptions dispensed in U.S. drugstores during 1991 and 1992.

17. Some analysts favor weaker rules for matching drugs, which permit comparing the average price in two countries of a given chemical entity, whether sold as a brand name or generic. For more details, see Danzon (1993).

18. In some cases, drugs could not be matched across countries for one or more of the following reasons: (1) the manufacturer did not sell the drug in the same dosage strength or dosage form in both countries; (2) the drug was sold by prescription in one country and over-the-counter in the other; (3) the drug sold in the United States was a generic product that was manufactured by a company that had no affiliate marketing it in the other country; and (4) the manufacturer selling the drug in the United States did not sell the drug in the other country. See GAO (1992), p. 10; GAO (1994), p. 18.

19. U.S. factory prices are taken from the Wholesale Acquisition Cost (WAC) listed in the Medi-Span Master Drug Data Base-Select. For the cash-paying outpatient market, the WAC measures the average transaction price that prevails when manufacturers sell to wholesalers. Canadian factory prices were obtained from either the Best Available Price (BAP) listed in the February 1991 Ontario Drug Benefit (ODB) Formulary or, for those drugs not listed on the ODB Formulary, directly from the manufacturers of the drugs or from a major Canadian wholesaler. U.K. drug prices are listed monthly in the *Chemist & Druggist Monthly Price List*. Because this listing contains wholesale prices rather than manufacturers' prices, factory prices are calculated by subtracting the standard 12.5% discount, which the drug manufacturers provide the U.K. wholesalers.

20. An ideal measure of the average price differential would weight each individual drug's price by its sales volume. While this is impossible with publicly available data, other measures of each drug's importance in the market can give some perspective on the average price differential. The U.S.-Canadian price differential for a market basket containing one prescription for each drug in the dataset would be 32% — the market basket would cost 32% more in the United States than in Canada. Alternatively, weighting each of these common prescriptions by the drug's rank in the *American Druggist's* list of the 200 most widely dispensed drugs yields an average U.S.-Canadian price differential of 29%.

21. Because these policies are expected to restrain prices in Canada relative to prices in the United States, the coefficient on these variables is expected to be positive. Therefore, evaluating their statistical significance calls for a one-tail test.

We specified the Ontario formulary variable as ODBDATE, which captures the age of drugs that are included on Ontario's formulary, because we believe the effect of the formulary is cumulative, increasing over time. In an alternative specification, where the effect of the Ontario formulary and age were measured separately, the formulary variable measure had an effect similar to that of ODBDATE and the time variable was not significant. In this specification, the regulatory variables were not jointly statistically significant at the .05 level, although two of them were individually significant.

22. Berndt (1993) discusses issues relating to specification of the generic variables. We adopt his specification of GENERIC-BOTH.

23. For example, Manning (1993) reported differences in product liability risk to be an important determinant of price differentials.

24. In contrast to the U.S.-Canadian comparison, sales volume data for each drug were available for computing weighted average price indexes for the U.S.-U.K. comparison. GAO (1994) presents additional analyses of the effects of manufacturers' discounts and generic drugs on other measures of average price differentials.

## References

*American Druggist* (1991) "The Top 200 Rx Drugs of 1990," February, pp. 56–68.

*American Druggist* (1992) "The Top 200", February, pp. 48–56.

Benn Publications Ltd. (1992) *Chemist & Druggist Monthly Price List*, Vol. 33, No. 5.

Berndt E (1993) MicroTSP Replication of GAO Study on US-Canadian Drug Prices. Sloan School of Management, unpublished manuscript.

Comanor W (1986) The political economy of the pharmaceutical industry. *Journal of Economic Literature* XXIV: 1178–1242.

Danzon PM (1993) International Drug Price Comparisons: Uses and Abuses. Prepared for the American Enterprise Institute Conference on Competitive Strategies in the Pharmaceutical Industry, Washington, DC.

GAO (U.S. General Accounting Office) (1992) *Prescription Drugs: Companies Typically Charge More in the United States Than in Canada.* GAO/HRD-92-110. Washington, DC: GAO.

——— (1993) *Prescription Drug Prices: Analysis of Canada's Patented Medicine Prices Review Board.* GAO/HRD-93-51. Washington, DC: GAO.

——— (1994) *Prescription Drugs: Companies Typically Charge More in the United States Than in the United Kingdom.* GAO/HEHS-94-29. Washington, DC: GAO.

Griliches Z and Cockburn I (1993) Generics and new goods in pharmaceutical price indexes. *American Economic Review* 84: 1213–32.

Gross D, Ratner J, Perez J, and Glavin S (1994) Prescription drug price regulations in France, Germany, Sweden, and the United Kingdom. *Health Care Financing Review* 15: 127–40.

Manning RL (1993) Products Liability and Prescription Drug Prices in Canada and the United States. Brigham Young University, unpublished manuscript.

Redwood H (1993) New drugs in the world market: incentives and impediments to innovation. *The American Enterprise* 4: 72–80.

Redwood H (1994) *New Horizons in India: The Consequences of Pharmaceutical Patent Protection.* Suffolk, England: Oldwicks Press.

Schulman SR (1994) The Canadian Patented Medicine Prices Review Board: new rules and new status. *Pharmacoeconomics* 6: 71–79.

Schulman SR and Gouveia W (1993) Therapeutic substitution as an option for cost-effective prescribing. *Pharmacoeconomics* 3: 257–59.

U.S. Senate, Special Committee on Aging (1989) *Prescription Drug Prices: Are We Getting Our Money's Worth?* Washington, DC: U.S. Government Printing Office.

# 9

# The Professional
# and Corporate Context:
# Trends in the United States

J. WARREN SALMON

Pharmacological treatment remains at the heart of medicine; drugs are prescribed in most medical encounters. Pharmacists are usually the dispensers of prescribed drugs, the bulk of which are manufactured by multinational corporations based in six advanced industrial nations. This situation places the profession of pharmacy in a position to mediate the conflicting interests of patients, prescribers, and pharmaceutical manufacturers. In addition, pharmacists are subject to rules and regulations frequently issued by public or private insurance programs and public or professional regulators.

At this juncture in the history of pharmacy in the United States, it is instructive to examine forces influencing some 190,000 practicing pharmacists who find themselves undergoing myriad changes. Inside the profession, its leadership is attempting to professionalize. These efforts run parallel to those of nursing and other allied health professions, which seek to upgrade credentialing and expand their respective realms of responsibilities. Pharmacists have been advocating a role broader than the dispensing function in clinical relationships with patients, beyond the drug sales transaction, to promote more rational drug therapy (Rucker, 1987; Kusserow, 1990) and to ensure optimal patient outcomes (Hepler, 1985).

In addition, the increasingly corporate character of the practice of medicine over the past 25 years imposes a new set of dynamics on patient care activities (Salmon, 1994). Proprietary hospital and nursing home systems and managed care organizations (e.g., health maintenance organizations, preferred provider organizations, hospital physician organizations) now dominate the overall delivery system; the so-called not-for-profit providers mimic their for-profit brethren, offering virtually indistinguishable organizational behaviors in the competitive health marketplace (Salmon, 1990a). This change in ownership, purpose, and control of health care has drastically altered professional relationships.

Meanwhile, pharmacy has undergone a simultaneous corporatization itself with professionals as employees of consolidating national firms. The "community pharmacy"—quite a misnomer today—has yielded to regional and nationwide chain drug stores, where actual pharmacy operations are but a small part of their mass merchandising (National Association of Chain Drug Stores, 1993). Likewise, national mail order pharmacy and pharmacy benefits management (PBM) firms, now consolidating under the control of selected pharmaceutical manufacturers, are eclipsing their corporate chain predecessors.

With the professions of medicine and pharmacy subject to this ongoing corporate transformation, the realities of clinical practice, including both pharmaceutical prescribing and dispensing, exhibit a vastly different context. Skewed more toward overall corporate objectives than toward health promotion and health restoration in the entire population, the priorities of delivery organizations and the looming power of consolidating pharmaceutical manufacturers together deserve critical review.

This chapter examines recent developments in the pharmacy profession related to ongoing changes in the U.S. health care system. It is intended to be instructive about dynamics in other national systems facing corporatization trends and privatization policies, or at least useful for delineating political, economic, social, and ethical implications to heed elsewhere. The corporatization of medicine and pharmacy in the U.S. is summarized, and the main related directions of the pharmaceutical industry are described.

## The Corporatization of Medicine

Dramatic alterations in medical practice emanate from within the health care marketplace. These changes had been antecedent to, and were racing forward in anticipation of, national health reform by the Clinton administration and the U.S. Congress. With the defeat of health reform, these trends are set to intensify.

### From Old to New Medical Industrial Complex

Beginning in 1965 with the massive infusion of federal subsidies under Medicare and Medicaid, the provision of health care in the United States has become an extremely profitable endeavor (Turshen, 1976). The growth in health care (now 14% of the Gross National Product) fashioned a medical-industrial complex, including commercial insurance companies and a host of corporate manufacturers that supplied products and services to a then generally public and not-for-profit delivery system (Salmon, 1990a).

While delivery of care in the United States remained chiefly within not-for-profit and public institutions into the 1970s, corporate suppliers collectively gained enormous economic power (McKinlay, 1984). Physicians stayed in individual and small group practices, retaining traditional relationships with their patients, as well as community and teaching hospitals. Most observers of the health care scene seemed unalarmed by the size of this *old* medical industrial complex in the finance and supply functions, generally assuming these entities to be essential to modern health care.

However, as for-profit forces began to deliver medical services, an alarm over the *new* medical industrial complex rang out (Relman, 1980). Proprietary entry into the hospital, nursing home, psychiatric, home care, and other business lines in health care saw a rapid advance in most local markets. Their prolific spread nationwide was fostered by federal policies under the Reagan and Bush administrations, admidst profit opportunities in competition with traditional providers (Light, 1986).

The subsequent rise of regional and later national for-profit hospital chains became an epiphenomenon to Nixon's health maintenance organization (HMO) strategy, which had encouraged private investment to restructure the health care system (Salmon, 1984). As the market ethic replaced professional altruism and charitable institutional mission, health care delivery has taken on a new and different character (Relman, 1992).

## Employer Purchaser Pressures

Employers have not been satisfied with the value of the costly medical benefits they purchase for their employees (Donkin, 1989). Along with federal and state governments and private insurers, employers are demanding more accountability for their climbing outlays, which means more information on costs, usage, and quality of the services they buy. Cost containment for retiree health benefits has led to contracting with mail order pharmacy firms and, as prescription costs for them climbed, even greater employer purchaser pressures to hold down drug costs.

Managed care has recently become dominant, strongly supported by corporate and governmental purchasers. Essentially, this mode of delivery is a prepaid benefits package for a set annual premium, which necessitates provider controls on services rendered for greater cost effectiveness. Managed care organizations in the United States have grown rapidly as purchasers and payers of care have sought to eliminate unnecessary tests and operations. They have mounted substantial efforts to persuade physicians to prescribe cheaper and more cost-effective drugs and to lessen the use of ancillary, diagnostic, and surgical procedures. Moreover, technological introductions are being highly scrutinized before being adopted and dispersed throughout the health care system.

The managed care arena is controlled extensively by for-profit forces, be they national provider systems or the six largest commercial insurers (see Tables 9-1 and 9-2). Metropolitan areas all across America have been targeted selectively by these corporate powers, while smaller regional provider systems rapidly amalgamate into networks (Salmon, 1995). The economics of managed care necessitate utilization management through primary care "gatekeeping" and eliminating inappropriate later-stage interventions. As such, the emphasis on cost containment has led to integration into ever-enlarging organizational entities. Managers have sought to arrange for, or take over, a continuum of providers. Large corporate provider networks require the

TABLE 9-1.  Top Corporate Health Provider Systems, 1993[a]

| Company | Sales in Billions $ | Profits, in Billion $ | Margin, in Percent | Business Line |
|---|---|---|---|---|
| American Medical | 2.3 | 0.07 | 3.2 | Hospital management |
| Beverly Enterprises | 2.8 | 0.06 | 2.1 | Nursing homes |
| Cardinal Health | 2.3 | 0.04 | 1.7 | Managed care |
| Caremark International | 1.8 | 0.08 | 4.4 | Physican practices/mail order pharmacy |
| Columbia Health Care | 10.3 | 0.58 | 5.6 | Hospital management |
| FHP International | 2.3 | 0.05 | 2.3 | Managed care |
| Foundation Health | 1.8 | 0.08 | 4.5 | Managed care |
| Health Trust | 2.4 | 0.14 | 5.8 | Hospital management |
| Humana | 3.1 | 0.09 | 2.8 | Managed care |
| Manor Care | 1.0 | 0.07 | 6.4 | Nursing homes |
| Medical Care America | 0.4 | 0.01 | 1.4 | Home care |
| National Medical Enterprises | 3.4 | 0.17 | 5.0 | Hospital management |
| Oxford Health Plans | 0.3 | 0.01 | 4.8 | Managed care |
| PacifiCare Health Systems | 2.4 | 0.07 | 2.8 | Managed care |
| Physician Corp. of America | 0.5 | 0.04 | 7.3 | Physician practices |
| United Health Care | 2.5 | 0.19 | 7.7 | Managed care |
| U.S. Health Care | 2.6 | 0.30 | 11.3 | Managed care |

Source: Business Week, March 28, 1994, pp. 64–144.

[a]Not including subsidiaries of conglomerates or non-publicly held corporations.

development and implementation of clinical performance standards, now accomplished through advanced information systems capabilities (Feinglass and Salmon, 1994).

While no other nation in the world saw such a phenomenal rise in health expenditures as the United States, nowhere else is there such a for-profit presence in any delivery system, nor an enjoyment of such magnanimous returns in health care (Roemer, 1988). This corporate takeover has bountiful implications for professionalism in medicine, pharmacy, and the other health professions (Haug, 1976; Light and Levine, 1994; Salmon, White, and Feinglass, 1994). Clearly, the United States is

TABLE 9-2.  Top Six Health Insurance Firms, 1993

CIGNA
Prudential Insurance Co.
Aetna Life Insurance Co.
Travelers Companies[a]
MetLife Insurance Co.[a]
Blue Cross-Blue Shield[b]

[a]Recently announced combination for managed care concentration.

[b]Federation of approximately forty state and regional plans.

witnessing the twilight of the physician known since the Flexner reforms in medical education. Conditions of medical practice are undeniably changing, with historic roles being redirected by corporate managers, not practitioners.

## The Corporatization of Pharmacy

The corporatization of retail pharmacy was initially represented in the rise to dominance of the national chain drug store. These entities overtook independent pharmacies in the late 1970s. The proliferation of mail order pharmacy, engulfing pharmacy use under managed care organization ownership, and other forms where pharmacy services are subsumed under pharmaceutical manufacturer integration, constitutes a nascent but revolutionary development in the 1990s (Miller, 1992; Weber, 1994). While the professional practices of medicine and pharmacy will be profoundly affected by these specific marketplace dynamics, the bulk of each profession remains generally unaware of their potential outcomes, nor equipped to successfully resist them.

### Prescribing Process Under Managed Care

The process of obtaining medical care including drug therapy involves a tedium of events following the patient's perception of illness. Much has been said about the concentration of clinical decision making in the hands of the physician (Kronus, 1976), but conditions of managed care are altering this power (Winslow, 1992). Subject to restrictions of manager superiors (or insurance payers), physicians are no longer secure in their autonomy, either concerning working conditions or, increasingly, therapeutic decisions (Salmon, White, and Feinglass, 1994).

Monitoring physician prescribing behavior has not yet become as extensive, or intrusive, as restraints on performing costly diagnostic or surgical procedures to address variations in medical practice (Eddy, 1984; Wennberg, 1986; Eisenberg, 1987). However, the use of restrictive formularies within hospitals and health maintenance organizations, institution of prospective drug use review, and the profiling of physician prescribing patterns all may lead to limitations on practitioners' choices over drug therapy. Moreover, computerized health information management (HIM) systems (Feinglass and Salmon, 1994) may guide prescribing for both cost and therapeutic benefits. Where one institution automated its medical records and linked them to computerized drug and test ordering, overall costs declined 13% (Winslow, 1993). Savings from such electronic connectivity has attracted the attention of insurers, employers, and provider managements (Gaudemans, 1994). Other managed care attempts to control prescription drug expenditures, although not widely adopted, include strengthening pharmacy and therapeutic committees, generic and therapeutic interchange by pharmacists, volume purchasing discounts, and demands for demonstration of economic value for drug products. Such conditions fostered the advent of pharmacy benefits management.

## Pharmacy as a Profession

The profession of pharmacy has yet to achieve full professional status and authority (Birenbaum, 1982). Adamcik et al. (1986: 1187) described it as "a profession in transition . . . characterized by considerable ambiguity and uncertainty concerning its status as a health profession." While significant enlargement in scope of practice has occurred for clinical pharmacists in certain tertiary institutions (Hepler, 1987), several observers express the need for unilateral acts of exerted expertise beyond the physician, for example, prescribing authority and greater shared authority for substitution or altering dosages and regimens.

Within the last decade, professional leaders claimed that the pharmacist is often the most accessible health professional in the ambulatory system and, being underused, argued for empowerment to provide pharmaceutical care (Strand, Cipolle, and Morley, 1992). Revealing that 50 to 70% of all prescriptions are improperly taken (Whitney et al., 1993), patient compliance studies point to the neglect in patient counseling in drug therapy (Sherbourne et al., 1992). Needless to say, payment for pharmacy services may be the only way to create incentives for retail pharmacists to counsel patients fully and consistently (Cardinale, 1993).

Pharmacy leaders have been proclaiming a new mission for the profession to assure optimal therapeutic outcomes (Hepler, 1985). Patient counseling is integral to this new desired role. Whether pharmacists want to do it or not, the federal Omnibus Budget Reconciliation Act of 1990 (OBRA-90) mandates counseling (National Association of Boards of Pharmacy, 1993). State Boards of Pharmacy promulgated new pharmacy practice acts to urge pharmacists to become effective in their communication of drug information to patients and/or caregivers. This major change expands ordinary happenings in retail pharmacy, but it has not been without strong opposition from rank and file pharmacists and, more vehemently, from their corporate chain owners.

The increasingly complex conditions of drug therapy have led the pharmacy profession down a road mimicking medicine by establishing specialty practices. The national Board of Pharmaceutical Specialties has four current certifications, with new areas, and now subspecialties, being advocated. These directions remain limited to non-retail practice, where academic and hospital pharmacists have long been the leading force in professional advancement. In the evolving inpatient setting, clinical pharmacists, like advanced practice nurses (Masters prepared), may eventually be granted therapeutic interchange, if not prescribing authority along critical algorithms, and take over tasks that house staff and attending physicians have historically performed. Automated dispensing devices and robotics are at various stages of refinement; their anticipated impact in both the retail and hospital settings (beyond what mail order pharmacy has made possible) portends dramatic future role shifts.

## Obstacles to Professionalization

Francke (1969: 163) maintained that pharmacy will remain a marginal profession because the commercial setting of pharmacy where the majority practice "debases the profession of pharmacy in America." A similar argument regarding professional conflicts can be levied whenever and wherever bottom-line dictates take precedence over patient well being.

Though it continues to be used as a term with nostalgia, "community pharmacy" no longer appropriately characterizes retail dispensing of drugs. The Norman Rockwell painting on the cover of the *Saturday Evening Post* of the neighborhood pharmacist compounding a family's prescriptions, while the kids sip chocolate pop at the soda counter, has not portrayed real life for a long time.

Retail pharmacy in America today is solidly corporate (see Table 9-3). In chain drug stores, the pharmacy is almost always placed in the back of a 50,000-plus square foot building containing multiple rows of products unrelated to health. In fact, the pharmacy is often positioned in a store environment with items detrimental to health (e.g., tobacco and alcohol products); the best connection to health enhancement may be groceries in some retail outlets. Rarely are other professional services offered by mass merchandisers, though they may attempt to diversify with an investment and insurance trade, or vision care services. But like pharmacy, the vision care service is centered mainly around selling the eyeglass product, and inducing other product purchases.

Over time this world of corporate practice has reduced the retail pharmacist to employee status, paid on an hourly basis increasingly under flexible part-time arrangement. Work within the chain drug stores is geared for production under management control (see Table 9-4). Pharmacists are usually the only credentialed persons in the store environment among minimum wage retail clerks. The supervising

TABLE 9-3. Top Corporate Pharmacy Operations, 1993[a,b]

| Company | Sales in Billion $ | Profits, in Billion $ | Margin, in percent |
|---|---|---|---|
| Bergen Brunswig | 5.0 | 0.06 | 1.2 |
| Caremark International | 1.8 | 0.08 | 4.4 |
| Hook-SupeRx | 2.0 | 0.03 | 1.5 |
| Kmart[c] | 34.1 | −0.32 | 0 |
| Longs Drug Stores | 2.5 | 0.05 | 2.0 |
| McKesson | 12.2 | 0.15 | 1.2 |
| Medical Care America | 0.4 | 0.01 | 1.4 |
| Merck-Medco | 10.5 | 2.17 | 20.6 |
| Revco | 2.4 | 0.02 | 0.9 |
| Rite Aid | 4.2 | 0.13 | 3.0 |
| Value Health | 0.6 | 0.008 | 1.4 |
| Walgreen | 8.5 | 0.25 | 2.9 |
| WalMart[c] | 67.3 | 2.30 | 3.5 |

*Source: Business Week*, March 28, 1994, pp. 64–144.

[a]Not including subsidiaries of conglomerates (such as food distribution chains) or non-publicly held corporations.

[b]May include retail chain drug store, home infusion therapy, wholesale pharmacy, or mail order operations.

[c]Includes entire retailing operation beyond pharmacy.

TABLE 9-4.   Differences Between the Working Conditions of Pharmacists in the United States Around 1950 and Today

| Key Prerogatives of an Occupational Group | Pharmacists in Small-Scale, Independently-Owned Stores (1950) | Pharmacists in Corporate Chain Drug Stores (1994) |
|---|---|---|
| 1. Criteria for entrance | Almost exclusively middle- and working-class white ethnic males | Increasingly multi-ethnic and predominately female |
| 2. Content of training | Largely dictated by the professional societies | Outside interests affecting content and scope of curriculum |
| 3. Autonomy over the terms and content of work | Work typically more generalized and controlled by the individual pharmacy owner | Work typically routinized and directed by store manager in accordance with organizational constraints (profit) |
| 4. The object of labor | Patient usually regarded as the pharmacist's neighbors | Patients are customers purchasing other store merchandise and/or tied to managed care organization through Rx payment plan; value added counseling service becoming a possibility |
| 5. The tools of labor | Drug store and equipment typically owned or leased by the pharmacist, and employees are hired by the pharmacist | Potential for automation in dispensing owned by employing store and operated by other corporate employees |
| 6. The means of labor | The physical setting is typically owned or rented and operated by pharmacists themselves | The store is owned and operated in the interest of the organization (profit) |
| 7. Remuneration for labor | The hours worked, the level of use, and the fees charged are pretty much determined by the individual pharmacist | Work schedules and salary levels determined by employing chain drug store |

Source: Adapted from McKinlay and Stoeckle (1990).

store manager may very well not even hold a baccalaureate degree. In fact, other than perhaps MBAs and attorneys in the central office, Pharm.D. pharmacists are the only advanced degree holders within the entire regional or national chain. Most aspects of the work conditions are decided centrally by upper management. It is no wonder then that pharmacists often become frustrated with conditions surrounding performance of their technical, let alone professional, functions in the retail setting.

## Imperatives For Change

Interestingly, this mode of market-driven provision of drug products evolving over the last three decades was not in response to the pharmaceutical care needs of or demands by the American populace. This corporatization of pharmacy chains came in the midst of an ever-increasing complexity of pharmaceutical agent entities, now numbering over 8,000 in the U.S. market. The need for greater knowledge on the part of pharmacists to adequately perform the drug dispensing function leads to rapid obsolescence after their educational experiences. State-mandated continuing education for pharmacy remains less demanding than for medicine and nursing, and hospital pharmacists pursue it more vigorously than those in retail due to institutional requirements and reimbursement for it.

Accompanying clinical imperatives, to which the pharmacy leadership has worked to respond, are policy initiatives, about which practitioners appear less sanguine. The profession was granted inordinate attention through the federal OBRA-90; this legislation's significance lies beyond its mandate for patient counseling by pharmacists with each Medicaid prescription dispensed. It required that state drug utilization review (DUR) programs be set up to monitor physician and pharmacist activities. Again, these public policy directions run parallel to private sector initiatives, all part of what Relman (1988) called the "new era of assessment and accountability."

Managed care organizations require new behaviors and relationships for pharmacy. They have favored chain drug stores or kept pharmacy operations in-house for better management control. Moreover, directions by pharmaceutical manufacturers to take over pharmacy benefits management reveals a horizon of phenomenal integration. As public policy makers, employer purchaser benefits managers, and managed care executives realize that it is more cost effective to provide comprehensive pharmaceutical care, the character of pharmaceutical manufacturers merits consideration.

## The Pharmaceutical Industry

The U.S. pharmaceutical industry has been the world leader in the development of new prescription drug products and therapies. While the introduction of many new products has been extremely costly, pharmaceuticals have helped to extend life expectancy and relieve suffering for many people with multiple disease conditions. Prescription drugs have been widely shown to be better alternatives to more expensive treatments, such as surgery and hospitalizations.

The industry held a competitive edge in world trade across the 1980s (Ballance, 1996). In 1992, nine of the top 15 companies worldwide (sales for each firm at least $3.5 billion) were U.S.-based (see Table 9-5). However, most top firms in terms of R&D expenditures as a percentage of sales are smaller companies below the top 20. In terms of actual R&D expenditures on pharmaceuticals in 1992 among the top seven world firms, Bristol-Myers Squibb was the sole American one (Anonymous, 1994a).

From the late 1960s on, the pharmaceutical industry has proven resistant to the larger U.S. economy's stagnation and intermittent recessions. Return on equity for the pharmaceutical industry averaged above 20% for the late 1980s. However, the current decade has seen dramatic corporate restructurings in response to increasing research and development costs, growing sales of generic drugs, and as mentioned above, increased (and yet-to-come) government regulations. OBRA-90 mandated

TABLE 9-5.  Top U.S. Pharmaceutical Manufacturers, 1993[a,b,c]

| Company | Sales in Billion $ | Profits, in Billion $ | Margin, in Percentage |
|---|---|---|---|
| Abbott Laboratories | 8.4 | 1.39 | 16.6 |
| American Home Products | 8.3 | 1.47 | 17.7 |
| Amgen | 1.3 | 0.37 | 27.3 |
| Baxter International | 8.8 | −0.27 | 0 |
| Bristol-Myers Squibb | 11.4 | 1.96 | 17.2 |
| Eli Lilly | 6.4 | 0.49 | 7.6 |
| Johnson and Johnson | 14.1 | 1.79 | 12.6 |
| Marion Merrell Dow | 2.8 | 0.36 | 12.8 |
| Merck-Medco | 10.5 | 2.17 | 20.6 |
| Pfizer | 7.5 | 0.66 | 8.8 |
| Rhone-Poulenc Rorer | 4.0 | 0.42 | 10.5 |
| Schering-Plough Pharmaceuticals | 4.3 | 0.83 | 19.0 |
| Syntex Pharmaceuticals | 2.1 | 0.40 | 18.6 |
| Upjohn | 3.6 | 0.40 | 11.0 |
| Warner Lambert | 5.8 | 0.29 | 4.9 |

Source: Business Week, March 28, 1994, pp. 64–144.

[a]Not including subsidiaries of conglomerates or non-publicly held corporations.

[b]Includes firm's medical supply, generic, and pharmacy benefit management subsidiaries and related operations.

[c]Foreign owned corporations not included, most conspicuously Glaxo, SmithKline Beecham, Roche, Burroughs-Wellcome, and about six others with an obvious presence in the U.S. market.

price rebates on pharmaceuticals reimbursed under the Medicaid program. Now manufacturers must offer Medicaid the best price with rebates ranging to a maximum of 25%. Beyond Medicaid, other federal purchasing programs have followed suit through similar legislative mandates for rebates. Medicaid rebates by manufacturers under OBRA-90, user fees to FDA for new drug applications, discounts to Veterans Affairs Hospitals, and the Clinton budget of 1993 were estimated to cost the industry $14.46 billion from FY 1993–98 (Price Waterhouse, 1993).

## Policy Influences

The U.S. pharmaceutical industry has been facing more profound change in the 1990s than ever before, even in an industry that has gone through varying stages since the turn of the century (Walker, 1971; Murray, 1974). Clearly, congressional discussions, invigorated Food and Drug Administration actions, and the (failed) Clinton health plan proposal—which would have necessitated controls over future price rises—together introduce a new regulatory era. This anticipates not just greater toughness on the drug approval process, but inclusion of cost effectiveness criteria for new pharmaceutical introductions. In 1985, the FDA recategorized investigational new drugs (INDs) to ease the regulatory review, and in 1988 another change was made in the approval process for drugs that treat life threatening and severely debilitating illnesses, mainly propelled by AIDS activists and other consumer constituencies.

FDA new drug approvals are the most rigorous in the world. The Center for the Study of Drug Development at Tufts University maintained that U.S. pharmaceutical firms take an average of 12 years and $231 million (in 1987 dollars) to bring a new medicine from the laboratory to the pharmacy shelf (DiMasi et al., 1991). While such costs are attributed by the industry to the strict regulatory environment, there are also increasing legal costs growing out of product liability and medical malpractice suits that affect development costs (Shikles, 1992), which incidentally have less relevance to "me too" formulations and generics.

Under Reagan Administration economic and health policies, pharmaceutical manufacturers initiated rapid rises in drug prices, increasing them at twice the rate of other consumer prices. The National Association of Chain Drug Stores (1993) claimed that the average prescription rose from $6.62 in 1980 to more than $25.00 in 1993.

A U.S. Senate committee (Special Committee on Aging, 1992) reported that the highest prescription price inflation occurred in drugs on the market for several years. Research and development costs should have been already recovered, but it was clear that market position enabled manufacturers to reap higher returns, rather than to discount prices to the benefit of consumers and payers.

From the late 1980s, the distribution of U.S. brand-name pharmaceutical sales by class of customer changed dramatically. Whereas in the past, wholesalers were the major buyers, now managed care entities, corporate hospital systems, and other group purchasing organizations (GPOs) contract for the bulk of drugs produced and sold in the country. Retail pharmacies do direct buying at a small percentage of total drugs sales. Manufacturers just cannot price according to past practices.

## Managed Care Influences

With treatment decisions increasingly lodged in the hands of corporate provider systems, pharmaceutical firms have rapidly established divisions to target the growing market segment of managed care. They have carefully designed promotional strategies to keep their products on formularies. Price reductions have been sought, and won, by major HMOs, as well as by hospital alliances and corporate hospital systems, to maintain a firm's line of products visible to prescribers. Larger managed care organizations have also extracted nonprice concessions from both manufacturers and wholesalers by capitating therapeutic classes (that is, providing a standard charge for all diagnosed patients in a particular treatment category). Similar risk sharing initiatives by pharmaceutical manufacturers are with hospital chains and alliances.

Moreover, these ever-enlarging centralized GPOs are becoming clearinghouses for data on costs per member of the GPO, conducting technology assessments, and assisting with development of measures of health outcomes and clinical guidelines. Besides reducing the clout of national and local pharmacy wholesalers, these GPOs pose a severe challenge to pharmaceutical manufacturers who fail to adapt to the rapidly changing market.

Manufacturers refer to the practice of multitier pricing of drugs as discretionary pricing, while aggrieved retail pharmacists call it discriminatory pricing. Manufacturers grant price breaks to different purchasers, often allowing larger provider buyers substantial reductions beyond simple volume discounts. Needless to say, independently-owned pharmacies cannot compete for special discounts, adding another pressure on their economic viability.

In addition, generic drugs now account for 30% of total prescriptions written (Anonymous, 1994b). Direct-to-consumer advertising for patented drugs has likewise greatly increased. Additional promotion and marketing expenses have also driven up manufacturers' costs. During the next five years, it is expected that $8 to $12 billion worth of brand-name drugs are set to come off patent. Cost-cutting efforts by providers, as well as the federal and state governments, will likely further crimp profit levels in the pharmaceutical industry.

In the wake of Clinton's proposals for national health reform, pharmaceutical manufacturers made drastic cuts in their workforces and underwent huge corporate restructurings. Most firms announced cuts between 1,500 and 4,000 employees (mostly in sales and marketing), with a few firms scrambling to shore up their business in the face of discounting to large buyers, government pressure on prices (both here and abroad), and anticipation of new policy strictures. Most firms streamlined their manufacturing, distribution, and administrative infrastructures. Among the forms of consolidation occurring in the industry are mergers and acquisitions, joint ventures, strategic alliances, licensing agreements, and cooperative marketing arrangements. Firms are also forming alliances to bundle products to sell to large provider systems. A variety of combinations will be vigorously pursued, while downsizing and refocusing continues.

## Pharmacy Benefits Management

Just as independent pharmacies were overtaken by national chain drug stores, the entity of community pharmacy is being eclipsed by pharmacy benefits management firms, originating for the most part as mail order pharmacy, and then utilization management. The not-for-profit mail order firms were quickly overtaken by for-profit entities by the turn of this decade. The most notable mail order firms, Medco and Caremark (together 60 to 70% of the present market) grew rapidly to billion-dollar operations in the early 1990s, built upon dispensing automation and business client contracts to lower employer prescription drug outlays. Annual mail order prescriptions grew to over $5 billion in 1993, with several chain drug stores (Walgreens, Eckard, Long's, Thrift, Revco, WalMart, and American Stores) and subsidiaries of HMOs now partaking in this business line. Mail order pharmacy accounts for 7.2% of total prescription sales (Laskoski, 1993).

Pharmacy benefits management firms arose in a parallel development as claims processors before enlarging their services to integrated managed care information systems for provider clients. Consequently, pharmacy services integration has come a long way quite rapidly. Pharmacy benefits management also comes directly from within individual HMOs and Preferred Provider Organizations (PPOs). The National Association of Chain Drug Stores formed Pharmacy Direct Network from 24 drug store chains (inviting participation from independent pharmacies too) to compete primarily with the PBMs of the manufacturers (Tanouye, 1994; Laskoski, 1994). Rhone-Poulenc Rorer, Pfizer and Bristol-Myers Squibb have established special ties to Caremark, and Glaxo was reported to be working to secure a special relationship with PCS, only to be scooped by the Eli Lilly $4 billion purchase in July 1994 (Burton and Tanouye, 1994; Hill, 1994).

The Merck-Medco merger of 1993 to provide for coordinated pharmaceutical care has shaken up both the industry and pharmacy profession. This merger represented an integration in the cycle from discovering compounds and developing drugs; to diagnosing, prescribing, and dispensing medicines and educating patients; through managing usage in its Coordinated Care Network by measuring outcomes and initiating pharmacoeconomic research on expenditure trends. While most larger U.S. pharmaceutical firms have over-the-counter divisions and subsidiaries for (or financial interests in) generic firms, this new Merck-Medco entity brings together both brand and generic manufacturing, research and development, group purchasing arrangements, mail order pharmacy, pharmacy benefits management, and a network of ties to 46,000 pharmacies, some independent, as well as chain stores.

## Future Implications

In a lead-off article entitled "Momentous week for industry" chronicling the Roche takeover of Syntex, Kodak selling Sterling, SmithKline Beecham's acquisition of Diversified Pharmaceutical Services, and Pfizer's diversification with Value Health, *Scrip World Pharmaceutical News* (Anonymous, 1994c: 1) predicted the pharmaceutical sector "by the end of the decade [would consist] of a handful of 'health conglomerates,' plus a plethora of niche companies and 'research boutiques'."

Clearly, this corporate pharmaceutical integration comes as a result of the increasing bargaining power of managed care buyers. Such vertical combinations will have a phenomenal impact on the chain of pharmaceutical care and drug distribution, including the professions of medicine and pharmacy. Such forward vertical integration will be pursued by multiple manufacturers perhaps in different forms than outright PBM purchase and operation. More likely, combinations to seek significant economic advantages may spur strategic alliances between provider systems and manufacturers to yield a variety of strange mixes, some of which may become highly unstable in performance and longevity. Already certain pharmaceutical firms have arranged to go at risk—that is, offer a discount if all patients in a therapeutic class are switched to their product—with HMOs and hospitals to handle the "disease state management" related to their product line. This highly-touted new model of care assumes an integrated services approach under a reimbursement scheme based on the natural course of a disease. The objective is to control total systems costs by managing health outcomes.

Either barred from entering a related market by law, or historically separated as provider, supplier, or insurer, present health care corporate endeavors are amalgamating into national and multinational constellations, whose size and shape were unforeseen (or even imagined) in America before this decade. It is now necessary to think hard about the powers that such vertically integrated combinations might wield. Will these new pharmaceutical firms seek to lock out rival suppliers, or will they decide that it is in their interest to be open on cost-effectiveness and quality of life indicators from studies conducted according to strict scientific principles?

It is right to question (as U.S. pharmacists are) whether some Merck-Medco customers (i.e., the real patients, not their provider systems) will end up with a limited choice of one preferred line of pharmaceuticals, to potentially suffer medically, beyond the economic effects of monopoly pricing. The Federal Trade Commission's investigation of the Lilly acquisition of PCS was concerned with this possibility.

It is also natural for the public to be wary of such PMB alliances among industrial giants with histories of practices attuned more to profit accumulation in the marketplace than to the public's overall health advancement.

Policy makers have yet to investigate implications of giant horizontally-integrated corporate provider systems. For example, the political and national market influences of the Columbia Health Care System, the largest provider system at $10.3 billion sales (1993), is larger than the top 15 academic health centers in the nation combined, as well as every one of the individual U.S. pharmaceutical manufacturers, except Johnson and Johnson, Bristol-Myers Squibb, and Merck.

To ponder the more worrisome implications of PBMs associated with nationwide provider systems, consider the situation of adverse drug events associated with the use of pharmaceuticals in society. Adverse drug events can be largely attributed to existing governmental regulatory practices and the tendency of pharmaceutical manufacturers to overstress benefits from their products, while playing down potential risks—akin to the cost-effective quality outcomes promised from manufacturers' newly developing disease management programs. In the past, firms have often failed to provide adequate and timely warnings about untoward side effects on selected drug products. Some regulation by the industry and the medical profession has over the years demonstrated "a startling capacity for prejudice and denial, and a corresponding problem when it came to learning from mistakes" (Medawar, 1992: 215).

Government reporting systems in the United States now provide a distorted reflection of only a small fraction of significant adverse drug effects. As new pharmaceutical biotechnological agents are brought to market, longer-term monitoring (post-marketing surveillance) will be necessary to generate important adverse drug reaction data. But pharmacoepidemiology must achieve widespread application to understand more about the impact of our population's general drug consumption over 50 years with so many agents brought to market, prescribed by the medical profession, and consumed by patients. While managed care organizations linked to PBMs may possess a theoretical ability, through advanced health information management systems, to facilitate population-based tracking, is it reasonable to expect to get data from privately-held corporate entities within a tangled world competitive environment?

Government inactivity over drug distribution has been, and will likely continue to be, largely determined by political and economic forces rather than by strict scientific considerations. Particularly when it comes to substances introduced into the body, American medicine still does not focus on information to consider gross risks, which may not be noticed for years to come. The highly touted mission of outcomes management remains nascent in its development; methodological frameworks for proper measurement will continue to be controversial for policy purposes.

Though highly regulated in advanced nations, the pharmaceutical industry, as one of the most powerful sectors in the world economy, benefits from the ever-increasing growth in health care expenditures across all nations. Nevertheless, it is not understood by practitioners in medicine and pharmacy how precarious their own practice futures may be, given the above-described directions by this multinational health industry.

Across all national health systems, privatization and market reforms are being introduced with fervor. Not only are nations importing American medical technologies, pharmaceuticals, and other health care products, but they are often equally eager to adopt the social technology of ideas, forms of care delivery, computerization schemes, and payment mechanisms to redirect the course of social development for their respective health sectors (Salmon, 1990b).

Changes under corporate health care are entirely reshaping the social purpose of the health care enterprise in the United States, with its marketplace reorientation affecting practitioners' values, choices, and behaviors, including clinical decisions on behalf of their patients. Of course, the outcomes will depend on how the new corporate ownership patterns promote their pursuit of profits vis-à-vis regulatory constraints and consumer preferences (Muirhead, 1994), with some socially beneficial results being reasonably predicted. Nevertheless, multinational megacorporate health entities seeking high returns do not portend a public health-oriented system of care in the United States. Without the latter, implications for the population's health appear pernicious.

## Acknowledgments

My deep appreciation to Agatha Gallo, Stephanie Crawford, and T. Donald Rucker for comments on an earlier draft, as well as to Peter Davis. Special thanks to Maggie Garcia for extensive work in preparation of the manuscript.

## References

Adamcik BA, et al. (1986) New clinical roles for pharmacists: a study of role expansion. *Social Science and Medicine* 23: 1187–200.

Anonymous (1994a) 2% growth forecast for U.S. industry. *Scrip* (January 28), No. 1892, p. 16.

Anonymous (1994b) Generic dilemma for brand name firms. *Scrip* (April 22), No. 1916, p. 15.

Anonymous (1994c) Momentous week for industry. *Scrip* (May 6), No. 1920/21, pp. 1–2.

Ballance R (1996) Market and industrial structure. In: Davis P (ed.) *Contested Ground: Public Purpose and Private Interest in the Regulation of Prescription Drugs*. New York: Oxford University Press, pp. 000–000.

Birenbaum A (1982) Reprofessionalization in pharmacy. *Social Science and Medicine* 16: 871–78.

Burton TM and Tanouye E (1994) Eli Lilly to buy McKesson unit for $4 billion. *Wall Street Journal* (July 12), p. A3.

Cardinale V (1993) Getting paid for services: building pharmacy's case. *Drug Topics* (December 13), pp. 86–89.

DiMasi JA, Hansen RW, Grabowski HG, and Lasagna L (1991) Cost of innovation in the pharmaceutical industry. *Journal of Health Economics* 10: 107–42.

Donkin R (1989) Medicine's search for "what works": what it means to employers. *Business and Health* (May), pp. 18–25.

Eddy DM (1984) Variations in physicians practice: the role of uncertainty. *Health Affairs* 3: 74–89.

Eisenberg JM (1987) How will changes in physician payment by Medicare influence laboratory testing? *Journal of the American Medical Association* 258: 803–8.

Feinglass J and Salmon JW (1994) The use of medical management information systems to increase the clinical productivity of physicians. In: Salmon JW (ed.) *The Corporate Transformation of Health Care, Part II: Perspectives and Implications.* Amityville, NY: Baywood Publishing Co., pp. 139–62.

Francke DE (1969) Let's separate pharmacy and drugstores. *American Journal of Pharmacy* 141: 161–76.

Gaudemans J (1994) The case for local budgeting. *Health Affairs* 13: 243–46.

Haug M (1976) The erosion of professional authority: a cross-cultural inquiry in the case of the physician. *Milbank Memorial Fund Quarterly* 54: 83–106.

Hepler CD (1985) Pharmacy as a clinical profession. *American Journal of Hospital Pharmacy* 42: 1298–306.

Hepler CD (1987) The third wave in pharmaceutical education: the clinical movement. *American Journal of Pharmacy Education* 39: 369–85.

Hill GC (1994) There's a life after selling PCS, McKesson's chief vows. *Wall Street Journal* (July 12), p. B6.

Kronus C (1976) The evolution of occupational power: a historical study of task boundaries between physicians and pharmacists. *Sociology of Work and Occupation* 3: 3–37.

Kusserow RP (1990) *The Clinical Role of the Community Pharmacist.* Washington, DC: U.S. Department of Health and Human Services, Office of the Inspector General.

Laskoski G (1993) Sleeping with the enemy. *American Druggist* (December), pp. 25–28.

Laskoski G (1994) A network of its own. *American Druggist* (May), pp. 11–16.

Light DW (1986) Corporate medicine for profit. *Scientific American* 255: 38–54.

Light D and Levine S (1994) The changing character of the medical profession: a theoretical overview. In: Salmon JW (ed.) *The Corporate Transformation of Health Care, Part II: Perspectives and Implications.* Amityville, NY: Baywood Publishing Co., pp. 163–80.

McKinlay JB (1984) Introduction. In: McKinlay JB (ed.) *Issues in the Political Economy of Health Care.* New York: Tavistock, pp. 1–19.

McKinlay JB and Stoeckle JD (1990) Corporatization and the social transformation of doctoring. In: Salmon JW (ed.) *The Corporate Transformation of Health Care, Part I: Issues and Directions.* Amityville, NY: Baywood Publishing Co., pp. 133–50.

Medawar C (1992) *Power and Dependence: Social Audit on the Safety of Medicines.* London: Social Audit.

Miller D (1992) Mail order pharmacy. *Newsletter* 34(33): 6 Pharmaceutical Manufacturers Association, Washington, DC, August 17.

Muirhead G (1994) How consumers see managed care. *Drug Topics* (May 23), pp. 40–54.

Murray MJ (1974) The pharmaceutical industry: a study in corporate power. *International Journal of Health Services* 4: 625–40.

National Association of Boards of Pharmacy (1993) *OBRA '90: Patient Counseling and the Pharmacist*. Nutley, NJ: Roche Laboratories.

National Association of Chain Drug Stores (NACDS) (1993) *Annual Report, 1992*. Alexandria, VA: NACDS.

Price Waterhouse (1993) *Financial Trends in the Pharmaceutical Industry*. New York: Price Waterhouse.

Relman AS (1980) The new medical-industrial complex. *New England Journal of Medicine* 303: 963–70.

Relman AS (1988). Assessment and accountability: the third revolution in health care. *New England Journal of Medicine* 319: 1220–2.

Relman AS (1992) What market values are doing to medicine. *Atlantic Monthly* 269: 99–106.

Roemer MI (1988) Foreign privatization of national health systems. *American Journal of Public Health* 77: 1271–72.

Rucker TD (1987) Pursuing rational drug therapy: a macro view a la the USA. *Journal of Social and Admininistrative Pharmacy* 5: 78–86.

Salmon J W (1984) Organizing medical care for profit. In: McKinlay JB (ed.) *Issues in the Political Economy of Health Care*. New York: Tavistock, pp. 143–86.

Salmon JW (ed.) (1990a) *The Corporate Transformation of Health Care, Part I: Issues and Directions*. Amityville, NY: Baywood Publishing Company.

Salmon JW (1990b) Possibilities for and constraints upon prevention under the health care market system in the United States. *Proceedings of The Challenge of Health: The New Role of Sickness Funds and Health Insurance Schemes*. Hamburg, Germany: International AOK/WHO Conference.

Salmon JW (ed.) (1994) *The Corporate Transformation of Health Care, Part II: Perspectives and Implications*. Amityville, NY: Baywood Publishing Company.

Salmon JW (1995) A perspective on the corporate transformation of health care. *International Journal of Health Services* 25: 11–42.

Salmon JW, White WD, and Feinglass J (1994) The futures of physicians: agency and autonomy reconsidered. In: Salmon JW (ed.) *The Corporate Transformation of Health Care, Part II: Perspectives and Implications*. Amityville, NY: Baywood Publishing Company, pp. 125–38.

Sherbourne CD, Hays RD, Ordnay L, DiMatteo MR, and Kravitz RL (1992) Antecedents to adherence to medical recommendations: results from the medical outcomes study. *Journal of Behavioral Medicine* 15: 447–67.

Shikles JL (1992) *Prescription Drugs: Changes in Prices for Selected Drugs*. GAO/HRD-92-128. Washington, DC: U.S. General Accounting Office.

Special Committee on Aging (1992) *Accessibility and Affordability of Prescription Drugs for Older Americans*. Serial #102-0. Washington, DC: U.S. Senate.

Strand L, Cipolle RJ, and Morley PC (1992) *Pharmaceutical Care: An Introduction. Current Concepts*. Kalamazoo, MI: Upjohn.

Tanouye E (1994) Pharmacy trade group creates firm to compete for prescription drug plans. *Wall Street Journal* (April 11), pp. A3–4.

Turshen M (1976) An analysis of the medical supply industries. *International Journal of Health Services* 6: 271–94.

Walker HD (1971) *Market Power and Price Levels in the Ethical Drug Industry*. Bloomington, IN: Indiana University Press.

Weber J (1994) Drug-merger mania. *Business Week* (May 16), pp. 30–32.

Wennberg JE (1986) The paradox of appropriate care. *New England Journal of Medicine* 314: 310–11.

Whitney HA, et al. (1993) Medication compliance: a health care problem. *Annals of Pharmacotherapy* 27, supplement.

Winslow R (1992) Prescribing decisions increasingly are made by the cost conscious. *Wall Street Journal* (September 25), p. A1.

Winslow R (1993) Hospitals wake up to the power of computers. *Wall Street Journal* (October 8), p. B1.

# 10

## Pharmacy in the Western World Health Care Systems

ALBERT WERTHEIMER
W. MICHAEL DICKSON
BECKY A. BRIESACHER

## Introduction

Mindful of the tremendous strides toward harmonization throughout the world, and especially within the European Union, health care systems continue as peculiar, paradoxical, and quite emotional enterprises. Within the Western world, health care systems differ enormously in virtually every aspect of organization, financing, operation, resource allocation, and management (Roemer, 1993). As Payer tells us, even the provision of personal health care services varies greatly from country to country (Payer, 1988: 27). This diversity affirms that health care delivery relies as much on social doctrine as on scientific discovery (Spector, 1979).

Trying to find a novel approach to the universal challenge of containing pharmaceutical costs is a common thread in many nations' policies on pharmacy and pharmaceuticals. Pharmaceutical services are one of the most visible, widely used, and expected benefits in virtually every health care system. Changes, especially if they cost the public more out-of-pocket, or decrease the extent of benefits, are usually met with singular protest and resistance. In recent years there have been attempts by many governments to constrain pharmaceutical expenditure through increased industry regulation, reduced benefits, or transferring more cost to consumers. Each country, however, addresses these objectives by devising its own method, which reflects the need to consider pharmaceutical benefits within the context of the existing cultural and regulatory environment. Before examining specific pharmaceutical distribution systems, and attempts to control pharmaceutical expenditure, it is necessary to review the general characteristics of the surrounding health care system (NERA, 1993).

For this chapter we have chosen to focus on four countries that represent diversity of philosophy, and significance as measured by market size. These countries (France, Germany, the United Kingdom, and the United States) have each developed different health care systems and approaches to regulating and providing pharmaceutical products and services.

Table 10-1 compares these four countries on selected demographic, economic, and health care statistics. The reader can easily conclude that there are vast differences among these countries on the variables shown. A careful reading will show that the European countries tend to be similar to each other, and, as a group, different from the United States. This is true for population, percentage of elderly population, Gross Domestic Product (GDP) per capita, health expenditure per capita, and health care expenditure as a percentage of GDP. The data on pharmaceutical expenditure does not follow this trend (final two rows in Table 10-1). Pharmaceutical expenditure per capita in the United States is similar to that for France and Germany, which are different from the United Kingdom, which is about one-half of the others. Finally, pharmaceutical expenditure as a percentage of total health care expenditure in the United States is about one-half that for France and Germany, but about the same as the United Kingdom. This inverse relationship is a function of health policy and will be discussed later in more detail (Spivey et al., 1992).

Table 10-2 shows a 10-year trend for the variables in Table 10-1. In contrast to the previous table, there is considerable diversity among the countries. Growth in population, GDP per capita, health care expenditure per capita, and pharmaceutical expenditure per capita are roughly similar across the four countries. The growth trends for percentage of elderly population, health care expenditure as a percentage of GDP, and pharmaceutical expenditure as a percentage of total health care expendi-

TABLE 10-1.   Summary of Selected National Statistics for 1990

|  | France | Germany | United Kingdom | United States |
|---|---|---|---|---|
| Health care model | NHI | NHI | NHS | Pluralistic |
| Population | 56,735,000 | 63,253,000 | 57,411,000 | 259,600,000 |
| Population, percent age 65 + | 14.0 | 15.3 | 15.7 | 12.6 |
| GDP per capita[a] | 17,311 | 18,289 | 15,943 | 21,051 |
| Health care expenditure per capita[a] | 1,528 | 1,522 | 988 | 2,600 |
| Health care expenditure, percent of GDP | 8.8 | 8.3 | 6.2 | 12.4 |
| Pharmaceutical expenditure per capita[a] | 256 | 325 | 98[b] | 210 |
| Pharmaceutical expenditure, percent of health care expenditure | 16.8 | 21.3 | 10.7[b] | 8.1 |

Source: Data are derived from OECD Health Data (CREDES), 1993.

[a]Financial data are expressed in Purchasing Power Parity (PPP)$ for comparison purposes.

[b]Data are for 1989.

TABLE 10-2.  Summary of Average Annual Growth Rates (%) from 1980–1990, Selected National Statistics

|  | France | Germany | United Kingdom | United States |
|---|---|---|---|---|
| Population | 0.52 | 0.27 | 0.19 | 0.99 |
| Population, percent age 65 + | 0.00 | − 0.13 | 0.52 | 1.09 |
| GDP per capita | 6.48 | 6.61 | 7.28 | 6.22 |
| Health care expenditure per capita | 8.14 | 6.49 | 8.05 | 9.35 |
| Health care expenditure, percent of GDP | 1.56 | − 0.11 | 0.72 | 2.95 |
| Pharmaceutical expenditure per capita | 8.74 | 7.88 | 7.52[a] | 8.62 |
| Pharmaceutical expenditure, percent of health care expenditure | 0.55 | 1.30 | − 0.48 | − 0.67 |

*Source:* Data are derived from OECD Health Data (CREDES) 1993.

Note: Table entries are average annual growth rates for 1980–1990.

[a]Growth rates for 1980 to 1989.

ture are very different across the countries. The elderly population in the United States, for example, is growing faster than the rate of growth in the population in general, whereas in Germany the trends are moving in the opposite direction. In all countries, GDP is growing faster than health care expenditure (as a percentage of GDP), but only in Germany is health care declining as a part of the GDP. Finally, pharmaceutical expenditure, as a percentage of health care expenditure, is declining in the United Kingdom and the United States, but growing slightly in France and Germany. Whether these are favorable must be interpreted within the context of each country (Schneider, 1992).

If viewed in terms of health care systems, each of these countries represents one of the major health care delivery models that can be found across the developed world. The models are described according to major subcategories that define an integrated system of drug product development, distribution, and reimbursement: drug list, product price determination, product reimbursement, margins and value added tax (VAT), and generic market. While the details of these subcategories and models may be specific to the countries chosen, readers should find general themes that are useful for classifying health care systems in most other countries.

## Overview of the National Health Insurance Model

National health insurance (NHI) schemes operate throughout large portions of the world. Most were introduced during the early part of the twentieth century. At that time, when governments assumed responsibility for financing access to personal health services, the insurance approach did the least alteration to the existing system of providers. Government provided a method for organizing and defining a health benefit and raising the money to pay for it. Services were provided by the existing private sector. From such modest beginnings, NHI programs became monopsonists with huge market power that they used to initiate policy, set standards, and establish payment limits for providers.

France and Germany both have the national health insurance model, but with slightly different methods of implementation. In an NHI model, providers of service may be entrepreneurs or employed by the state. Providers include private physicians, government clinics, community owned hospitals, and so forth. Such a system includes the obligation of citizens to purchase health insurance according to the mechanisms available in a particular country. A brief review of the health care systems in France and Germany contrasts two versions of the same model.

## French System

France's social welfare system, including health care, is funded by a special tax on employers and employees. Most industries have their own regimes (insurance carriers). The System General is for everyone not in a special regime. Health care and retirement benefits are different across the regimes, but there is a movement to harmonize the benefits (Eschenbach, 1992). The social security system (Securité Social) is managed by boards of employers and employees but controlled by the government.

Participation in the social security system is mandatory for everyone, but there are voluntary systems (usually a non-profit insurer called a mutuelle) designed to provide additional health care and retirement benefits. The voluntary decision to purchase some form of supplementary insurance is at the group level (usually an employment group). Currently over 90% of the population have some additional coverage.

### Drug List

In practice there is no list of products approved for reimbursement because nearly all prescription products are reimbursed, but technically there are two lists. The first is for products used for outpatients, and the second is for hospital drugs. In recent years the government has used *delisting* (removing products from the reimbursement list) to enforce various pharmaceutical regulatory provisions, such as those governing promotional expenditure. The listing is important because it determines the method of pricing and reimbursement, discussed below.

### Product Price Determination

Prescription drug prices have been regulated in France since 1945. Between 1945 and 1980, prices were based on production (i.e., ex-factory) drug costs. In 1980 a transparency commission was instituted to establish the reimbursement level for products and to set prices according to a principle of improved medical care (IMC) and certain industrial conventions (e.g., exports, investment, employment, etc.). Between 1986 and 1993, a price was set for every prescription drug product once it received marketing approval (SNIP, 1992).

In January 1994 a new system of pricing was instituted as the result of criticism that the specific product pricing system failed to control pharmaceutical expenditures, even though French pharmaceutical prices were among the lowest in Europe. The French pricing system was modified to constrain pharmaceutical expenditure through a medical approach to the rational use of pharmaceutical products consistent with the recently adopted agreement with physicians known as good medical practice guidelines. Both interventions are designed to reduce pharmaceutical consumption. Thus, the new pricing system contains the following components (Anonymous, 1994a):

- a specified annual rate of increase (maximum allowed) in spending for reimbursed prescription products
- a policy of setting new drug prices that recognizes improvements in therapy
- faster pricing decisions
- agreement on medically justified volumes
- a decrease in overall industry promotional spending
- a commitment to develop pharmacoeconomic studies
- the option of multiyear contracts by companies

The intent of the new system is to provide companies with some pricing freedom through multiyear contracts that may include pricing flexibility (Anonymous, 1994b). The government has adopted the view that expenditure can best be reduced through more rational prescribing which, in this case, has been interpreted to mean reducing the volume of consumption. The new medical practice guidelines directly target prescribing practices for certain conditions. The effectiveness of the new guidelines is not yet clear.

## Product Reimbursement

In addition to decisions on pricing, the transparency commission also determines the rate of reimbursement for outpatient products by placing each in a reimbursement category. The possibilities are:

- Products for special diseases: reimbursed at 95% (at 100% until 1994).
- Products without scientific merit, including products for colds, allergies, other types of symptomatic relief, vasodilators, and homeopathic remedies: reimbursed at 35% (40% until 1994).
- All other products. This group constitutes the majority of products: reimbursed at 65% (70% until 1994).

When a prescription product is dispensed from an outpatient pharmacy, the patient pays for it, and submits reimbursement forms to the social security agency. If the patient also has mutuelle insurance, the unreimbursed portion is then submitted to that company. In practice, there is little out-of-pocket expenditure for prescription products. The natural consequence of this arrangement is that consumers are relatively insensitive to prescription prices. Physicians feel little pressure to reduce prescribing or use less expensive products. The absence of an economic stake in prescription use is thought to be the basic cause for high consumption in France.

## Margins and Value Added Tax

Prices for reimbursed products are controlled from the producer to the retailer. The location and number of pharmacies are regulated to insure proper distribution and an adequate trading area for each pharmacy. Much of the revenue in a pharmacy comes from prescription sales because general merchandise is strictly limited. These constraints at the retail level should be recalled when considering the margins that appear below. The following are average margins, although specific products will vary (Dickson, 1994: 90):

- Wholesalers, 6.8%
- Retailers, 30.4%
- VAT, 2.5%

## Generic Market

France has one of the lowest rates of generic drug penetration in Europe. This condition is the result of several market attributes. First, pharmaceutical prices are very low compared to other European countries. Consumers have no incentive to purchase generics (see above section on product reimbursement). Physicians lack an incentive to prescribe generics since they regard all prices as legitimately set by the government. Finally, there is a general perception that generics are not of good quality. These forces, taken together, have kept generics to less than 5% of the French market.

With 75% of the French market going to branded pharmaceuticals that are off patent, the government is eager to reduce spending on health care by encouraging greater generic use. In addition, because pharmacists are reimbursed on a margin system they have no reason to recommend less expensive products. Development of a truly robust generic market will require significant changes in these obstacles.

## Summary

The French pharmaceutical market is at the threshold of change. There is great hope that the new pricing system and practice guidelines will improve the quality of prescribing as well as slow the rate of pharmaceutical expenditure. The government and mutuelles have expressed interest in the development of a generic market, but the feasibility is not clear. Pharmacists probably will not support a larger generic market so long as their reimbursement is tied to product price. Finally, the industry is adjusting to the new pricing system with the expectation that greater pricing freedom will create greater efficiencies and sufficient revenue margins to support more research.

## *German System*

In Germany, health insurance is obtained through regional health insurance agencies called Krankenkassen (sickness funds). The system is largely financed by public pay-roll taxation. About 92% of the population must participate in this system. Cost of the system is shared equally between employers and employees. Another 4% of the population is public employees with their own system for financing health care. It is common practice for public employees to carry additional private insurance for noncovered medical expenses. The remaining 4% of the population has only private insurance. This group generally includes the self-employed (except farmers and artists, who each have their own sickness fund). The unemployed also are covered in the general system. Thus, 100% of the population has health insurance (Spivey et al., 1992).

In contrast to France, the German system does not regulate individual product prices. Until July 1989, ex-factory pharmaceutical prices were unregulated. In July 1989, a reference price system was introduced in response to rapidly increasing health care expenditure. Further changes were made in 1993 in response to new financial pressures on the system (Arnold, 1991).

## Drug List

Germany's sickness funds use a negative list to exclude selected products from reimbursement. However, the exclusions are minor by comparison to some other countries. For example, exclusions include syrups for adults and oral contraceptives. A large part of the negative list is composed of drugs for minor conditions such as colds and motion sickness. The list also contains products marketed prior to the current drug approval law. All these products were grandfathered for a period of time while they were evaluated for effectiveness. Approved products became eligible for reimbursement, but all others were moved to the negative list. The negative list is set by the national association representing physicians and sickness funds. All other products are eligible for reimbursement.

## Product Price Determination

Producers are free to set any price for their products in Germany. However, the reference price system establishes the maximum level of reimbursement that will be made by the sickness funds for selected product groups (BPI, 1991). The relevant legislation states that a reference price must guarantee a sufficient economic supply of good quality products, exploit the potential for savings, induce effective price competition, and give good value for money to the public. In practice, this means that reference prices are set above the lowest priced product, but just enough to meet the savings criterion. Reference prices are set for three groups of products:

- Selected generic categories
- Pharmacologically similar products (not generically equivalent); a reference price does not apply for products in this group if the product has a novel contribution to care (e.g., a lower side-effect profile)
- Products with similar actions (therapeutic categories)

Products in each of the major groups are subdivided into more homogeneous subgroups. For example, nitroglycerin (a generic group) could be separated into subgroups based on dosage form (e.g., sublingual and patch). A reference price is set for one package size in each of the subgroups, usually the most commonly used size.

Once the reference price is set for the standard package size, the others are determined according to statistical methods that will yield a similar cost per day.

### Product Reimbursement

All products are eligible for reimbursement (including homeopathic remedies and OTCs if written on prescription) except those on the negative list. The reference pricing system instituted in 1989 was changed in 1993 to make the system more uniform and institute some emergency cost saving measures. The current reimbursement system requires that consumers pay 3 deutsche marks (DM) for each small package size prescriptions, 5 DM for medium size packages, and 7 DM for large packages. Physicians are reluctant to prescribe products priced above the reference price because patients must pay the difference.

### Margins and Value Added Tax

The margins and VAT are set for wholesalers and retailers by the government, which uses a sliding digressive scale, but the averages are shown below (Dickson, 1994). Also note that pharmacies are required to give the sickness funds a 5% discount on the drug retail price, which is not included in the schedule shown.

- Wholesalers, 13.8%
- Retailers, 30.9%
- VAT, 14.0%

### Generic Market

There is an incentive for physicians to prescribe generic products because the sickness funds regularly audit prescriber performances to determine their economic impact on the fund. There is a fixed amount for the pharmaceutical budget which, if exceeded, exposes the physician to auditing. If prescribers' weighted average prescribing costs exceed the budget by 15% they can be asked to provide an explanation. If the amount is 25% above the average, physicians are at risk for repayment ("claw-back" provision).

### Summary

The German system has recently experienced significant changes that are too new to assess adequately. It is clear that the rate of growth in pharmaceutical expenditure is decreasing and consumers are being asked to assume more of the financial burden. Physicians have reacted with caution (reduced prescribing) due to uncertainty regarding the new regulations in 1994. Prescribing volumes now appear to be returning to the pre-1994 rates.

## Overview of the National Health Service Model

In a national health service (NHS) model, health care costs and responsibility for management of the system reside with the government. The government owns most of the health care facilities (e.g., hospitals, clinics, offices, etc.), and employs the providers of service. As the main purchaser of health care, the government can set regulations on prices, and make decisions on resource allocation that affect the availability of services. This is in contrast to the NHI system in which resource allocation is done in the private sector, facilities are largely privately owned, and service providers have greater influence on health policy.

## British System

Britain's National Health Service is an example of the NHS model. The system was founded in 1948 by the Labour Party with the intent of providing free health care for all citizens. The NHS provides comprehensive care with universal coverage of the population. Most hospitals are owned by the NHS, and specialists working in hospitals are paid a salary; however, they may choose to devote part of their time to private private practice (Basch, 1990). Pharmacists are a part of the private sector. They are reimbursed for their services by a formula based on the prescriptions dispensed. The NHS is funded largely by general taxation with employed people paying a sliding percentage of wages (0 to 9%) to a national insurance fund, and only a modest additional amount for some services (Eschenbach, 1992).

### Drug List

All licensed medicines in Britain are prescribable within the NHS as long as they are not on the *Selected List*. This is a negative list established in 1985 that currently includes 16 categories of products that will not be reimbursed by the NHS. These products, such as cold remedies, vitamins, and mild analgesics, are generally for minor ailments. Most, but not all, products on the *Selected List* are available as OTCs. The economic problems of the 1980s required changes in the British system, which established the foundation for changes in medical practice (Day, 1991).

### Product Price Determination

The Pharmaceutical Price Regulation Scheme (PPRS) has operated since 1957 based on a voluntary agreement between the Department of Health and Social Security (DHSS) and the pharmaceutical industry, represented by the Association of the British Pharmaceutical Industry (ABPI). In principle, this six-year renewable agreement covers all branded products and vaccines regardless of their patent status. Generics are not included in the PPRS. In practice, the NHS monitors only those firms with annual sales to the NHS of at least £500,000. These firms (about 100) must submit annual financial data to the DHSS. The financial reports are used in negotiations between individual companies, and the DHSS sets the target profit for the firm. Prices for NHS hospitals are negotiated separately, and OTC prices are not regulated (ABPI/DHSS, 1986).

The PPRS is unique among European countries because it is the only national system that regulates pharmaceutical firm profits (product prices are not regulated). Firms subject to the PPRS negotiate a target profitability that is in the range of 17 to 21%. A profit in excess of the target may be kept by the company under certain conditions as long as the margin does not exceed 50%. The most recent agreement

(October 1993) between the DHSS and ABPI modified the target profitability concept by imposing a 2.5% price reduction (with a three-year freeze), which effectively reduces the return on capital by about 1.5% (ABPI, 1994).

Firms are free to set the price of new products (NCEs) for the first five years of marketing, being constrained only by the negotiated target profit. Prices on existing products may be raised only with the permission of the DHSS. Generally, this requires that the company demonstrate that it will fall far short of its profit target without the price increase.

## Product Reimbursement

The NHS requires a £5.25 copayment for each prescription as of April 1, 1995. However, over 80% (by monetary value) of outpatient prescriptions do not include a copayment. The rate is quite high because there are numerous exemptions, including the elderly, pregnant women, children, and others. It also is possible to pay a one-time flat fee for all prescriptions for the year. The result is that consumers in the United Kingdom, like those in France, pay very little out of pocket when prescriptions are received.

## Margins and Value Added Tax

Producers supply medicines to wholesalers at a discount as shown below, to cover the costs of distribution. Within this margin, wholesalers compete on the level of discount they pass on to the retail pharmacy. A typical discount would be in the range of 9%, though it is quite variable. The Department of Health conducts a regular survey of average discounts obtained by pharmacies for the purpose of adjusting their NHS reimbursement. Thus, pharmacies have a strong financial incentive to achieve discounts greater than the average. The average margin structure is:

- Wholesalers, 12.5%
- Retailers, 20.0%
- VAT, 0.0% (OTCs have 17.5% VAT)

## Generic Market

General Practitioners (GPs) in Britain are strongly encouraged to prescribe generic products. The NHS exhorts GPs to establish their own formularies (most GPs practice in groups) in which price is one consideration. The NHS publishes a monthly *Drug Tariff* that includes the prices of generic drugs. There also are sources of prices on branded products for prescribers. Currently, about 43% of prescriptions are written generically and 37% are dispensed that way (some generic prescriptions are available only as brands). GPs also receive monthly PACT (Prescription and Cost Analysis) reports that compare each medical group's prescribing to its peer groups. Research shows these educational efforts can pressure "outliers" to adjust their prescribing toward the norm.

A new, but important, force for increasing generic use is the government's fund holding concept for GPs. This concept provides groups of GPs with capitated payments for services (that is, payment per enrolled patient), but allows certain funds to be reallocated (Spivey et al., 1992). If there are savings, that portion of the budget may be shifted to selected other services. Thus, if the prescribing budget (the cost of the prescriptions written by the GPs) is reduced through the use of generics, the group can reallocate savings. Generic prescribing encourages GPs to save on their budget since the pharmacist must dispense as the prescription is written. However, many GPs worry that the payments do not properly consider their patient mix.

## Summary

Revisiting Tables 10-1 and 10-2 will remind the reader that the United Kingdom has the lowest per capita expenditure on health care and pharmaceuticals of any of the countries shown. Growth rates for the pharmaceutical component also are low. While it is difficult to assign causality, we should note they have accomplished this without price controls on new pharmaceutical products. These policy decisions are not always popular because many believe they contribute to the waiting lines for health care services. Support for private medicine in the United Kingdom is gaining popularity and political visibility, since over 500,000 people are on waiting lists (for as long as three years) for nonurgent operations. The British government does grant some tax relief to those paying for private health insurance, but still demands payments to the NHS. Currently about six million Britons are covered by private insurance (Eschenbach, 1992).

There also are signs of stress on the DHSS and ABPI voluntary agreement. The last negotiation between these groups came to a stalemate at one point, but was ultimately resolved. One point of contention is the 9% sales cap on promotional expenditure. Smaller and newer companies claim this will place them at a competitive disadvantage to firms with more sizable revenue. However, this arrangement is unusual, if not unique, and certainly must be considered as a reflection of the political process in the United Kingdom.

## Overview of a Pluralistic System

Pluralistic is a term used to define health care systems that do not fit more appropriately into the NHI and NHS models. The United States is the largest market with this characteristic, and perhaps one of the few existing among developed countries. Since pluralistic can mean many things, the U.S. system reviewed below is seen as an example, but not a prototype, for this group of health systems.

### United States System

Historically, the U.S. experience with health care has been a gradual shift in responsibility from individuals to governments at the local, state, and federal levels. In 1993 about 39% of health expenditure was from private sources (34% insurance and 5% other private), 43% came from various government sources, and the remainder was out of pocket (Levit, 1994). There currently is no single system of health care in the United States, but there has been a recent shift in the type of health insurance coverage from indemnity (reimbursement based on rendered services) to managed care (reimbursement based on managed relationships between patient populations and providers). In 1982 an estimated 13% of the insured population was covered by some form of managed care. In 1992 the total had reached 75%, and it is estimated to be nearly 90% by 1997 (APhA, 1994: 1). At the same time the number of un-insured continued to climb to a new high of 17.4%, or at least 40 million people in 1992 (Employee Benefit Research Institute, 1994: 145).

As of 1994, there were three major systems of care in the United States. The largest segment of the population has private insurance for themselves, and their families, through their places of employment. Many financing arrangements exist, but the most common is cost sharing of the premium between employers and employees. Most employers pay a high proportion of the premium cost as a benefit for their employees. Payment for pharmaceutical products is dependent on the policy of each payer. The second system is Medicare, which provides health insurance for elderly and disabled citizens. In 1993 36.3 million people were eligible for Medicare (Levit, 1994). About 29 million of the eligible population received benefits in 1993, which accounted for 19.3% of total personal health care expenditure. The program is funded by employer and employee contributions while the individual is working, and small annual premiums when coverage is received. Outpatient prescription drugs are not covered by Medicare. However, some managed care organizations have begun to offer Medicare recipients an outpatient prescription drug benefit as induce-ment to join their plan.

The third system is Medicaid, a federal and state jointly funded program, which provides health care coverage for the poor and unemployed. In 1993 there were 33.4 million Medicaid recipients, which accounted for 14.4% of total personal health care expenditure (Levit, 1994). Eligibility requirements are different across states, but there are federally mandated minimums for eligibility (related to the income poverty level in each state), and the services to be provided (Fincham and Wertheimer, 1992).

The most recent data for the United States (1993) indicates that total health care expenditure was $884.2 billion; an increase of 7.8% from 1992, which is below the rate shown in Table 2 for the 1980s (Levit, 1994). The vast majority of this (89%) was for personal health care, which also grew more than 7% since 1992. By all measures, health expenditure in the United States continues to grow at a substantial rate. Most health care expenditure (about 42% of personal health care expenditure) went to hospitals, which are the site of the most intensive care and the focus of medical education.

The recent trend toward managed care has profoundly influenced changes in the provision of hospital, physician and pharmaceutical services. The hospital sector is consolidating to create larger institutions or networks. Physicians are also joining networks as well as facing more constraints on prescribing through the use of formu-laries and prior authorization programs. Pharmaceutical services are being restruc-tured to help keep patients out of hospitals and in ambulatory care settings. Most health insurance plans require that patients enter the health care system by first seeing a primary care provider who determines whether a specialist is necessary. In the community environment, the managed care organizations are seeking alliances with large pharmacy chains.

## Drug List

Because there is no single health care system, the United States has no one drug list, although managed care and hospital formularies are becoming more common and more restrictive. Medicaid pharmaceutical benefits are not required to use a formulary, but many state schemes have either a positive or negative list. The Omnibus Budget Reconciliation Act of 1990 (OBRA-90) created doubt about the ability of Medicaid to use formularies, but they are still routinely used in conjunction with prior authorization programs (Gagnon, 1979; NPC, 1994).

## Product Price Determination

Product prices are not controlled by the government but by marketplace forces. With the widespread use of managed care, there has been a substantial restructuring of the prescription drug marketplace in terms of customers and their influence on prices. The presence of large buyers and closing formularies have created price concessions based on exclusive and quantity-purchasing contracts. The market discipline imposed by managed care is often cited as the reason for moderating pharmaceutical prices in the last two years.

## Product Reimbursement

In general, public and private prescription plans do not cover OTCs (there are some exceptions when written on prescription). For prescription items there are two main reimbursement strategies to control costs. The first, differential cost sharing, provides for a consumer copayment that is lower for generic products. Mail order service is the second method for exercising reimbursement control. Plans typically impose higher charges if the consumer chooses to use a local pharmacy rather than the mail order service. This is yet another force restructuring the community pharmacy market, and creating a more difficult operating environment for independent pharmacies.

Medicaid does not mandate consumer cost sharing (although some state programs impose a charge on those who can afford it), but there are guidelines for reimbursement to pharmacies and rebates from manufacturers. The Maximum Allowable Cost (MAC) and Estimated Acquisition Cost (EAC) programs were instituted to set limits on product reimbursement for multisource and single-source products respectively. The concept is similar to a reference price in that it places an upper limit on reimbursement. Pharmacists generally do not support this system because manufacturers can raise prices faster than the MACs or EACs are raised, which places a squeeze on their margins. In 1990, OBRA-90 required rebates from manufacturers on their products sold to Medicaid patients. The rebate currently stands at about 15% for branded prescription products.

## Margins and Value Added Tax

As noted earlier, prices are not set by the government for prescription products. Thus, margins are not fixed, and VAT does not exist in the U.S. market. It also was noted above that Medicaid uses MAC and EAC to set reimbursement limits, but these are not fixed margins. The same is true for private health plans that set specific reimbursement prices for pharmacies. Since the pharmacist's purchasing price is not set, the retail margin also is not fixed.

## Generic Market

There is a substantial generic market in the United States because of the price constraints imposed by payers (private and public), and the competitive nature of the marketplace. Furthermore, in most states, pharmacists are permitted to make generic substitutions on equivalent multisource products. These conditions make for a sizable generic market, which in 1993 was estimated to be $3.5 billion dollars for retail pharmacies. This is a 25% increase over the 1992 level. For the same time period, generically written prescriptions increased by 16% (Chi, 1994). The managed care movement and talk about health care reform will continue to push these figures higher.

In the United States, as in some other countries, a generic product may not be marketed until the patent has expired, which is 17 years. Much controversy surrounds this number since most patents are filed upon discovery of the compound, and the road to FDA marketing approval is long and costly. It is not uncommon for a product to have less than 10 years of patent life remaining when it receives marketing approval (Fincham and Wertheimer, 1992).

## Summary

The U.S. market is continuing the movement toward managed care. All present indications are that health care will remain a part of the private sector. Competition will continue to discipline the market, and further consolidation among provider and payer groups will create larger blocks of selling and purchasing power. Prescription pharmaceuticals occupy a relatively small part of the total health expenditure picture, but they are high on the list of items to control because many consumers are without significant insurance coverage for pharmaceuticals. It is estimated that about 30% of outpatient prescriptions are covered by an insurance plan (Goldberg, 1986).

Two other significant characteristics of the U.S. health care system are the American preference for highly technical care, and the substantial labor force engaged in health care. The health care industry is the largest U.S. private profession, accounting for more than 5% of the nation's total labor force (Williams, 1988). Like their European colleagues, American physicians are among the highest paid professionals, and as a group they account for approximately 20% of total U.S. health care expenditure (Fincham and Wertheimer, 1992).

## Discussion

This chapter has attempted to capture the diversity of pharmaceutical systems as part of selected models of health system organizations. Each system was presented in the context of the culture in which it was developed and applied because a society's attitudes toward health care largely form its national pharmaceutical care policies. The overall theme of this discussion is the multitude of approaches (many seemingly comparable) to containing pharmaceutical costs, and improving the quality of phar-

TABLE 10-3.  Health Care Coverage of the Population in Selected Countries, 1991

| | NHI | | NHS | Pluralistic |
|---|---|---|---|---|
| Trait | France | Germany | United Kingdom | United States |
| Percentage of population in public health care scheme | 99% enrolled in mutuelles | 89% enrolled in statutory insurance programs | 99% | 30%[a] enrolled in a government-funded program |
| Percentage of population with private insurance | 66% for only supplemental coverage | 19% for only supplemental coverage | 11% for only supplemental coverage | 55% |

*Sources*: Eschenbach, 1992; Fincham and Wertheimer, 1992.

[a]1990 data.

maceutical services. Four of the more sophisticated and integrated strategies are represented by the four countries covered in this chapter.

At this point it will be useful to review Table 10-3, which summarizes health care coverage for all the countries reviewed in this chapter. The European countries cover virtually all their populations. The United States has adopted a different system, which from Table 10-3 shows a lower percentage of the population with insurance coverage for health care. Table 10-4 summarizes the various cost containment strategies employed in each country. It shows, again, that the U.S. market is quite unlike

TABLE 10-4.  Pharmaceutical Cost Containment Strategies, 1993

| | NHI | | NHS | Pluralistic |
|---|---|---|---|---|
| Trait | France | Germany | United Kingdom | United States |
| Formulary | State list based on therapeutic groups | Yes | British National Formulary is prescriptive but not restrictive | Varies by program |
| Price Controls | State list of reimbursable drugs Price/volume tradeoffs Pricing committees Multiyear contracts, est. 1993 | Rebates and reference pricing, est. 1989 | Unrestricted pricing for OTC and private drugs Tendering to hospitals Limited company profits, est. 1950s | Varies by program |
| Copayment | Illness-dependent, largely covered by coinsurance | Fixed amount | Fixed amount, 37% of population is exempt | Varies by program |

*Sources*: OECD, 1993.

TABLE 10-5.   Pharmacy and Pharmaceuticals, 1990

|  | NHI | | NHS | Pluralistic |
|---|---|---|---|---|
| Trait | France | Germany | United Kingdom | United States |
| Retail pharmacies | 21,452 | 18,029 | 11,400 | 62,000 |
| Pharmacists | 50,000 | 35,118 | 20,000 | 121,500 |
| Pharmaceutical manufacturers | 358 | 19 | 350 | 680 |
| Generics as percentage of national volume | 5% | n/a | 36% | 35% |

Sources: Eschenbach, 1992; Fincham and Wertheimer, 1992.

those of Europe. Finally, Table 10-5 provides summary data on the numbers of pharmacists, pharmacies, and pharmaceutical firms which, not surprisingly, are much higher in the United States than for the other countries. However, once the number of practitioners is expressed relative to population size and relative to the number of physicians, the U.S. rate is seen to be in the middle of the range (Table 10-6).

In summary, the government in France has adopted the view that expenditures can best be reduced through more rational prescribing which, in this case, has been interpreted to mean reducing consumption. The government plans to reduce this consumption by constraining pharmaceutical promotion and limiting annual growth in pharmaceutical expenditure. Therapeutic equivalence of generic products is not well promoted, and patients are largely unaware of the prices of their prescriptions.

Producers in Germany are free to set any price for their products, but reimbursement levels are set to give good value for money to the public. The physician is responsible for prescribing patterns that adhere to average prescribing costs. Patients pay standard copayments by package size and are aware of prices only when they exceed the government's reference pricing.

As the major employer, purchaser, and facilities owner in the health care system, the British government wields enormous control. This is the only national system that regulates pharmaceutical manufacturer profits. Consumers pay a small copay-

TABLE 10-6.   Practicing Pharmacist Data for Selected Countries

|  | France | Germany | United Kingdom | United States |
|---|---|---|---|---|
| Total practitioners | 51,983 | 35,181 | 36,779 | 167,000 |
| Number per thousand population | 0.9 | 0.6 | 0.6 | 0.7 |
| Number per hundred physicians | 34.2 | 18.7 | 47.0 | 30.7 |
| Year reported | 1990 | 1989 | 1988 | 1986 |

Sources: OECD, 1993; Noyce and Howe, 1992.

ment if any at all. Physicians may manage an allocated drug budget for their patients and may reallocate any savings for other medical services.

The United States is the most fragmented system, with many levels of coverage, copayments, and price determinations. There are informal mechanisms for constraining pharmaceutical prices but market forces influence most schemes. Managed care is a growing trend that has evolved through market competition and that is currently causing great consolidation and networking between vertical and horizonal components of the health care system (Smith, 1975).

Despite all this variety, two trends transcend the diversity; governments are more willing than ever before to apply reimbursement controls, and more willing to consider borrowing techniques that appear to be successful in other countries. The challenge for all of these systems is to measure and determine success. For most health care analysts, pharmacoeconomics offers the only methodology and tools to address these issues. The rather remarkable development of this new discipline and its influence on regulatory structure indicate the concern payers (especially governments) have for the cost of pharmaceuticals. As the earlier discussion has described, pharmaceuticals are a relatively small portion of total expenditure, but growth is substantial, and there is a desire to obtain value for money. The developments in pharmacoeconomics are a leading indicator of the future in other service sectors in health care.

# References

ABPI (1994) Pharmaceutical industry and Department of Health agree guidelines for the economic analysis of medicines. Press release (May), London: ABPI.

ABPI/DHSS (1986) *The Pharmaceutical Price Regulation Scheme*. London: ABPI and DHSS.

Anonymous (1994a) SNIP presents new French price system. *Scrip* No. 1984, pp. 2–3.

Anonymous (1994b) French contract signing speeds up. *Scrip* No. 1991, p. 2.

APhA (American Pharmaceutical Association) (1994) *Opportunities for the Community Pharmacist in Managed Care*. Washington: APhA.

Arnold M (1991) *Health Care in the Federal Republic of Germany*. Cologne: Deutscher Arte-Verlag.

Basch PF (1990) *Textbook of International Health*. New York: Oxford University Press.

BPI (Bundesvergand der Pharmazeutischen Industrie e.v.) (1991) *Fixed Amounts, Research and Medicine*. (March). Frankfurt am Main, Germany: BPG.

Chi J (1994) Spurred by demand, generics continue blistering pace. *Drug Topics (August 22) Supplement*, pp. 12s–15s.

Day P and Klein R (1991) Britain's health care experiment. *Health Affairs* 10(3): 39–59.

Dickson M (1994) Paying for prescriptions in Europe. In: Poullier J-P (ed.) *Health: Quality and Choice*. Paris: OECD, pp. 83–109.

Employee Benefit Research Institute (EBRI) (1994) *Sources of Health Insurance and Characteristics of the Uninsured*. Washington, DC: EBRI.

Eschenbach D (ed.) (1992) *In Focus: The Health Systems and Pharmaceutical Markets in 16 Countries*. New-Isenburg, Germany: Arzneimittle Zeitung.

Fincham JE and Wertheimer AI (eds.) (1992) *Pharmacy and the U.S. Health Care System*. Binghamton, NY: Haworth Press.

Gagnon JP and Jang R (1979) *Federal Control of Pharmaceutical Costs: The MAC Experience.* Nutley, NJ: Hoffmann-La Roche.

Garattine L, et al. (1995) A Proposal for Italian Guidelines in Pharmacoeconomics. *Pharmacoeconomics* 7(1): 1–6.

Goldberg T, et al. (eds.) (1986) *Generic Drug Laws: A Decade of Trial—A Prescription for Progress.* (June). Washington, DC: National Center for Health Services Research.

Levit K, et al. (1994) National Health Expenditures, 1993. *Health Care Financing Review* 16(1): 250–65.

NERA (National Economic Research Associates) (1993) *Financing Health Care with Particular Reference to Medicines.* (May). New York: NERA.

Noyce PR and Howe JA (1992) United Kingdom. In: Spivey RN, Wertheimer AI, and Rucker TD (eds.) *International Pharmaceutical Services: The Drug Industry and Pharmacy Practice in Twenty-Three Major Countries of the World.* Binghamton, NY: Haworth Press, pp. 557–601.

NPC (National Pharmaceutical Council) (1994) *Pharmaceutical Benefits Under State Medical Assistance Programs.* Reston, VA: NPC.

OECD/CREDES (1991) *OECD Health Data. A Software Package for the International Comparison of Health Care Systems.* Paris: OECD/CREDES.

Payer L (1988) *Medicine and Culture.* New York: H. Holt & Co.

Roemer MI (1993) *National Health Systems of the World.* Vol. 2. New York: Oxford University Press.

Schneider M, Dennerlein RK, Kose A and Schaltes L (1992) *Health Care in the E.C. Member States.* Amsterdam: Elsevier.

Smith M (1975) *Principles of Pharmaceutical Marketing.* Philadelphia, PA: Lea and Febiger.

SNIP (Syndicat National de l'Industrie Pharmaceutique) (1992) *Regime Economique des Specialites Pharmaceutiques Remboursables.* Paris: SNIP.

Spector RE (1979) *Cultural Diversity in Health and Illness.* New York: Appleton Century Crofts.

Spivey RN, Wertheimer AI, and Rucker TD (eds.) (1992) *International Pharmaceutical Services: The Drug Industry and Pharmacy Practice in Twenty-Three Major Countries of the World.* Binghamton, NY: Haworth Press.

Williams SJ and Torens PR (1988) *Introduction to Health Services.* 3rd ed. New York: Wiley and Sons.

# III

# THE REGULATORY FRAMEWORK: INTERNATIONAL INNOVATION

# 11

## Pharmaceutical Policy and Regulation: Setting the Pace in the European Community

### LEIGH HANCHER

The pharmaceutical industry is viewed at the European Community (EC) level as one of Europe's best-performing high-technology sectors. It generates over 1% of the EC gross national product and has grown at an annual rate in excess of 6% between 1982 and 1992. Overall, the EC has a trade surplus with the rest of the world, except the European Free Trade Area (EFTA) countries and, to a lesser extent, the United States. The grouping of the current 12 Member States is also the world's largest market for drugs (amounting to 63.5 billion European Currency Units [ECU] in 1992).

Yet this potentially European-wide market remains partitioned along national lines. It is the primary goal of what might be termed European pharmaceutical industry policy to remove existing territorial barriers created by national legislation and to ensure that innovative European firms enjoy a sufficiently large market to fund rapidly growing research and development costs. The legal issues involved in the EC Commission's most recent attempts to fashion such a strategy are the main focus of this chapter.

Although the Community has concerned itself with different aspects of the pharmaceutical sector's activities for well over three decades, the need to design a broad industrial strategy for the sector is new. The Commission's first comprehensive policy statement (Commission, 1994) claims that this approach is necessary because the framework within which pharmaceutical companies operate has been profoundly shaken by rising research costs, the emergence of new technologies, and the international trend toward restructuring and mergers. Furthermore, the flow of funding for pharmaceutical research and development, the lifeblood of the industry worldwide, is threatened by health care reforms introduced by budget-conscious governments around the globe.

These developments are currently at the forefront of the EC Commission's concerns, and have forced it to conclude that "the European pharmaceutical industry needs a better integrated EC-wide market with more open competition to enable it to regain competitiveness and remain a world player" (Commission, 1994: 21). As the plans to achieve this aim make clear, creating an integrated EC-wide market will require considerable regulatory activity on the part of the Community. It is this regulatory activity—past, present, and to a lesser extent, future—with which this chapter is concerned.

## The Nature of Community Regulation

Before examining the process of regulation, some comments on the general EC executive process, and on the relationship between the adoption and the execution of legislation, are in order. In general, the Council of the European Union, in its capacity of legislative decision maker, leaves it to the individual Member States, or to the Commission, to execute the legislation adopted. The Member States have been described as "the mainstream executive branch of the Community government" (Lenaerts, 1993: 24). If a legislative act does not provide for any specific mode of execution, it will be for the member states to take the appropriate measures to ensure effective application and enforcement.

This institutional setup has been described (Frowein, 1986: 586) as a type of executive federalism, in which the division of powers between the central government and the component entities is not only defined in terms of areas in which each government holds substantive competence, but relates also to the division between the central government holding legislative power and the component entities holding executive power. It is within this general framework that the issue of Community pharmaceutical regulation and its impact at the national level must be situated. It must also be remembered that, where Community institutions have not enacted harmonizing legislation, the Member States themselves remain competent to regulate, as long as the resulting rules do not infringe the basic EC Treaty principles of free circulation and undistorted competition.

## Issues of Multiregulation

Given these peculiarities, regulation in the Community context can be characterized as a process of multiregulation involving both the Community and the Member States. Issues of multiregulation can be divided into four broad categories: (1) who should regulate; (2) what should be regulated; (3) what instruments of regulation should be selected; and (4) how should those instruments be enforced.

## Who Should Regulate?

The debate over where Community competence should begin and end, and the corresponding role of the Member States, has been given a new lease on life since the concept of "subsidiarity"—i.e., only legislate where necessary—was incorporated into the text of Article 3(b) of the Treaty of Union (TEU), adopted in Maastricht in December 1991 (Council, 1992). This concept raises issues of *vertical* multiregulation. The subsidiarity principle implies that the regulatory powers of either the Community or the Member States should be confined to a residual category. The question of which level enjoys primary powers and which level may only exercise residual powers in matters of pharmaceutical regulation is not always easy to resolve a priori, as we shall see below. The relationship between Community and national legislation is not a simple hierarchical one.

Community regulation of the pharmaceutical sector also raises questions of potential conflict between industrial policy and health and social protection policy objectives. The TEU has introduced new titles on health policy (Article 129) and on industry (Article 130), which are administered by separate Directorates-General (DGs) within the Commission. This raises problems of what may be termed *horizontal* multiregulation. Policy initiatives originating in various DGs must therefore be coordinated to some degree between DG III (internal market) and DG V (social security and health protection). This aim is often easier to state than to put into practice (Spierenberg, 1979).

The so-called integration principle, contained in Article 129(1) EC, requires the Community to take into account public health policy in its other policies. This requirement had an impact, as is apparent from the tone of the Commission's 1994 Communication on industrial policy for the pharmaceutical sector. Originally designed as a blueprint of future Community action and policy for the sector, the document in fact reflected a vaguely-worded compromise between the aims of DG III and those of DG V (Commission, 1994).

Thus the issue of who can regulate the pharmaceutical sector is not a straightforward one; numerous parties are involved and the relationship between resulting regulatory norms has both a vertical and a horizontal dimension. Furthermore, the Member States, as well as various lobby groups (including the well-organized pharmaceutical industry), have an important if less formalized input at the crucial negotiating and drafting stages.

## What Can Be Regulated?

Until the recent amendments introduced by the TEU, public health concerns had been recognized in Community law primarily in the context of national measures that could legitimately impede the free movement of goods, persons, or services. The Treaty recognizes strictly defined exceptions to these rights, which have been successfully invoked by the Member States to defend their policies regarding cost containment in the pharmaceutical sector.[1] Although a huge amount of Community legislation touches on public health matters, it has not been adopted expressly for this purpose. Instead, the main aim has been to harmonize national legislation to dismantle trade barriers within the market.

Article 3(o) of the EC Treaty, as amended by the TEU, charges the Community with contributing to a high level of health protection. Article 129, which spells out this obligation, marks the first express conferment of direct and active general competence for the Community in the field of public health. It is important to note that Community competence is clearly expressed to be supplementary only: It is to encourage national cooperation and is to be directed at the prevention of diseases, drug dependence, and so on, by the promotion of education and research (Article 129(1)). Community competence in the fields of public health finance and delivery is thus ancillary in nature (Commission, 1993).

Until the amendments were introduced into the Community legal order by the TEU, the Community had no explicit powers to adopt an industry policy. Article 3 of the EC Treaty now includes among the activities of the Community the strengthening of the competitiveness of Community industry. Article 130 specifies the Community industrial objectives, expressed as guidelines for the Commission. The emphasis is on convergence and coordination of national policies.

## What Instruments of Regulation Are To Be Chosen?

The current debate surrounding the Commission's proposed plans for the internal pharmaceutical market revolves around the issue of reconciling a market-based or pro-competition approach to the industry with a more regulatory approach based on concepts of solidarity and social provision. The Community obviously faces a difficult task if it aims to impose convergence on such diametrically opposed national priorities.

The recent debate over subsidiarity has also prompted discussion of whether the Member States should be given more freedom to select the types of instruments with which to pursue Community goals. In principle, the most widely used instrument in Community legislation, the *Directive*, confers considerable discretion on Member States in implementing Community objectives in their own legal systems, although they must guarantee implementation of the goals of Community measures (Commission, 1990).

A *Regulation*, however, is automatic and self-executing at the national level. In the pharmaceutical sector the Council has adopted two Regulations. Regulation 1768/92 creates a supplementary protection certificate (SPC), which provides up to 15 years of protection from the date of first marketing authorization in the Community.[2] This Regulation is intended to address the problem of effective patent protection and operates to supplement intellectual property protection once the original patent has expired. Regulation 2309/93 sets up the European Medicines Evaluation Agency and, with it, a centralized procedure for authorizing the marketing of new products. This is discussed below.

## How Is Regulation To Be Enforced?

It is probably in the sphere of regulatory enforcement that the interplay of Community and national regulation has long been most evident. At the Community level, and outside the field of competition or antitrust law, the possibilities for enforcement are limited; this task is left to the competent authorities of the Member States themselves. In addition, private individuals and companies may enforce their Community legal rights in their national courts, and the latter are obliged to give effect to those rights. Sanctions, such as damages for financial loss for breach of Community norms, are imposed at national, not Community, level.

Even in terms of monitoring national enforcement practices, the Commission has, in general, very limited resources and must rely on the cooperation and goodwill of what are often the very targets of Community regulation – the governments of the Member States. In recent years efforts have been made to reinforce the Community's monitoring function. In some cases this has led to the establishment of specialized Community bodies, but such Community agencies as the European Agency for the Evaluation of Medicinal Products (discussed below) are the exception, not the rule. The recent Council Directive 92/25 on the wholesale distribution of medicinal products for human use promotes cooperation between the relevant authorities by allowing for mutual access to national records (see below).

In conclusion, and to emphasize a point already made, we cannot treat the issue of multiregulation in the Community context as a simple hierarchical process in which regulatory norms stipulated at Community level will automatically displace national norms. Multiregulation must be seen as a complex polydimensional process, with different levels of policy input and output. Moreover, and especially in the current political climate within the Community, regulation may increasingly take the form of nonbinding instruments that are merely declaratory or exhortatory in nature. This is particularly true of the health and social security sectors where cooperation at the national level, gradually converging toward a series of Community nonbinding targets, is the most that is aimed for.[3]

## Some Consequences of Multiregulation

These features of multiregulation have a number of consequences for the development and practice of regulation in the pharmaceutical sector, which are now examined in the context of pricing and reimbursement policy, and policy on parallel imports.

### Pricing and Reimbursement

The almost exclusive competence of the Member States to determine their own levels of public health care and social security protection, as well as the means of financing these systems, would appear to be firmly established.[4] This does not mean that Member States may freely choose to discriminate against products coming from other EC markets in their efforts to cut back their health care budgets. Such a strategy would clearly be in direct conflict with the principle of free movement of goods, one of the cornerstones of the EC Treaty. It remains up to the individual country, however, to determine how much it will spend on health care in general, and on pharmaceuticals in particular. If it chooses to reduce the level of spending, and in doing so purchases a reduced volume of drugs, or will only buy lower-priced products or generic products, there is nothing in EC law that can prevent it from doing so, as long as imported products are not put at a disadvantage.

One may temporarily conclude that, in respect of pricing and cost containment policies, the regulatory relationship between the Community and Member States can be characterized as vertical—but it is clearly the former that plays the residual role. This is further reflected in the actual content of the only Community measure that regulates national price regulations and cost containment policies. This Directive, adopted in 1989, is discussed later in the chapter.

## Parallel Imports

Parallel trade occurs within the EC because of the considerable price differences for identical branded products in different EC markets. Prices have been strictly regulated and held at low levels in countries that have high volumes of drug consumption, such as Portugal, Spain, Greece, France, and Italy. These countries are the main sources of parallel exports to the high-price countries, particularly the United Kingdom and the Netherlands (Commission, 1992: 16).

There are two forms of parallel trade in pharmaceuticals. *Classical* parallel import occurs when a drug is manufactured in two or more EC countries and sold ex-factory at significantly different prices, and is eventually exported to the high-price country where it is sold to a local wholesaler, hospital, or pharmacist at a price below that of the same drug supplied from domestic manufacture. Parallel *reimport* occurs when a drug is exported by the manufacturer from a high-price country, but at a lower price than it commands in the domestic market. This means that the manufacturer has accepted a low price imposed by the national health authority in the export market. The drug reaches an importer or wholesaler in the low-price market, who then ships it back to the high-price market where it can still be sold at a lower price than the identical drug through the standard distribution system.

No official statistics exist for parallel trade, but the Commission has estimated that the total value of parallel trade in the EC can be estimated at between ECU 370–435 million, or about 2% of the prescription market. Assuming the continuation of price differentials and regulatory and commercial factors, studies for the Commission estimated that parallel trade in the EC could grow at an annual rate of 5 to 12% between 1990 and 1995.

Interestingly, the Commission devotes only a few lines in its 1994 Communication to the issue of parallel imports. It recognizes that parallel imports, along with generics, are important for multisource competition (Commission, 1994: 19). Given that the Court of Justice has always maintained that parallel imports are legal, irrespective of the factors that determine price differences, it would be impossible for the Commission to oppose this form of trade. If parallel trading is to be eliminated, or at least reduced, it would be necessary for the Commission to tackle the problem at its source: the wide variations that exist at national level in pricing and reimbursement policies. This would in turn require the adoption of far-reaching regulation.

# Consolidating the Internal Market for Pharmaceuticals

As already mentioned, one of the primary aims of European pharmaceutical industry policy is to remove barriers created by differences in national legislation and to ensure that pharmaceutical products can move freely from the place of production to the eventual place of consumption.[5] Indeed, this is a long-standing policy aim, one that has generated considerable Community regulation (Thompson, 1994). Nevertheless, progress has been uneven and the degree of harmonization of national controls is by no means uniform across the many aspects of pharmaceutical regulation. This section examines regulatory developments in the field of product licensing, distribution, and pricing.

## *Product Licensing*

Until recently the regulatory initiatives adopted in the field of pharmaceutical marketing requirements could be broadly placed in the category of vertical regulation. Under the terms of a series of directives adopted between 1965 and 1989, the Community attempted to implement the so-called decentralized approach to marketing authorizations. To ensure that products already authorized on one Member State's market were admitted to another's, the national authorities were required to recognize the existing product licenses.

This process of mutual recognition never quite worked in the way intended (Hancher, 1990). Although the intention was to create a hierarchical relationship, with Community norms taking precedence over national rules, the decentralized approach to pharmaceutical product licensing was eventually judged to be a failure. National differences remained and each Member State was reluctant to recognize and automatically endorse licenses granted by another national authority. Products were subjected to further tests and clinical trials before being admitted to the market.

In terms of the categories of regulation outlined earlier, the most recent regulatory initiatives adopted by the Community exhibit a tendency to move away from the multiregulatory form based on this vertical division of competences at Community and national levels, to a *unitary* form of regulation centralized at the Community level. Community regulation effectively displaces national regulation, at least with respect to certain types of pharmaceutical products.

This process is at its most evident in the arrangements for the functioning of the new European Medicines Evaluation Agency. In European terms this is a unique regulatory institution. Consensus on its creation and functions was by no means easy to obtain.[6] The latest legislation provides for a new marketing authorization system for medicinal products for human and veterinary use, and at the same time establishes the new agency.[7] Firms wishing to gain access to the European market within 300 days are able to choose one of two procedures:

A centralized procedure, leading to a single authorization or license valid across the whole EC. This procedure is reserved for certain new, high-technology medicinal products. It is mandatory for all products derived from biotechnology.

A decentralized procedure, designed for the majority of medicinal products. This procedure is based on mutual recognition of national marketing authorizations. Where disputes arise, they will be settled by a compulsory, binding Community arbitration procedure.

## The Centralized Procedure

Under the new centralized procedure, the Member States will lose their powers to license or refuse to license products derived from biotechnology. If the manufacturer so chooses, the national authorities will no longer exercise any control over the admission of high-technology products to their markets. They may refuse access to their markets for a product licensed by the Agency only in exceptional circumstances. However, experts from the national regulatory authorities will be used by the Agency to provide the necessary scientific support.[8] It will be for the Agency, and eventually the EC institutions, to act on these scientific evaluations, and to grant the requisite Community-wide licenses.

## The Decentralized Procedure

Even under the decentralized procedures, as amended by the 1993 Directives, the individual Member States have lost a substantial degree of control over marketing authorization policy. In its ruling in Case C83/92 *Pierrel v Ministero della Sanita*,[9] the court held that the existing pre-1992 Directives represented a high degree of harmonization. Member States could no longer withdraw a product license, except on the basis of the criteria stipulated in the relevant Community measures. Any other national criteria had become redundant.

In the early case 104/75 *De Peiper*[10] the court held that, until Community harmonization in the area of pharmaceutical product licenses had been fully achieved, national product licensing regimes were not contrary to Article 30 EC, which prohibits quantitative restrictions or measures of equivalent effect. The court stated that national licensing procedures could be permitted under Article 36 EC, as long as their operation was in line with Treaty objectives. The *De Peiper* case concerned the parallel importation of a product, Valium, which had been licensed in both the exporting country (the United Kingdom) and the importing country (the Netherlands) by its original manufacturer. The court interpreted Articles 30 and 36 to require only less onerous procedures for the licensing of such products, and not automatic acceptance of a product licensed elsewhere in the Community.[11]

In the recent case C347/89 *Freistaat Bayern v Eurim-Pharm GmbH*,[12] the court was asked to consider the legality of certain aspects of the German law on medicinal products of 1976, and in particular a requirement that medicinal products imported from other Member States should be labeled and accompanied by a package insert in conformity with the German law on medicines at the time of importation. The court ruled that these additional restrictions on importation were not required for the effective protection of human health and life. This was already guaranteed by the requirement that producers should hold manufacturing and marketing authorizations.

The principle of effective protection has been further applied by the court in case C62/90 *Commission v Germany*, which concerned the legality of a German provision banning the importation by post by a private person of medicines lawfully prescribed by a doctor and dispensed by a pharmacist in another Member State.[13] The court had no difficulty in concluding that the various measures harmonizing marketing authorizations for medicines, as well as the directives harmonizing qualifications in the medical and pharmacy professions, combined to produce an effective guarantee that the public health was adequately protected, and that the ban on importation by post served no justifiable purpose.

It remains to be seen whether, once the reinforced decentralized procedure is fully implemented as on 1 January 1995 by the Member States, the court will be prepared to consider that a sufficient level of harmonization has been achieved to protect the public interest and therefore require automatic mutual recognition of marketing legislation.

## Regulation of Distribution

The Commission hopes, perhaps optimistically, that the creation of the new Agency will help to reduce the diversity in pharmaceutical distribution. In the meantime, the so-called rational use package of directives was adopted in 1992. The directive on wholesale distribution of medicines[14] will facilitate and stimulate intra-Community trade, while ensuring the integrity of transactions, regulating recall of defective products, and deterring counterfeit products. Two related directives, on medicines advertising[15] and on labeling and leaflets,[16] will standardize and improve information for patients, limit waste and unnecessary duplication, and impose requirements on promotion to health professionals. Both these measures make it compulsory to mention in all relevant information the common designation, or generic name, of the product. Finally, Council Directive 92/26 on classification harmonizes, at least at a minimum level, classification criteria for medicinal products that may only be obtained on medical prescription.[17]

Member States still enjoy considerable scope to determine what goods are sold on prescription, as well as what products are available only in pharmacies. Access to so-called over-the-counter (OTC) products varies significantly from one EC country to another. The Community has not begun to tackle the regulation of retail distribution, never mind the thorny issues of the very different margins pharmacists can earn on prescription and nonprescription products. The European Court of Justice also has proved reluctant to attack pharmacists' monopolies over a wide range of pharmaceuticals and parapharmaceuticals (that is, homeopathic and traditional preparations).[18] Given the considerable differences in the way all these matters are regulated at national level, the EC pharmaceutical market remains firmly divided on national lines.

## Pricing and Reimbursement

If considerable progress has been achieved on product licensing, and at least a start has been made on distribution, the Community has been less successful in its attempts to reduce price differentials. In the absence of Community legislation, Member States retain considerable discretion to adopt various types of price or profit control measures and cost containment strategies. The Court of Justice has been reluctant to denounce such controls as contrary to the EC Treaty rules of free movement of goods.

Although national laws do not usually have to be overtly discriminatory and block imports in order to fall foul of Article 30 EC, the Court of Justice has consistently refused to rule that price controls automatically constitute measures having an effect equivalent to quantitative restrictions on imports. Material discrimination or concrete proof that imported products have been put at a disadvantage must be demonstrated.[19] Similarly, profit controls will not infringe Community law provided that producers remain free to determine their own retail prices and could thereby adapt their prices to their own cost structures.[20]

In the important case 238/82 *Duphar*, the court considered the legality of a so-called negative list that excluded certain expensive products from reimbursement by health insurance institutions, and held that such schemes may be compatible with Article 30, hence recognizing that Member States have a legitimate interest in controlling drug budgets. Given this cautious attitude of the Court of Justice, it would seem that further progress can only be achieved by the adoption of harmonizing regulations at Community level.

## Community Controls

In 1989 the Council adopted a Directive relating to the transparency of measures regulating the pricing of medicinal products for human use and their inclusion in national health insurance schemes.[21] This measure began a process whereby disparities in price and reimbursement regulatory schemes are to be gradually eliminated. The controls themselves were not to be eliminated. The Directive merely requires a certain amount of transparency or openness in the way pricing and related decisions are taken by the relevant national authorities. In addition, the Directive requires that national authorities respond within 90 days to applications for prices for new products or price revisions for existing products, and review any imposed price freeze at least once a year.

By making controls more transparent, the basic objective is "to enable all concerned to verify that the requirements of Community law are being respected by laying down a series of rules regarding time limits, the reasoning and publication of decisions, and so on, which would be directly effective so that those concerned may defend their interests in the national courts" (Commission, 1986).

## Attempts at Reform

In a Discussion Document published in mid 1991, the Commission considered two alternative strategies that might be pursued at this second stage (Commission, 1991b):

> To deepen the transparency of the policies and measures taken by the Member States
>
> To seek an alignment of these policies by harmonizing a number of their aspects

The first option would have required strengthening existing vertical regulation, as well as requiring Member States to take measures to ensure more transparency in the way pharmaceutical companies calculated costs and determined prices. The second option, which sought harmonization of national policies, would have had more far-reaching regulatory effects, but would have been difficult to realize, especially as national reimbursement regimes are becoming more complex and their cost-containment policies more finely tuned. Several Member States, including the Netherlands and Germany and, to some extent, the United Kingdom, have devised and subsequently refined ways of limiting expenditure on reimbursable medicines by the introduction of reference pricing systems.

The Commission also considered whether harmonization of reference price systems eventually might be necessary. Given that there is no objective reason why therapeutic classification should vary from one Member State to another, the adoption of a common therapeutic classification was contemplated. Precedents for common classifications already exist; namely the anatomical-therapeutic-chemical (ATC) classification adopted by the Nordic Council and practiced by the World Health Organization.

Obviously the introduction of a centralized system of therapeutic classification at the Community level would lead to a considerable concentration of vertical regulatory power. Not surprisingly, it was opposed by most of the Member States who commented on the Commission's discussion document (Commission, 1991a). The European Federation of Pharmaceutical Industry Associations (EFPIA) have taken the view that reimbursement is a national rather than an EC matter, and that questions of subsidiarity may arise in the future. At the same time, the European pharmaceutical industry has persistently claimed that reference pricing distorts clinical decision making, deprives patients of a choice of treatment, and removes incentives to conduct research into new medicines.

Progress on amending the 1989 Directive proved problematic. In late 1991 the Commission prepared draft amendments intended to impose greater transparency on marketing costs for reimbursable medicines and to make it compulsory for Member States to give it advance notice of any draft new law relating to prices. Following discussions, in December 1992 the Commission announced that it would not proceed with the proposed legislative measure at all, but that it would press ahead with the creation of a Community-wide database.[22]

A draft Recommendation was planned that would aim to reconcile national concerns about the rising cost of health care and free circulation of medicines with the necessity to promote R&D on new medicines as the basis of a high level of health protection. Although Recommendations are legally nonbinding, the Commission's early drafts provoked adverse reactions from both the Member States and the industry, and the tone of the proposed measure was further weakened. The draft was subsequently abandoned, and the Commission indicated that the proposals would eventually reappear as part of a package on industrial policy for the industry. It was this policy document that eventually appeared in March 1994.

## Toward a Community Industry Policy

At around the same time that negotiations over the amendments to the 1989 Directive were taking place, and apparently out of concern about the EFPIA's warnings over the European industry's long-term future, the Commissioner responsible for industrial policy matters set up a special advisory task force comprising experts from the leading European companies and Commission officials working together to produce a draft directive aimed at guaranteeing free pricing for new products, a phasing in of more general price liberalization, and increased patient co-payment (EFPIA, 1992).

As already indicated, the industry's views were not allowed to prevail. Whereas DG III (internal market) had originally planned to address its industrial policy aims to the most serious concerns of the European drug companies—the increasingly severe national controls on pricing and reimbursement—the final version of the 1994 Communication abandoned the deregulation of pricing controls recommended in earlier drafts by DG III and backed by the industry (*Financial Times*, 1994). The Commissioner responsible for social security affairs made it clear that national health services would not be asked to adapt to the needs of the drug industry. As a result of all the horse trading between the various parts of the Commission, the so-called Community strategy has been very much diluted.

The Member States are the ultimate beneficiaries of this infighting. They retain almost unconditional autonomy to manage their own health care budgets, including pharmaceutical pricing and reimbursement regimes. The Commission expresses an optimistic hope that these national policies can eventually converge, if loosely directed at Community level.

The 1994 Communication makes it equally clear that although the Commission expresses a commitment to fostering the advantages of multisource competition—that is, generics and parallel imports—the Community will not enact any regulatory measures or other incentives to do so. The Community's role will be to ensure that the 1989 Directive is complied with and that no discrimination occurs.

## Conclusion

This chapter has focused primarily on the development of, and contrast between, two different aspects of multiregulation in the European Community. It has indicated that substantial progress toward removing the complex barriers to the creation of an internal market will require the transfer and unique centralization of regulatory power in a new Community agency. However, the latest package of directives, adopted in 1992, establish little more than a minimal level of harmonization. Member States still retain a substantial degree of autonomy to regulate the marketing, distribution, and dispensing of medicines. In the crucial area of pricing and cost containment, the Member States retain almost full autonomy, and the regulatory role of the Community is, at most, residual. Indeed, national policies appear to be diverging rather than converging.

The Commission's latest attempt to reconcile the growing problem of divergent national regulatory policies with its objective of creating a more conducive regulatory environment for the European drug industry, as expressed in its 1994 policy document, has been to try to fashion a broader policy framework in which to address the various dimensions of pharmaceutical policy and health care. The new Medicines

Agency will serve as a focal point for enhanced cooperation among the Member States in matters of R&D, with the aim of avoiding duplication of projects. Enhanced cooperation in the industry at the level of research and development is also being encouraged through the provision of funding, particularly in biotechnology.[23]

It is unlikely that the Community will ever achieve sufficient political consensus to impose a centralized system of price and reimbursement regulation on its member states. In the current political climate, with its emphasis on subsidiarity, this would prove an impossible task. Therefore, one may ask whether the Community will have to seek an alternative to the traditional forms of multiregulation via harmonization, which has been its dominant strategy in the past. The 1994 policy document indicates a preference for a Community convergence of aims within a broad policy framework and the subsequent coordination of national regulation.

This writer would suggest, however, that the removal of barriers through harmonization, and hence through regulation, is still the Community's major task. A shift toward convergence and cooperation is not sufficient to achieve a single market for pharmaceuticals. The problems and consequences of multiregulation will not disappear. Perhaps the only feasible solution is for both the Member States and the Community institutions to recognize these problems and to attempt to find more efficient ways of dealing with them.

## Notes

1. These exceptions are to be found in Article 36 EC and allow Member States to restrict free movement of goods if this is justified in the interests of public policy, public security, public order, or on public health grounds. See generally, case 238/82 *Duphar v Netherlands* [1984] ECR 523 (reimbursement policy).

2. *Official Journal of the European Community* (O.J.) 1992 L182/1.

3. See Resolution of the Council and the Ministers for Health, Meeting with the Council of 11 November 1991, O.J. 1991, C304/5; Council Recommendation 92/442 on the convergence of social protection objectives and policies, O.J. 1992 C245/49. See most recently the Commission's White Paper on Health (1993).

4. See also Council Recommendation 92/442/EEC of 27 July 1992 on the convergence of social protection objectives and policies in the Member States, O.J. 1992 L245/49.

5. The report on the "Cost of Non-Europe for Pharmaceuticals," which was sponsored by the EC Commission, estimated that the opportunity cost for the pharmaceutical industry of remaining barriers to trade in these products could be between ECU 160 to 533 million, equivalent to 0.6 to 2.1% of sales.

6. *Agence Europe* (a daily newsheet of EC developments) of 6/7 July 1992, pp. 11–12 for a description of the various positions taken by the Member States at the Council meeting of June 1992.

7. Regulation 2309/93 and Directives 93/39, 93/40 and 93/41 (O.J. 1993 L214/1).

8. The Agency's management is to be entrusted to an administrative board that will consist of two representatives from each Member State, two representatives of the Commission, and two representatives appointed by the European Parliament—Article 56(1) of the Regulation.

9. Judgment of December 7, 1993.

10. [1976] ECR 613.

11. See also case 32/80 *Kortmann* [1981] ECR 1098. The Commission subsequently issued a Communication on Parallel Imports, offering guidelines on how *Centrafarm* might be complied with. Several countries, including the Netherlands, Ireland, and the United Kingdom have adopted simplified procedures for parallel imports.

12. [1991] ECR I-1747.

13. [1993] ECR I-2601.

14. Council Directive 92/25, O.J. 1992 L113/1.

15. Council Directive 92/28, O.J. 1992 L113/13.

16. Council Directive 92/27, O.J. 1992 L113/8.

17. O.J. 1992 L113/5.

18. Case C369/88 *Delattre* [1991] ECR 1-1487; case C60/89 *Monteil* [1991] ECR I-1547; case C271/92 *LPO v UNSOF* [1993] ECR I-2919. Its latest ruling in case C292/92 *Hunermund*, (15.12.93, not yet reported) confirms this cautious position.

19. For a detailed explanation of the Court's approach to the interpretation of Article 30, see further, White (1989).

20. Case 78/82 *Commission v Italy* [1983] ECR 1995; case 231/83 *Cullet*, op. cit.

21. Directive 89/105, O.J. 1989 L40/8.

22. At the request of the European Parliament, the Commission will endeavor to develop in close cooperation with the Member States a European databank on medicinal products— ECPHIN, the European Community Pharmaceutical Products Information Network. This will contain data of a therapeutic nature, information on price, cost of treatment, eligibility for reimbursement, classification, etc.

23. Biotechnology Research for Innovation Development and Growth in Europe, BRIDGE, was established for three years in 1990 and had a budget of 100 million ecus. Promotion and coordination of R&D efforts in the pharmaceutical sector is one of the priority objectives of the fourth Community framework program for research and development 1994 through 1998.

# References

Commission of the European Communities (1986) *Report on the Implementation of the Transparency Directive 89/105*. Brussels.

Commission of the European Communities (1990) *The Rules Governing Medicinal Products for Human Use in the EC*. Vol. I, II, III, and IV, plus Addendum no. 1 (1990) and no. 2 (1992). Luxembourg.

Commission of the European Communities (1991a) Compilation of responses to the discussion document on the elaboration of the proposal referred to in Article 9 of Directive 89/105. Brussels.

Commission of the European Communities (1991b) Discussion Document on the Elaboration of the Proposal Referred To in Article 9 of Directive 89/105/EEC. III/3001/91. Brussels.

Commission of the European Communities (1992) *Impediments to Parallel Trade in Pharmaceuticals within the EC*. Brussels.

Commission of the European Communities (1993) *Communication of 24 November 1993 on a Community Strategy in the Field of Public Health*. Com (93) 559. Brussels.

Commission of the European Communities (1994) *The Outlines of an Industrial Policy for the Pharmaceutical Sector in the EC*. Com (93) 718, final. Brussels.

Council of the European Community (1992) *Treaty on European Union, 7 February 1992*. Luxembourg: Office of Official Publications of the EC.

EFPIA (European Federation of Pharmaceutical Industry Associations) (1992) *Memorandum on an Industrial Policy for the European Pharmaceutical Industry*. Brussels: EFPIA.

*Financial Times* (1994) March 23, p. 8.

Frowein JA (1986) Integration and the Federal Experience in Germany and Switzerland. In: Cappelletti M, Seccombe M, and Weiler J (eds.) *Integration Through Law*. Berlin: De Gruyter, pp. 300–304.

Hancher L (1990) *Regulating for Competition*. Oxford: Clarendon Press.

Lenaerts K (1993) Regulating the regulatory process. *European Law Journal* 18: 23–49.

Spierenburg D (1979) *Proposals for the Reform of the Commission and its Services*. Report made by an Independent Review Body under the Chairmanship of Mr. D. Spierenburg, Sept. 1979. Luxembourg: EC Commission.

Thompson R (1994) *The Single Market for Pharmaceuticals*. London: Butterworths.

White E (1989) In search of the limits of Article 30, *Common Market Law Review* 26: 235–51.

# 12

# The Liberalization of Access to Medication in the United States and Europe

PAULINE VAILLANCOURT ROSENAU
CHRISTINE THOER

Access to prescription medication is being liberalized widely in the industrialized nations. In this chapter, we seek to understand and assess it in the context of larger currents and as influenced by ongoing social, political, and economic events. Liberalization takes different forms and involves several mechanisms, including: switching medication from prescription to over-the-counter (OTC) availability, crossing borders to obtain medication restricted in one country but not in another, and employing medication for purposes other than those for which it was approved (so-called off-label use).[1]

Liberalization of access may be defined in a number of ways, encompassing financial, legal, and therapeutic availability. While the direction of greater access may be clear, the forces that drive it are not the same in every country. Differences between Europe and the United States are of special interest here. We examine how liberalization of access is influenced by government strategy, individual interests, political philosophy, policy goals, and professional concerns. We analyze these factors and conclude with some reflections for the future.

## The State

A key player in the liberalization of access to medication is the state, since governments have the power to define prescribing rights and control access to medicines in various ways. A number of sometimes conflicting currents are at play in this arena.

## Cost Containment in the United States

In both Europe and North America, governments have attempted in recent years to control drug expenditures. One way to save is to encourage self-care, which reduces both doctor visits and the use of expensive prescription medications (Fleming et al., 1984; Deletraz-Delporte, 1992). The *New England Journal* suggests "that providing medical consumers with information and guidelines about self-management can lower rates of use of services, often by 7–17 percent" (Fries et al., 1993: 322). Governments wishing to reduce health care costs by encouraging self-care must increase access to prescription medication. If the general availability of OTCs makes self-care viable, switching prescription medication to OTC status encourages it even more.

In the United States during the 1980s, more than 200 drugs were switched from prescription to OTC (Segal, 1991: 8).[2] The Nonprescription Drug Manufacturers Association (NDMA) estimates that more than 400 OTC products now use ingredients or dosages available only by prescription 15 years ago (NDMA, 1991; Newton et al., 1994).[3] The medications now available on demand are not just those that "relieve symptoms of minor, self-limiting conditions." They include medications of substantial importance that "prevent diseases" and "manage chronic conditions" (Young, 1988: 6).[4]

The impact of switching on the medication practices of citizens and on doctor-patient relations is tremendous. Neither are the financial dimensions of the prescription to OTC switch trivial. Switched drugs have improved the profit margin of pharmaceutical manufacturers (Rosen, 1991). All but one of the ten best-selling OTC drugs introduced since 1975, including Advil, Nuprin, Sudafed, and Benadryl, was a switched drug (NDMA, 1991; Cope, 1991: 7). It is estimated that nearly $50 million in payments for doctor visits was saved in 1989 alone when cold remedies were switched from prescription to OTC status (Temin, 1990: 3). One third of a billion dollars was saved when .5% hydrocortisone was switched (NDMA, 1991). By the year 2000, the savings are expected to be nearly $20 billion (Proprietary Association, 1988: 17).

## Cost Containment in Europe

All European countries are presently facing escalating expenditures and sometimes efforts to contain costs actually reduce financial access to medication. The number of medicines switched from prescription to OTC to contain costs varies from country to country in Europe. Some European governments are trying to ease the switching process for pharmaceutical companies. The need to adopt a uniform registration system in Europe will certainly reinforce this trend. In 1992, the British government authorized an annual timetable of switching for 1993 to speed the process. This meant that switching could be accomplished within a year.

The prescription to OTC switch does not always prove as profitable to companies in Europe as in the United States. In the United Kingdom, the introduction in 1985 of the Black List, a list of drugs not reimbursed, did not result in a subsequent growth of the OTC market. In Denmark, where many prescription medicines were switched in 1984 and 1989, including ulcer treatments such as Tagamet (Cimetidine) and Zantac (Ranitidine), the increase of consumption was, in most cases, relatively limited (Juul, 1991). For the same reason, and because the French view reimbursement status as a "label of quality," when patent medications (tonic phials) were delisted in the early 1990s and became available to the public without prescription, their sales dropped rapidly (Jolly, 1993).

There are few studies of the savings and safety of switching drugs from prescription to OTC status. In Denmark, where the switch movement is well advanced, the experience was generally positive (Juul, 1991; Bagger-Hansen, 1991). In 1989, 80 products based on 20 prescription ingredients were switched to OTC status. However, the switch process was guided by very strict principles; to be considered for a switch a drug had to be safe in ordinary use, possess no risk of overdose or abuse, be indicated for minor ailments that do not require the diagnosis of a physician, require no professional supervision, and have been on the market for a long time. Careful estimates established that the National Health Care Insurance system saved US$1.5 million annually—in addition to savings from the diminished number of doctor visits. Switching appears relatively safe even in the case of $H_2$ Blockers, causing minimum serious adverse drug reactions (Juul, 1991).

One major force for liberalization of medication in Europe is the unification envisioned by the European Economic Community. Different countries have different rules regarding medications (Burstall, 1991). Harmonizing regulations regarding medications is desirable because without border surveillance between countries, as is now the case within the EEC, such rules are unenforceable. But strong forces oppose interfering with national pharmaceutical regulations, including the regulatory bodies in each country and the pharmaceutical industry (Orzack et al., 1992).

## Supranational Trends – Harmonization in the European Community

The European Commission recently proposed pharmaceutical legislation to provide for the movement of medicinal products in the EC. The European Community adopted four key directives regarding wholesale distribution, classification, labeling, and advertising of drugs. The EC is also discussing a community-wide registration system under which a drug approved in one country would be registered in other countries through mutual recognition, thereby speeding up the marketing process throughout the EC. A sole European drug agency, which will start operating in 1995, would be in charge of the registration of biotechnical drugs and would arbitrate differences in the mutual recognition process. Mutual recognition will be required for OTCs, but if a member state does not recognize the marketing authorization issued by another country, the European Agency for Medicine Evaluation (EAME) will be responsible for mediating differences and producing a binding decision (De Guili, 1992).

The EC's classification directive (92/26/EEC) is the most important with regard to the increasing availability of prescription drugs. The EC classification lists should stimulate harmonization of drug classification and may lead to a growth in switching, especially in countries where the OTC market is still underdeveloped. Indeed, governments that have maintained a strict regulatory policy might consider switching a drug if they realize that it is being sold OTC in other European countries without ill effects (De Guili, 1992).

Forces against harmonization certainly exist, and for many reasons complete harmonization will not be achieved in the short run (Burstall, 1991: 167). Medications are used for different purposes in the various EC countries (Mela, 1992). Also, the medical culture of the EC is quite diverse. Classification deals with the public health policies of each country and involves matters such as the practice of medicine, methods of treatment and diagnosis, and prescribing habits of physicians, all of which are influenced by culture (Payer, 1988). Such cultural factors are very slow to change.

Distribution patterns vary in the EC and this slows harmonization. One EC directive addresses wholesale distribution; increasing the availability of drugs implies expanding the distribution network. In France, the Public Health Code is interpreted very strictly and products defined as medications, that is, having therapeutical effects (Art. L 511 of Public Health Code), are available only in pharmacies where they are stored behind the counter and must be requested from the pharmacist (Fielding and Lancry, 1993; Umbrecht, 1992). This is likely to change since French consumers associations and grocery chain stores are lobbying for liberalization, asking that the pharmacists' monopoly on OTCs be eliminated and that nonpharmaceutical outlets, such as supermarkets, be allowed to sell parapharmaceutical products.[5]

## The Decline of State Control in the United States and Europe

In the United States, as in Europe, the state has its own needs that affect the rate and timing of liberalization of access. To the extent that making prescription medication more easily available is viewed as a cost-containment measure, it is likely to be supported. But the cost-containment potentials of liberalized access to medication are complex and results vary from medication to medication and from person to person.

In the United States over the last decade there has been a growing suspicion about the competence of government bureaucracy and the legitimacy of state intervention. The trend to switch from prescription to OTC parallels the desire to reduce government's role. In the 1930s the spirit of regulation received broad approval and the government's monitoring of unsafe medication to protect citizens was viewed as appropriate (Temin, 1980: 55). Efforts to reduce the power of the FDA in order to accord freer access to medication began in the mid 1970s (Wardell and Lasagna, 1975). By the 1980s, sentiment grew for allowing citizens to assume their own risks, not just in the case of medication but in all areas of life (Temin, 1980).

Disenchantment with government has not been the same in Europe as in the United States. Here it reflects concerns arising from a different experience (Huttin, 1992). In most European countries universal comprehensive health care coverage has been considered a basic right. However, this view is being challenged by those who attribute the increasing health expenditures in their countries to government intervention. As in the United States, they argue that the state's overwhelming and paternalistic involvement in the health care sector has produced an inefficient system by removing individual responsibility.

In Europe, where confidence in market mechanisms is less than in the United States, concern with pharmaceutical prices has led to direct government control – price restrictions and limitations on doctors' prescribing power – rather than switching medication to OTC and eliminating the state's responsibility to reimburse for it. The role of the state as protector, responsible for individual welfare, has not been challenged to the same extent that it has in the United States. Revision of prescription status is certainly occurring, but more to serve the needs of the state in its new form (the EC) than to diminish its influence.

## The Consumer

In the United States, liberalization of access to medication is part of a larger societal trend toward individual rights, human rights, civil rights, and the "public acceptance of the notion of rights as applied to health care" (Beauchamp, 1990: 148; see also Cope, 1991). Democracy and participation trends are on the rise globally and the liberalization of access to medication is in line with this trend as well.

### The Medically Empowered Individual – The United States

A number of assumptions are associated with the advocacy of increased access to medication. Consumers of health care are thought to be analytically skilful and consequently able to make decisions about their own health (Silverman, 1987: 1; Blishen, 1991: 146).[6] Highly educated citizens gain confidence in their own medical knowledge (Fleming and Andersen, 1976: 49). Self-medication was practiced widely at the beginning of the century before the medical community gained recognition for expertise, and empirical studies report that self-medication is once again making gains. Citizens have "demanded more freedom to self-medicate and to exert control over their own health" (Cope, 1991: 4).

American individualism, expressed as the desire to have control over one's destiny, reinforces the trend toward self-medication. Self-medication has been assumed to be a "God-given right" (Silverman and Lee, 1974). A moderate assessment argues that patients in the United States have forgone significant health benefits because of regulatory delays in return for only modest benefits from their reduced exposure to risk (Grabowski and Vernon, 1983). Extremists go so far as to contend that people even have the right to kill themselves with home remedies if they so desire (Silverman and Lee, 1974: 211). Prescription status of drugs is assumed to interfere with self-medication (Temin, 1979), while the greater availability of powerful OTCs encourages it.

Prescription status implies a model of medicine in which a patient consults a doctor and complies with instructions without questioning or requiring much explanation. Patient power is on the rise and doctors are increasingly expected to negotiate treatment with patients and to relate to them as equals (Beauchamp, 1990: 145). Some even suggest the professional MD's new role will be that of an advisor or partner, except in instances where the patient is unconscious (Blishen, 1991: 147). Patient preference plays an increasing role in medical decisions and researchers suggest ways of presenting risk data so that patients can assess whether they want to accept the diagnosis and treatment recommended by their doctor (Chassin et al., 1987: 2457). Physicians are encouraging patients to make medical decisions where efficacy of alternative medical treatments are in doubt (Kolata, 1994). Self-medication advocates even argue that "consumers will be the primary practitioners in the new health care system" (Ferguson, 1992: 9; see also Gordon, 1993).

Self-treatment implies self-diagnosis followed by self-medication, and the means necessary for both are increasingly available, at least in some states. Manuals to assist lay individuals in interpreting the results of medical tests are available (Sobel and Ferguson, 1985). In California today, consumers can initiate self-tests that in the past only physicians could order. They may request a blood test given by a commercial enterprise in a drug store or supermarket, pay for the test, and obtain the results, without ever consulting a physician. Flu shots are sold at the local grocery store in many states (Smothers, 1993). In many cases the medication necessary for treatment of the self-diagnosed illness is available OTC.

## Social Movements and Industry Needs

Political activism in the form of social movements and the expansion of individual rights has contributed to the liberalization of access to medication. The legitimacy of such political and social actions rests on questioning modern scientific medical knowledge. Challenges to medical expertise are not without a basis and this explains why they have been so successful and why access has increased. The present state of science does not allow for "the selection of a unique 'best drug'" (Temin, 1980: 8–12). Drug effectiveness is vaguely defined and poorly measured. Side effects vary from person to person. Studies of these phenomena are expensive and difficult. Most doctors lack the technical skill to evaluate drugs in every case (Temin, 1980). Prescription drug choices, as it turns out, are often customs sustained by the local medical community rather than a designation of the best drug available. The broad distribution of information about liability suits, medical mistakes, and the suggestion of widespread inappropriate use of medical procedures (Wenneker et al., 1990: 1259), have also made the public more critical and suspicious of medical expertise (Lambert, 1978; Blishen, 1991: 146).

At the same time, allowing politics to dominate science does not always produce a better outcome. Political pressure to stop tests of AZT in the United States in 1989 meant that the drug was made available to all those HIV positive. In Europe, where health officials were far less likely to be responsive to advocacy groups and political pressure, the tests were continued and it was discovered that the benefits were not nearly as great as those manifest in the short-term U.S. studies. Prescription patterns and medical recommendations for use have been dramatically modified as a result of the longer tests (see summary in Altman, 1993). But it would have been politically impossible to have continued the AZT drug trials in the United States.

Social movements seeking liberalized access to medication are constructed on any number of bases. International linkages have been established around a specific disease facilitating drug provision by mail or by personal transportation designed to circumvent government regulation in one country for a drug that is available in another country (Johnson, 1991). The impossibility of controlling access across international boundaries puts governments on the defensive and makes the task of regulatory agencies very difficult.

Some of the political activity initiated to liberalize access to medication makes for unexpected and unconventional alliances. The pharmaceutical industry has worked with AIDS support groups in the United States to lobby government to liberalize access to experimental medications for AIDS patients. The political efficacy of small, extra-parliamentary groups such as Act Up have made them a model of effective political organization for change. The *New York Times* revealed that the prescription drug industry created and financed a consumer organization called The Coalition for Equal Access to Medicines, which is made up of "poor people, minority members, and public health advocates." The issue that prompted the manufacturer's gesture was the Congressional proposal to contain costs of drug reimbursement by using formularies for Medicaid programs. Both low-income individuals and the prescription drug industry share the goal of having government continue to pay for whatever medications are prescribed by physicians, no matter what the cost (Pear, 1993: A1, A12).

## The Industry

Pharmaceutical companies are concerned with the liberalization of access to prescription medication largely to the extent that it affects their profit potential. The distinction between prescription and OTC producers is breaking down. As drugs are switched the marketing strategy for a medication includes sale, first as a prescription medication, and later as an OTC. Prescription companies establish divisions that will take charge of the OTC distribution.

In the United States the pharmaceutical companies' enthusiasm for the liberalization of medication is conflicted. On one hand they favor removing government regulation across the board on ideological grounds (Young, 1988: 24). On the other hand, pharmaceutical companies receive substantial financial assistance from the government to develop new drugs. They favor government intervention in this aspect of pharmaceutical research and drug development.

Another major concern of the pharmaceutical industry is legal liability. While liberalization in many cases promises greater profits, it would not be attractive if it led to greater risks of legal problems because of the misuse of the more easily available medications.

In Europe pharmaceutical companies generally favor prescription to OTC switching. They view it as a way to escape strict government price controls and scale back generic competition (Ball, 1992). However, some national companies have mixed feelings since the switched drugs have not always proved as profitable in Europe as they have in the United States. The PAGB (Proprietary Association of Great Britain), on the other hand, has actively worked to encourage a climate of opinion that would favor switching.

## The Professions

The medical community appears divided on the advisability of liberalization of medication in the form it has taken in the United States, but ironically they have acted to expand it even though such action is, arguably, not in their self-interest. Prescription to OTC switching, for example, reduces physicians' income and diminishes their power vis-à-vis the patient.

### The Changing Medical Profession in the United States

Physicians have failed to defend their professional interests for several reasons. The prestige of the medical profession has been on the decline in the United States. MDs find themselves with less autonomy because payer organizations monitor their performance, question their diagnoses, and challenge their treatment protocols. This has meant, perhaps for psychological reasons alone, that they have been demoralized and that they are less effective in defending their own interests.

A consensus in the medical profession is lacking on greater access to medication. Liberalization appears undesirable to older members of the medical profession, but new members seem to accept it. For example, older, male, well-established solo practitioners seem less likely than younger, female specialists with low-volume practices to have a preference for switched drugs (Madhavan and Gore, 1994).

In the United States the medical profession plays another role in liberalization with the off-label use of prescription medications. In this instance, it retains control and enhances its own gatekeeper function. Off-label use involves a physician prescribing a drug already tested and licensed for treatment of one disease, for a different condition, disease, or illness. The prescription of beta blockers for performance anxiety is an example. There is widespread tolerance of physicians experimenting with such medication in ways not approved by the FDA. Flexibility for the physician may empower patients, to the extent that the physician is sensitive to patient input. At the same time, off-label use may be the result of patient pressure on the physician.

Physicians are also sensitive to the expanding legal rights of patients. Physicians know that accountability and responsibility for treatment ultimately depend on compliance, which is in the patient's hands. At the moment, under a competitive, largely private, health care system, the patient retains some flexibility. If a patient is not satisfied with a physician, he may change physicians. This too makes physicians sensitive to patients and their requests for access to medication.

### The Role of Pharmacists

Physicians also experience the threat of professional rivalry from pharmacists. For example, in Great Britain citizens are urged to consult a pharmacist about whether they really need to see a doctor. The pharmacist is asked to be involved in diagnosis and in the selection of an appropriate medication. This change is reflected in the more stringent training requirements for pharmacists. Pharmacists' professional organizations call for a more central role for pharmacists in the health care system (Ball, 1992) and for the development of common and complementary strategies among health professionals (Li Wan Po, 1991). The success of this strategy has varied from country to country and is strongly influenced by history and tradition.

Pharmacists ease switching and facilitate the liberalization of access to medication. They expand the options available to policy makers and regulators. In the United States medication is either prescription or OTC, but in some European countries prescription medication can be made available on request or after consultation with a pharmacist. In some cases medication is not on public display and the customer must ask the pharmacist for it. Some medication can be sold only in a pharmacy. The pharmacist contributes to liberalization through education and counseling.

Pharmacists generally favor the liberalization inherent in switching, to the extent that it has a positive impact on pharmacies in the long run (Ball, 1992). Professional representatives of pharmacists in some European countries, especially Denmark and Great Britain, have successfully lobbied government for a larger role in health care. Manufacturers have joined this group in their request for switching medications to OTC status. But the pharmacist, unlike the manufacturer, also lobbies for "pharmacy only" sales.

In the United States the pharmacist's role has remained restricted to traditional dispensing functions. But even here the prescription to OTC switches have resulted in the pharmacist playing a more important role in health care as customers voluntarily, and on their own initiative, consult with them about former prescription medications that are now available without a doctor visit.

## Summary and Conclusions

Forces for the liberalization of access to prescription medication are stronger in the United States than in Europe. In the United States there has been greater attention to ensuring legal access (that is, the removal of the requirement that a physician prescribe). Financial access—the ability of the patient to pay—remains an important determinant of access, however. In Europe financial access historically has been higher than in the United States. Direct and indirect price controls have increased financial access by keeping prices low (GAO, 1994). However, barriers to access through restriction of reimbursement to formularies have not been popular with patients. Neither has increased legal access, achieved by switching medications to OTC status, been welcomed by patients, because it is associated with increased financial barriers due to out-of-pocket payment.

Liberalization may be the logical result of the interconnection of all nations. International pharmaceutical companies lobby for reduced restrictions and for direct access to markets, even though at the same time some of their national divisions may be seeking protected markets for their own products. Information about new drugs discovered and tested in one country seems immediately available in other countries, and this increases demand for the medication and for the rescinding of any legal and regulatory hindrances to distribution.

A combination of expedited approval, the so-called off-label use of current prescription drugs, and a major switch from restricted to over-the-counter availability, has changed the dynamics of consumer access to medications. This reflects a better educated, more articulate, participatory citizenry in industrialized countries. It also is an indicator that the prestige and authority of the family physician is on the decline, at least in the United States.

The distinction between prescription and OTC is not a hard and fast boundary. Given the increasing complexity of prescription pharmaceuticals, a series of different levels of access is likely to develop as the simple bipolar division of the world into doctors and patients breaks down at both ends, and as medical specialization becomes more complex and patients more sophisticated. The rise of new biotech pharmaceuticals and the new gene technology contribute to this trend and may mediate for tighter regulation of some drugs, while others become more available.

Fiscal crises experienced by nations worldwide mean that the role of a government vis-à-vis its citizens has not remained constant over the years. While during some time periods, and for some countries, government has been interventionist and protective of its citizens, in other times and places minimal intervention has been the pattern. Today, governments faced with budgetary deficits have hard choices to make.

Liberalization touches many other aspects of health care as well. We have observed that the role of health professionals, especially pharmacists, has changed with increased liberalization of access. Social movements have pointed to the political role of access. The patient-practitioner relationship has been influenced and complicated in several different directions.

There is much speculation, little concrete knowledge, and few studies about the ultimate consequences of liberalization. It is neither positive nor negative in any absolute sense. If the trend toward liberalization continues, the need to communicate accurate information about medications in a form that can be easily understood and evaluated by the general population must be available. This will not be easy because even for the less complicated OTC products, labels often mislead. If misinformation is too prevalent or if information is not available, then the risks for dangerous drug reactions, drug toxicities, and treatment failures are great.

The history of pharmaceutical legislation suggests that restriction follows major mistakes resulting in large numbers of deaths or serious injury. The forces in favor of liberalized access are great today and their effectiveness in influencing government has been impressive. But this could end abruptly if liberalization were to result in a major mishap involving the widespread loss of life.

## Notes

1. Off-label use involves a physician prescribing a drug that is already tested and licensed for treatment of one disease for different conditions, diseases, or illnesses. The prescription of

beta blockers for performance anxiety is an example. In the United States there is widespread tolerance of physicians experimenting with medication in ways not approved by the Food and Drug Administration (FDA).

2. From 1976 to 1983, 29 ingredients moved from prescription to OTC (U.S. Congress, 1983: 4).

3. Switching a medication from prescription to OTC represents increased access as well as a substantial revision of opinion about the character and qualities of the drug in question (Kaplan, 1982). Switching at the level observed in the United States suggests that the original definition of prescription no longer stands and has been informally, but substantially, revised (Rosenau, 1994). Thus it appears that the criteria formally used to designate a drug prescription are no longer being applied. Prescription has come to signify a preliminary trial status, necessary until experience accumulates. Today, a drug is designated prescription for the time needed to demonstrate that it is relatively safe for self-administration and has a favorable benefit-to-risk ratio. While toxicity and potential harmful effects are still a consideration, potential benefits may outweigh these considerations. "A low margin of safety may be appropriate for particular OTC drugs (where the benefits to be obtained are high)" (Rachanow, 1984: 205). When this can be established, the medication is switched to OTC status. The reasons for a prescription assignment today are not that a drug is inherently unsafe, as the definition of prescription long assumed. It is rather that there is not enough knowledge about it (U.S. Congress, 1983: 30).

4. Peter Temin (1982: 21) concluded that even penicillin could pass the cost-benefit analysis test and should be available OTC. He dismisses the possibility that resistant strains of bacteria might develop, the argument that most authorities use to preclude OTC penicillin.

5. Grocery chain stores such as Leclerc and Carrefour are already selling parapharmaceutical products such as vitamins and hygiene products. But this matter, especially regarding the sale of vitamins, is currently in litigation because pharmacists are lobbying to maintain their monopoly.

6. Self-medication has a long history in the United States and Western Europe (Berridge and Edwards, 1981).

## References

(92/26/EEC) Directive on Classification for the Supply of Medicinal Products for Human Use, *Official Journal of the European Communities*, L2/113/5.

Altman LK (1993) AIDS study casts doubt on value of hastened drug approval in US. *New York Times* (Medical Section) April 6: C3.

Bagger-Hansen A (1991) Switching of prescription products: the Danish experience. *Swiss Pharma* 13(5a): 83–85.

Ball J (1992) European self-medication—time for expansion: European reimbursement—A common thread for expansion. *Swiss Pharma* 15(5-S): 37–40.

Beauchamp T (1990) The promise of the beneficence model for medical ethics. *Journal of Contemporary Health Law and Policy* 6: 145–55.

Berridge V and Edwards G (1981) *Opium and the People; Opiate Use in Nineteenth-Century England*. London: Allen Lane/St. Martin's Press.

Blishen B (1991) *Doctors in Canada: The Changing World of Medical Practice*. Toronto: University of Toronto Press.

Burstall ML (1991) Europe after 1992: implications for pharmaceuticals. *Health Affairs* 10: 157–71.

Chassin M et al. (1987) How coronary angiography is used: clinical determinants of appropriateness. *Journal of the American Medical Association* 258: 2543–47.

Cope JD (1991) *You* Can *Do Something About the Weather: 12 Suggestions on How to Change the Climate*. Presentation to the World Federation of Proprietary Medicine Manufacturers, October 18th, Seoul, South Korea.

De Guili C (1992) European self-medication—time for expansion: the EC classification directive—how it will influence national law. *Swiss Pharma* 15(5-S): 41–44.

Deletraz-Delporte M (1992) Issues in harmonization of classification of medicines available on prescription only. In: Huttin C and Bosanquet N (eds.) *The Prescription Drug Market: International Perspectives and Challenges for the Future*. Amsterdam: Elsevier Science Publishers B.V., pp. 13–40.

Ferguson T (1992) Patient, heal thyself; health in the information age. *The Futurist* 26(1): 9–13.

Fielding JE and Lancry PJ (1993) Lessons from France—vive la difference. The French health care system and US health system reform. *Journal of the American Medical Association* 270: 746–56.

Fleming G and Andersen R (1976) *Health Beliefs of the U.S. Population: Implications for Self-Care*. Chicago IL: University of Chicago, Center for Health Administration Studies.

Fleming, G, Giachello A, Andersen R, and Andrade P (1984) Substitute, supplement, or stimulus for formal medical care services? *Medical Care* 22: 950–64.

Fries J et al. and the Health Project Consortium (1993) Reducing health care costs by reducing the need and demand for medical services. *The New England Journal of Medicine* 329: 321–25.

GAO (Government Accounting Office) (1994) *Prescription Drugs: Companies Typically Charge More in the United States than in the United Kingdom*. GAO/HEHS-94-29. Washington, DC: U.S. Government Printing Office.

Gordon JS (1993) Taking a holistic approach to health care reform. *Washington Post National Weekly Edition*, Sept. 6–12: 25.

Grabowski H and Vernon J (1983) *The Regulation of Pharmaceuticals*. Washington, DC: American Enterprise Institute.

Huttin C (1992) More regulation or more competition in the European pharmaceutical market. In: Huttin C and Bosanquet N (eds.) *The Prescription Drug Market: International Perspectives and Challenges for the Future*. Amsterdam: Elsevier Science Publishers B.V., pp. 78–105.

Johnson J (1991) *How to Buy Almost Any Drug Legally Without a Prescription*. New York: Avon Books.

Jolly F (1993) Pharmacist, personal interview communication, July.

Juul P (1991) Self-medication in the 21 century, prescription-to-OTC: is Denmark a model for the world? *Swiss Pharma* 12(11a): 100–104.

Kaplan A (1982) OTC and prescription drugs: the legal distinction under federal law. In: Proprietary Association, *Prescription OTC New Resources in Self-Medication, A Symposium*. Washington, DC: The Proprietary Association.

Kolata G (1994) Their treatment, their lives, their decisions. *New York Times Magazine*. April 24: 66, 100, 105.

Lambert EC (1978) *Modern Medical Mistakes*. Bloomington, IN: Indiana University Press.

Li Wan Po A (1991) Self-medication—role of health education in self care. *Swiss Pharma* 13(11a): 45–47.

Madhavan S and Gore P (1994) A multi-dimensional analysis of physicians' perceptions of prescription-to-OTC switched drug products. *Journal of Pharmaceutical Marketing and Management* 8: 3–28.

Mela S (1992) European self-medication—time for expansion: European perspectives for OTC medicinal products. *Swiss Pharma* 15(5-S): 45–6.

Newton G, Pray S, and Popovich N (1994) New OTCs: a selected review. *American Pharmacy* NS34(2): 31–40.

NDMA (Nonprescription Drug Manufacturers Association) (1991) *NDMA Fact Sheet on Rx-To-OTC Switch.* Washington, DC: NDMA.

Orzack LH, Kaitin KA, and Lasagna L (1992) Pharmaceutical regulation in the European Community: barriers to single market integration. *Journal of Health Policy, Politics, and Law* 17: 847–68.

Payer L (1988) *Medicine and Culture. Varieties of Treatment in the United States, England, West Germany, and France.* New York: Henry Holt and Company.

Pear R (1993) Drug industry gathers a mix of voices to bolster its case. *New York Times* July 7: A1, A12.

Proprietary Association (1988) *Self-Care Self-Medication in America's Future, A Symposium; Condensation of Papers and Discussions.* Washington, DC: The Proprietary Association.

Rachanow G (1984) The switch of drugs from prescription to over-the-counter status. *Food, Drug, Cosmetic Law Journal* 39: 201–10.

Rosenau P (1994) prescription to OTC switch movement. *Medical Care Review* 51: 431–69.

Segal M (1991) prescription to OTC: The switch Is on. *FDA Consumer,* 25(2): 8–11.

Silverman HI (1987) What lies ahead for prescription-to-OTC switches. *Drug and Cosmetic Industry,* August: 1–4.

Silverman M and Lee PR (1974) *Pills, Profits, and Politics.* Berkeley and Los Angeles: University of California Press.

Smothers R (1993) Attention shoppers: in aisle 1, flu shots (supply is limited). *New York Times* October 23: A1.

Sobel DS and Ferguson T (1985) *The People's Book of Medical Tests.* New York: Summit Books.

Temin P (1979) Origins of compulsory drug prescriptions. *Journal of Law and Economics* 22: 91–105.

Temin P (1980) *Taking Your Medicine: Drug Regulation in the United States.* Cambridge, MA: Harvard University Press.

Temin P (1982) Costs and benefits in switching drugs from prescription to OTC. In: Proprietary Association, *Rx OTC New Resources in Self-Medication, a Symposium.* Washington, DC: The Proprietary Association, pp. 15–21.

Temin P (1990) Realized benefits from switching drugs. Paper prepared for the NDMA (Nonprescription Drug Manufacturers Association). Washington, DC.

Umbrecht B (1992) A la frontiere du medicament. *MGEN,* 141: 19–23.

U.S. Congress (1983) Hearings before the Subcommittee on Oversight and Investigations of the Committee on Energy and Commerce, House of Representatives, Ninety-Eighth Congress, *First Session on The Food and Drug Administration's Policies and Procedures in Switching Drugs from Prescription to Over-The-Counter Status.* Washington, DC: U.S. Government Printing Office.

Wardell W and Lasagna L (1975) *Regulation and Drug Development.* Washington, DC: American Enterprise Institute for Public Policy Research.

Wenneker M, Weissman J, and Epstein A (1990) The association of payer with utilization of cardiac procedures in Massachusetts. *Journal of the American Medical Association* 264: 1255–60.

Young FE (1988) A theme in three parts: science; society; the economy. In: Proprietary Association, *Self-Care Self-Medication in America's Future, A Symposium.* Washington, DC: The Proprietary Association.

# 13

## Developments in Economic Evaluation: The Subsidization of Pharmaceuticals

MICHAEL ARISTIDES
ANDREW S. MITCHELL
DAVID A. HENRY

There are two broad types of choices in health care (Drummond et al., 1987): first, choosing the best interventions for a particular patient (choices usually made by the health care professional and patient) and, second, choosing the best interventions for the whole community. Economic evaluation contributes to this second choice and can direct or influence the general use of health care's scarce resources. Its primary aim is to maximize health gains to the community by providing decision makers with measurements of costs and health outcomes for alternative interventions.

At a time when governments are attracted to ways of gaining the best outcomes with increasingly limited resources, a systematic and formal process has been developed in Australia in which drug companies are required to submit economic evaluations according to a set of guidelines when applying for government subsidy (Commonwealth of Australia, 1992). Other countries, such as Canada, are considering similar initiatives (Detsky, 1993).

In choosing whether a drug should be subsidized, the techniques of economic evaluation are used to inform decision makers of its value for money, or economic efficiency, compared to other interventions (usually other drugs that are already subsidised). The guidelines promote a rigorous quantitative comparison of health outcomes, and the construction of an economic evaluation around this comparison.

Economic evaluation also helps decision makers by identifying parameters to which the estimates of efficiency are most sensitive, and patient subgroups for whom treatment is better value for money.

This chapter will outline the application of economic evaluation to questions of drug subsidization, drawing on the recent experience in Australia and other countries where this methodology is being developed.

## The Economic Evaluation of Drug Treatments

The fundamental rationale for economic evaluation is that the assessment of interventions in health care, such as drug treatments, should extend beyond their clinical effects to their economic efficiency. It relates the outcomes of interventions to the resources consumed in an explicit and quantitative fashion. Therefore, economic evaluation has been defined as "the comparative analysis of alternative courses of action in terms of both their costs and consequences" (Drummond et al., 1987).

### The Limited Use of Economic Evaluation

Yet, for all its potential, economic evaluation has only been used sporadically in health care decision making. It has assisted sporadically with single major decisions, such as that for mammographic screening for postmenopausal women in Australia (Breast Cancer Screening Evaluation Steering Committee, 1990), and in the addition of low osmolar contrast agents in the United States (Eddy, 1992), but its use has not been systematic.

It has been suggested that the main reason for this limited use is that few formal links exist between evaluators and decision makers (Drummond, 1987). Economic evaluators tend to be based in academic institutions, where they report their findings in academic journals rather than directly to decision makers.

Other reasons are provided by a recent survey of 34 health care decision makers in Australia (Ross, 1994). Although there was a high level of awareness of economic evaluation, it was perceived that significant barriers to its usefulness exist. In particular, decision makers felt that their decisions needed to be made at short notice, before the results of an evaluation would be available, and that political imperatives were sometimes paramount. Often there were no data available on which to base an evaluation, and no expertise available to perform the evaluation. Another reason was low confidence in the methodology employed, including the use of poor-quality medical evidence.

Two recent reviews of published economic evaluations found that the quality of clinical or epidemiological evidence used was often poor. Gerard reviewed all cost-utility studies published in English between 1980 and 1990 (Gerard, 1991). Of the 51 studies found, only 12 (23%) were based on evidence from randomized controlled trials, and in 21 studies (41%) the source of clinical or epidemiological evidence was not clearly described. Salkeld et al. (1993) assessed published economic evaluations conducted in Australia since 1978. Of the 33 studies reviewed, the quality of the clinical or epidemiological evidence could be assessed in 22 (66%). Eighteen (81%)

were considered to include inadequate evidence of effectiveness or of the relevant epidemiology. The most common deficiency was failing to take into account selection bias and other sources of confounding. Moreover, most of the studies used point estimates of effectiveness measures without considering statistical measures of uncertainty. These reviews also highlight other areas of methodological weakness, including limited use of sensitivity analysis and poor justification of the selection of the comparator intervention.

## Basic Concepts

Economic evaluation is a decision-making tool that can be used to improve the health status of the community with available resources. To achieve this, more emphasis needs to be given to proven cost-effective interventions, generating more health benefits for the health care dollar. For example, if two drugs are shown to have equal clinical outcomes but have different costs (whether due to different prices or costs of administration), then the drug associated with the lowest cost is the most efficient. A recent randomized clinical trial showed no clinically relevant differences between a standard formulation of atenolol and a controlled-release formulation of metoprolol (Walle, 1994). Evidence of this nature justifies use of the cheaper drug.

Alternatively, if one drug is more effective but incurs a greater cost, then the incremental cost per unit of health outcome (say, the cost per life-year gained) should be considered as an estimate of the efficiency of the alternative drug or the usual treatment. For example, the cost effectiveness of treating high cholesterol with cholestyramine, compared with no drug treatment, was assessed in the United States (Oster et al., 1987). The incremental cost per life-year gained was estimated according to the age at initiation of therapy and pretreatment cholesterol levels.

A key concept in evaluation is economic cost or *opportunity cost*, which refers to the consumption of a resource that could be used in another beneficial intervention. This is often distinct from financial cost. For example, although a hospital bed-day saved may have little or no impact on the hospital budget, as many of the financial costs are fixed, it represents a valuable resource for a waiting patient, since it can be valued as the sum of the staff, capital inputs, and consumables that make it up.

Furthermore, the impact of health care interventions on resource use can go beyond that of the health care provider (direct costs to health care). It can also include the costs to individuals undergoing care (private costs) and, outside the health care system, the impact on the production of goods and services (indirect costs). Together, these categories of costs represent *social costs*, and it is usual to consider such social costs in an economic evaluation (Sugden and Williams, 1978).

## Types of Economic Evaluation

In health care there are commonly three forms of economic evaluation: cost-minimization analysis, cost-effectiveness analysis, and cost-utility analysis. Cost-benefit analysis is another, perhaps more controversial, form of economic evaluation in health care. It is less common, but has had a resurgence of interest (Johannesson, 1992; Morrison and Glydmark, 1992).

These forms of economic evaluation differ in the way the outcomes of interventions are measured. In the case of cost-benefit analysis, a monetary value is placed on health outcomes. Both cost-minimization and cost-effectiveness analysis measure outcomes in unidimensional natural units (e.g., life-years saved, or mean percent reduction in cholesterol). Cost-utility analysis, on the other hand, measures outcomes in multidimensional units of "utility." The preferences individuals have for particular states or dimensions of health are measured to derive estimates of quality of life or "utility weights" (Torrance, 1986).

In this last approach, the quality and quantity of life are combined to derive a composite measure such as the quality-adjusted life-year (QALY). The improvement in QALYs is taken to be the outcome of treatment. For example, if a treatment extends life by five years, but in a health state that is only 50% of full health, then the improvement is 2.5 QALYs ($5 \times 0.5 = 2.5$). The QALY represents a common unit of health and allows the benefits of different interventions to be compared within and across diseases. As this form of analysis is generally more costly and complex to perform, it should be reserved for cases where current clinical outcomes are inadequate—for example, where there are concerns about the quality of life in extensions of survival for end-stage AIDS sufferers. Also, where treatment generates a number of health improvements and adverse events, as in the case of schizophrenia, it is useful to be able to combine all outcomes into a single measure such as QALYs.

The main economic issue that arises from a new treatment concerns the evaluation of changes in resource use and health outcomes over an existing treatment. This is measured by the incremental cost-effectiveness/cost-utility ratio.[1] The ratio is defined as the difference in cost divided by the difference in outcomes. In the case of a more expensive but more effective intervention, the ratio conveys the extra cost per extra health outcome (such as the incremental cost per QALY gained).

This concept of incremental analysis leads to the definition of the appropriate comparator for an economic evaluation of a new drug as "the intervention most likely to be replaced by prescribers."[2] Measuring costs and outcomes of this therapy should reveal the main impact for efficiency. The identification of an appropriate comparator for the indication under consideration is critical for valid economic evaluation, but can be difficult in practice.

## Policy Objectives

Each of the following types of cost analysis can be linked to policy objectives in drug reimbursement.

Cost-minimization analysis seeks to identify the least costly alternative. If the drug under consideration is demonstrated to be therapeutically equivalent and there is no difference in the costs of administering it, it warrants no greater price or subsidy. This technique can form the basis of reference pricing. Here, the funder sets a price at which a given group or class of drugs will be subsidized, and the patient pays the difference between the subsidy and the price set by the company (Macarthur, 1992).

Hence, where a group of drugs is shown to be therapeutically equivalent, it would be most efficient to subsidize at the price of the cheapest drug.

Cost-effectiveness analysis seeks to identify the cost per unit of outcome, or the incremental cost effectiveness. This justifies a price premium over existing therapy.

Cost-utility analysis also forms the basis for justification of a price premium by considering the extra cost per QALY gained. It allows a comparison across the health care sector, but introduces an extra valuation step, the utility, which should be made transparent to the decision maker.

Cost-benefit analysis seeks to identify whether the social benefits are greater than the social costs. If so, there is an unambiguous gain in social welfare, and the intervention should be adopted. If not, funds should not be allocated to this intervention. This allows a comparison with resource allocation decisions outside the health care sector, but also introduces an extra valuation step—deriving monetary values for health improvements—which should be made transparent to ensure the sovereignty of the decision maker.

## Drug Subsidization Decisions

Economic evaluation can be used primarily to inform decision makers of the additional costs and health outcomes offered by a new drug over existing treatment. This information can then supplement the considerations of the decision maker. The primary policy objective is likely to be to assist the decision on whether to subsidize or purchase a particular drug, but this can involve the following additional features:

- To highlight critical areas of uncertainty in the evidence on effectiveness and cost
- To assist the negotiation of the price at which a drug should be subsidized
- To identify and target patients likely to benefit most

### Decisions on Selection for Subsidy

Whether in predominantly publicly-managed health care systems such as Australia and the United Kingdom, or in mixed systems such as the United States, where 41% of total health expenditure was publicly funded in 1990, drug expenditure is substantial and rising (OECD, 1992). Some mechanism of public funding of pharmaceuticals is common to most systems, and the funders often can choose which drugs will be subsidized. Even private third-party payers, such as the health maintenance organizations (HMOs) in the United States, can in principle choose which drugs will be subsidized for members (Schulman, 1993).

Information on the economic efficiency of a new drug under consideration by funders can, in principle, be used to assist the decision on whether the drug should be subsidized. This information should be relevant to the context of the funding decision: as discussed above, it should be in the form of a comparison either with an existing drug that is already funded or with a nondrug intervention such as surgery. If the drug under consideration represents unacceptable value for money in the funder's view, then the drug may be rejected from subsidy on this basis.

The funder may also consider other factors, such as equity concerns (access and affordability) and political imperatives. It is also possible to adopt other evidence-based approaches to assist decision making in health care. For example, evidence on clinical superiority alone could be used to ensure funding (asking the question "Is this drug more clinically effective?"). This would require an analysis of comparative— so-called head-to-head—clinical trials, and may also involve meta-analysis.[3] Less optimally, a comparative analysis can be conducted using placebo-controlled trials for both drugs.[4] However, it is important to emphasize that implicit value for money judgements are made in funding decisions even if they are not informed by an economic evaluation. Hence, in the above example of funding on the basis of clinical superiority, any health gain would have an implicit value of infinity, as the more clinically effective intervention would be adopted irrespective of cost.

## Areas of Uncertainty on Costs and Outcomes

Most estimates in an economic evaluation are surrounded by some uncertainty. For some of these it may be possible to derive statistical estimates of the uncertainty. A useful statistical measure, for example, is the 95% confidence interval (Braitman, 1991). Other estimates may come from expert opinion—on the rates of long-term compliance, for example—in which case the range of estimates could be used to characterize the uncertainty. However, not all the uncertainties are important to the final results. Sensitivity analysis can be used to identify those estimates to which the results are most sensitive by testing the impact of altering the value of parameters.

This technique presents an opportunity to focus on key variables for both evaluators and decision makers. For the evaluator, sensitivity analysis may be used to plan the economic evaluation—given that it can identify the most important variables and so make best use of the evaluator's own scarce resources. Decision makers should be aware of any important uncertainties so they may factor such risk into their decisions and also to identify what further information they may need. In particular, the decision makers can become aware of uncertainties that are sufficient to affect the decision on whether to fund.

## Negotiation of Prices

Where a drug is considered to represent poor value for money, an alternative for the decision maker may be to negotiate on the price of the drug. The economic evaluation can inform the decision maker whether the efficiency of the drug is sensitive to its price. If so, the efficiency for a range of drug prices lower than that proposed by the manufacturer can be presented, identifying prices at which funding can be considered acceptable.

## Identification of Patient Groups

As with other kinds of quantitative analysis, it is often possible to perform subanalyses that focus on areas of interest. An important potential focus for economic evaluation is the incremental effectiveness, and therefore incremental cost effectiveness, for patient subgroups. An improved response to a drug might be shown to strongly correlate, for example, with a particular prognostic factor in a patient. Restricting subsidy for use in such patients targets patients likely to benefit most from treatment, and is also better value for money. For this reason secondary prophylaxis, where a patient already has risk factors, can be more cost effective than primary prophylaxis, where a patient has no known risk factors. The extension of a patient's eligibility for subsidy could depend on the collection of data to demonstrate a change in a prognostic factor. For example, a complete tumor response to early cycles of a chemotherapy regimen could provide evidence that the prognosis for survival from continued chemotherapy is greater than it is in partial or nonresponders.

## The Australian Experience

Recent regulatory change in Australia concerns the use of economic evaluation to help determine whether a drug should receive government subsidy on its national formulary, the Pharmaceutical Benefits Scheme (PBS).

### Drug Subsidy Decisions

Since January 1993 pharmaceutical companies must submit an economic evaluation in their applications for their products to be reimbursed.[5] The economic evaluation should follow a set of guidelines that were written to assist companies to meet the new requirements (Commonwealth of Australia, 1992). Internationally, the implementation of this policy represents the first formal and systematic use of economic evaluation in health care decision making.

The PBS represents a second tier of drug regulation in Australia, the first tier being the approval of a drug for marketing by the Therapeutic Goods Administration (TGA). The TGA is analogous to the Food and Drug Administration in the United States and to the Health Protection Branch in Canada. Marketing approval is granted on the basis that a drug is safe, efficacious, and of acceptable quality. The PBS, by contrast, provides a selective list of drugs subject to government subsidy for use outside hospitals. A drug prescribed for any resident in Australia in accordance with this list can be dispensed at a subsidized price from a community pharmacy.

Pharmaceutical companies apply to the Pharmaceutical Benefits Advisory Committee (PBAC) to have their drugs listed for subsidy. The PBAC is an independent statutory body and its expert membership includes general practitioners, specialist physicians, clinical pharmacologists, and pharmacists. The PBAC historically has based its decisions for listing on the criteria of comparative effectiveness, comparative safety, and medical need. It recommends to the Minister of Health those drugs it considers should be subsidized, and advises the separate national Pharmaceutical Benefits Pricing Authority (PBPA) on their relative clinical importance to assist it in negotiating appropriate prices. Legislative change in 1987 required the PBAC to consider also the economic efficiency of drugs under application. In 1990 the PBAC released a set of draft guidelines for the inclusion of economic evaluations (Commonwealth of Australia, 1990) and companies were invited to submit economic evaluations during an optional phase-in period from 1991 to 1992. A revision based on this experience was released in August 1992, and submission of economic evaluations using the new guidelines became mandatory in January 1993 (Commonwealth of Australia, 1992).

Technical advice on applications to the PBAC is provided both by a team of officers within the federal health department and by an expert subcommittee of the PBAC. Both provide a rigorous assessment of clinical and economic claims and advise the PBAC on technical issues such as the choice of comparator, the assessment of clinical trial evidence, the measurement of costs, and the validity of models and assumptions in the evaluation.

## Focus of the Guidelines

The guidelines ask the company to base a submission on its marketing approval since it is the approved indications and doses that provide the constraints within which the PBAC can recommend reimbursement. The guidelines also encourage the company to focus on important issues. The underlying logic of the guidelines can be described as: (1) state the comparative clinical claims; (2) substantiate these claims with the best available evidence; and (3) perform an economic evaluation consistent with this evidence.

### State Comparative Clinical Claims

The drug's clinical place with respect to alternative therapies first must be clearly defined. This entails a statement of the main therapeutic claims of the drug (drug X) in terms of effectiveness and safety. Justification must be provided for the choice of the main clinical indication, the comparator (drug Y), and the primary measure of therapeutic outcome from clinical trials. This forms the basis for a statement such as "in prophylaxis against venous thromboembolism, drug X reduces the rate of deep vein thrombosis by 25% compared to drug Y, and is associated with similar safety."

### Substantiate Claims

These clinical claims must be substantiated with evidence. The best sources of evidence are either well-conducted randomized, head-to-head clinical trials of sufficient statistical power, or meta-analyses. This requires the application of biostatistical skills to assess available evidence on differences in outcomes and on the statistical variability around these estimates (the 95% confidence interval serves both functions). It is often appropriate to pool data from a number of trials to generate an overall estimate of effectiveness over the comparator therapy. This increases statistical power by narrowing the confidence interval and helps resolve conflicting trial results. It is also important to consider separately whether any statistical differences represent clinically important differences. For example, a 1% reduction in bone mineral density, or blood pressure, may not translate into a worthwhile reduction in the risk of hip fracture, or stroke, respectively. This example also illustrates the need to link intermediate outcomes measured in clinical trials to final outcomes.

Comparative clinical trials are an appropriate setting for the collection of quality of life and/or utility data (Guyatt and Jaeschke, 1990). Together with other measurements, such as survival, these can contribute to the generation of composite measures like QALYs or healthy-year equivalents.

A large number of analyses have been submitted to the PBAC in the framework of a cost-effectiveness analysis (arguing for price premiums on the basis of clinical advantages), but with only a theoretical argument in support of clinical superiority. These qualitative arguments are often due to a lack of empirical data, but small price premiums have been granted on occasion. For example, improved outcomes may follow better compliance associated with a reduction from twice daily dosage to once daily dosage. Evaluating officers in the federal health department now classify these claims as "pseudo cost-effectiveness analyses."

## Economic Evaluation

The economic evaluation should be built on the previous two steps. For both drugs in the relevant indication the costs of using the drug and associated resources must be estimated and then appropriately related to the clinical outcomes or utilities. In this way a cost-effectiveness ratio and an incremental cost-effectiveness' ratio can be estimated. To simplify the arithmetic, costs and outcomes are typically estimated per 100 hypothetical patients. The differences in costs between groups represent incremental (or marginal) costs. These costs may be negative if the new treatment saves sufficient resources. The PBAC has facilitated such costing by releasing a manual of prices of health care resources published alongside the guidelines in order to provide a source of standardized costs for the country (Commonwealth of Australia, 1993).

In the same way that clinical trials benefit from a prospective study design, economic evaluation in health care will be more scientifically rigorous if data on resource use and alternative measures of outcome are collected prospectively and concurrently (Drummond and Davies, 1991). Retrospective evaluation, sometimes referred to as desk analysis—occasionally including prospective data collection of some components—has been more common to date, but the piggy-backing of economic evaluation onto clinical trials is expected to increase.

Logistical advantages of this kind have been gained in the case of the economic evaluation instituted alongside the long-term intervention trial of pravastatin in ischemic disease (LIPID) (Davey et al., 1993). A battery of questionnaires was used, including a modified version of the York/Rosser questionnaire, to collect descriptive information on quality of life from patients with coronary heart disease. Other questionnaires used included items relating to time off work and patient-borne expenses such as nonprescription drugs.

## *Evaluations Submitted*

In the years 1991 through 1994 (inclusive) 133 economic evaluations have been submitted for new drugs, new formulations, new indications, and changes to prescribing restrictions. Release of detailed accounts of this experience is limited by the secrecy provisions of the legislation that authorizes the review of the submitted data, but preliminary observations have been published elsewhere (Aristides and Mitchell, 1994). In summary, the majority of submissions contained cost-effectiveness and cost-minimisation analyses. None contained a full cost-benefit analysis measuring health outcomes in monetary units. The more frequent deficiencies were in calculating the incremental cost-effectiveness ratio, understanding the economic criteria for the selection of the comparator, and a lack of consistency within various sections of the submission (most importantly, between the clinical and economic analyses). The standard of clinical data analysis and/or the quality of clinical evidence were sometimes very poor, with a high reliance on expert opinion.

## The International Experience

A number of nations, mainly in Europe, have created agencies for evaluating health care technologies, including pharmaceuticals, but the following discussion will be restricted to efforts relating to pharmaceuticals alone. In the four years since Australia first released its draft guidelines, rapid developments have taken place in other countries. This pace of development is likely to continue, given that virtually all countries are experiencing the same pressures that first motivated Australia's initiative.

Following Australia, the province of Ontario has released formal requirements from the Drug Quality and Therapeutics Committee (DQTC) for economic information to support applications for drug reimbursement (Province of Ontario, 1994). Ontario has a publicly-funded drug benefit program that covers 2.4 million people. The theoretical basis of these guidelines is consistent with that of the PBAC guidelines. For example, they focus on the measurement of incremental costs and outcomes, and they recommend that all sources of data be clearly identified and justified, and that sensitivity analysis be performed (Glasziou and Mitchell, forthcoming).

In the United States, each third-party payer of drugs operating a formulary system has a potential interest in the information provided by economic evaluations (Schulman, 1993). These payers include large federal systems such as Medicaid (in conjunction with each state), the Department of Veterans Affairs and potentially Medicare; they include large HMOs such as Kaiser-Permanente, and large health insurance companies such as the Blue Cross and Blue Shield plans and hospitals. Clearly, given so many private providers, the potential for duplication of studies is great.

In Europe, diverse regulatory structures are in place, but generally the issue of drug funding concerns the level of government subsidy rather than whether to subsidize. Economic evaluations can assist these decisions as well, but the application of this information would be different for benefit programs operating as selective formularies. Sweden, Finland, and Belgium directly control the price of drugs in price negotiations. All three countries now invite economic evidence from manufacturers in pricing negotiations, but have not issued any guidelines or mandatory requirements (Drummond et al., 1993). Germany and The Netherlands operate reference pricing systems, in which reimbursement is set in relation to other drugs in a particular class, but differences in effectiveness may not be reflected in differences in price. France encourages the submission of economic evaluations (Crampton, 1994), but has not released guidelines to indicate the information required or how it will be used. Drugs are listed for a period of only three years, and companies need to apply for a renewal at least six months before the expiration date. Updated clinical and/or economic data must support each application.

A unique regulatory structure applies in the United Kingdom, which controls the size of company profits rather than the price of drugs (Drummond, 1993). This applies to all licensed drugs, most of which are automatically subsidized under the National Health Service (NHS) (Bateman, 1993). However, recent changes to the NHS as part of the purchaser-provider split have granted some general practitioners the responsibility of budget holders to purchase specialist services, procedures, and drugs. This provides an incentive to use information from economic evaluation to select drugs that the budget holder would then preferentially prescribe (Maynard, 1988).

A possible source of information for the general practitioner is the Centre of Health Economics at the University of York. It has recently been given the responsibility to review and disseminate economic evaluations on various interventions for policy makers, health care professionals and managers (Sheldon and Chalmers, 1994). Also, guidelines defining the characteristics of acceptable economic evaluations have been agreed on by the Association of the British Pharmaceutical Industry and the Department of Health (Bottomley, 1994).

Other OECD countries such as Japan and New Zealand operate selective formularies similar in concept to those of Australia and the Canadian provinces. While these countries are likely to be receptive to economic evaluations, they have not yet formally requested them.

## Conclusion

The Australian experience and other international developments suggest that economic evaluations can be provided systematically to inform drug subsidy decision makers. This in itself is a significant development for the discipline of health economics. While it is too early to determine the full impact of this initiative on the decision making process, the fact that the provision of economic evaluations has been maintained, and indeed facilitated, indicates that the decision makers consider the information useful. It has been argued that the routine application of economic evaluation will make the generation and use of these studies more efficient (Hutton, 1994). This could be achieved by reducing duplication, by better targeting of the decision makers, and by development of data sources on costs.

The increasing interest of regulators and funders in the information provided in economic evaluations could have several impacts on the methodology used to generate the information. The development and release of guidelines in Australia and Canada helps bring a consistency, if not consensus, to the definition of acceptable methodological practice. They have also served to justify further methodological developments (Briggs et al., 1994; O'Brien et al., 1994).

Regulators and funders are also interested in asking for evidence to substantiate economic claims. If this is not available, the reluctance of regulators to accept claims should put pressure on sponsors and evaluators to collect better data.

To meet these expectations, more comparative trials should be conducted earlier in the development of new drugs than occurs at present. In addition, economic evaluations should be based on an assessment of comparative effectiveness under real-world conditions, and trial designs need to adapt to meet this need. At present, the randomized clinical trial provides the most rigorous environment (albeit a highly constrained one) for measuring the differences between treatments. The use of pragmatic randomized trials (Schwartz and Lellouch, 1967), measuring relevant health outcomes and costs and analysing data according to the principles of intention-to-treat,[6] is an approach encouraged in the Australian guidelines. This is intended to offer a balance between what appear to be the conflicting objectives of collecting data under real-world conditions and collecting data free of confounding factors.

The generation of data for economic evaluation also may be of importance to the sponsoring company. The research and development costs for new drugs are substantial. The criteria of value for money in subsidization decisions can, potentially, encourage more desirable innovation by directly influencing the revenue (price times quantity of sales) earned by pharmaceutical companies. Therefore, estimating economic efficiency early in the life cycle of a drug could help inform important investment decisions on its research and development.

Drugs that are perceived to represent poor value for money would be unlikely to obtain the price subsidy requested by companies, and a clear incentive would exist for companies to develop products that perform well against the criterion. Consider, for example, the possibility that at some stage during the development process, the new product is expected to be only marginally superior to the main incumbent drug. If the additional costs involved in developing this product imply that a relatively high price would be required relative to the incumbent drug, then, knowing the criteria for assessment, the company may choose to re-prioritize their commitment to this development. In principle, a framework exists to develop and promote efficient drugs when economic evaluation forms part of the basis for subsidy and/or pricing decisions.

## Notes

1. As there is no change in health outcomes in cost-minimization analysis, it does not apply in this case.

2. The comparator need not be a drug intervention.

3. A meta-analysis is a systematic process for finding, evaluating, and combining the results of sets of data from different clinical and scientific studies.

4. A placebo-controlled trial measures endpoints in two groups of patients. One group takes the drug, the other group takes an inactive formulation. Patients and investigators cannot distinguish between the formulations.

5. Except in the case of applications for generic drugs, for which evidence on clinical equivalence has already been assessed and so the same or a lower price is negotiated.

6. Intention-to-treat analysis is performed by using all patient data according to which group they were randomly allocated—regardless of how their health conditions might progress in the course of the study.

# References

Aristides M and Mitchell A (1994) Applying the Australian guidelines for reimbursement of pharmaceuticals. *PharmacoEconomics* 3: 196–201.

Bateman DH (1993) The selected list: diversion rather than threat. *British Medical Journal* 306: 1141–42.

Bottomley V (1994) Minister for Health, press release. London, UK: Department of Health, 19 May.

Braitman LE (1991) Confidence intervals assess both clinical significance and statistical significance. *Annals of Internal Medicine* 114: 515–17.

Breast Cancer Screening Evaluation Steering Committee (1990) *Breast Cancer Screening in Australia: Future Directions*. Report to the Australian Health Minister's Advisory Council. Canberra, ACT: Australian Institute of Health.

Briggs A, Sculpher M, and Buxton M (1994) Uncertainty in the economic evaluations of health care technologies: the role of sensitivity analysis. *Health Economics* 3: 95–104.

Commonwealth of Australia (1990) *Draft Guidelines for the Pharmaceutical Industry on Preparation of Submissions to the Pharmaceutical Benefits Advisory Committee: Including Submissions Involving Economic Analyses*. Canberra, ACT: Department of Health, Housing and Community Services.

Commonwealth of Australia (1992) *Guidelines for the Pharmaceutical Industry on Preparation of Submissions to the Pharmaceutical Benefits Advisory Committee: Including Submissions Involving Economic Analyses*. Canberra, ACT: Department of Health, Housing and Community Services.

Commonwealth of Australia (1993) *Manual of Resource Items and their Associated Costs: For Use in Submissions to the Pharmaceutical Benefits Advisory Committee Involving Economic Analyses*. Canberra, ACT: Department of Health, Housing, Local Government and Community Services.

Crampton R (1994) Pharmacoeconomics: a new kid on the block. *Inpharma* 921: 7–8.

Davey P, Hall J, and Seymour J (1993) *Cost-effectiveness of Pravastatin for Secondary Prevention of Ischaemic Heart Disease – Feasibility and Pilot Study*. Centre for Health Economics, Research and Evaluation, Discussion Paper No. 17, Westmead Hospital, NSW, Australia.

Detsky A (1993) Guidelines for economic analysis of pharmaceutical products: a draft document for Ontario and Canada. *PharmacoEconomics* 3: 354–61.

Drummond MF (1987) Economic evaluation and the rational diffusion and use of health technology. *Health Policy* 7: 309–24.

Drummond MF and Davies L (1991) Economic analysis alongside clinical trials: revisiting the methodological issues. *International Journal of Technology Assessment in Health Care* 7: 561–73.

Drummond MF, Rutten FFH, Brenna A, Gouveia Pinto C, Horisberger B, et al. (1993) Economic evaluation of pharmaceuticals: a European perspective. *PharmacoEconomics* 4: 173–86.

Drummond MF, Stoddart GL, and Torrance GW (1987) *Methods for the Economic Evaluation of Health Care Programmes*. Oxford: Oxford Medical Publications.

Eddy DM (1992) Applying cost-effectiveness analysis: the inside story. *Journal of the American Medical Association* 268: 2575–82.

Gerard K (1991) *A Review of Cost-Utility Studies: Assessing their Policy Making Relevance*. Health Economics Research Unit, Discussion Paper (November), Aberdeen, UK.

Glasziou P and Mitchell A (forthcoming) Use of pharmaeconomic data by regulatory authorities. In: Spilker B (ed.) *Quality of Life and Pharmaeconomics in Clinical Trials*, 2nd ed. New York: Raven Press.

Guyatt G and Jaeschke R (1990) Measurements in clinical trials: choosing the appropriate approach. Spilker B (ed.) *Quality of Life Assessments in Clinical Trials*. New York: Raven Press, pp. 37–46.

Hutton J (1994) Economic evaluation of healthcare: a half-way technology. *Health Economics* 3: 1–4.

Johannesson M (1992) The contingent valuation method–appraising the appraisers. *Health Economics* 2: 357–60.

Macarthur D (1992) *Pharmaceutical Pricing and Reimbursement in the Single European Market: Consensus or Conflict*. Richmond, UK: Scrip, PJB Publications.

Maynard A (1988) *Whither the National Health Service?* Centre for Health Economics, NHS White Paper Occasional Paper Series No. 1, University of York, UK.

Morrison G and Glydmark M (1992) Appraising the use of contingent valuation. *Health Economics* 1: 233–43.

O'Brien BJ, Drummond MF, Labelle RJ, and Willan A (1994) In search of power and significance: issues in the design and analysis of stochastic cost-effectiveness studies in health care. *Medical Care* 32: 150–63.

OECD (Organization for Economic Cooperation and Development) (1992) *US Health Care at the Crossroads*. Paris: OECD.

Oster G and Epstein AM (1987) Cost-effectiveness of antihyperlipemic therapy in the prevention of coronary heart disease: the case of cholestyramine. *Journal of the American Medical Association* 258: 2381–87.

Province of Ontario (1994) *Ontario Guidelines for Economic Analysis of Pharmaceutical Products*. Toronto: Ontario Ministry of Health.

Ross J (1994) *The Use of Economic Evaluation by Health Care Decision Makers–an Australian Study*. Centre for Health Economics, Research and Evaluation, Discussion Paper No. 24, Westmead Hospital, NSW, Australia.

Salkeld G, Davey P, and Arnolda G (1993) A critical review of health-related economic evaluations conducted in Australia since 1978. *Economics and Health: 1993*. Proceedings of the Fifteenth Australian Conference of Health Economists. University of Monash, Victoria, Australia.

Schulman KA (1993) The use of evaluation in pharmaceutical reimbursement decisions in the United States. In: Schubert FS (ed.) *Canadian Collaborative Workshop on Pharmacoeconomics: Proceedings*. Princeton, NJ: Excerpta Medica, pp. 19–23.

Schwartz D and Lellouch J (1967) Explanatory and pragmatic attitudes in therapeutic trials. *Journal of Chronic Diseases* 20: 637–48.

Sheldon T and Chalmers I (1994) The UK Cochrane Centre and the NHS Centre for Reviews and Dissemination: respective roles within the information systems strategy of the NHS R&D programme, coordination and principles underlying collaboration. *Health Economics* 3: 201–3.

Sugden R and Williams A (1978) *The Principles of Practical Cost-Benefit Analysis*. Oxford: Oxford University Press.

Torrance GW (1986) Measurement of health state utilities for economic appraisal. *Journal of Health Economics* 5: 1–30.

Walle PO et al. (1994) Effects of 100 mg of controlled-release metoprolol and 100 mg of atenolol on blood pressure, central nervous system-related symptoms, and general well-being. *Journal of Clinical Pharmacology* 34: 742–47.

# 14

## The Self-Regulation of Pharmaceutical Marketing: Initiatives for Reform

JOEL LEXCHIN
ICHIRO KAWACHI

The pharmaceutical industry spends heavily promoting its products to physicians. Next to the cost of producing the drugs, the companies spend more money promoting their products than on anything else: $10 billion a year in the United States versus just over $7.1 billion for research and development (Drake and Uhlman, 1993). There is good evidence to show that this investment pays off in increased sales (Montgomery and Silk, 1972; Walton, 1980; Parsons and Abeele, 1981; Krupka and Vener, 1985; Healthcare Communications Inc., 1989), helping to make the pharmaceutical industry among the most profitable in the world (Drake and Uhlman, 1993).

If all promotion did was to increase sales of a product, there would not be that much concern about regulating it. However, promotion also affects the quality of prescribing. Studies from a number of countries have consistently shown that the more physicians rely on promotion for their information about drugs, the less appropriate they are as prescribers (Becker et al., 1972; Linn and Davis, 1972; Mapes, 1977; Haayer, 1982; Ferry et al., 1985; Blondeel et al., 1987). Even prescribers who think they rely on scientific literature for their knowledge can be influenced by promotional sources without being aware of it (Avorn et al., 1982; Greenwood, 1989).

Pharmaceuticals also differ from ordinary products in that the person who orders the medication is not the person who consumes it or pays for it. This unique characteristic of pharmaceuticals, plus the adverse effects of promotion on the quality of prescribing, help explain why it is a candidate for some form of regulation. In most countries with a free-market economy, voluntary self-regulation has been the norm for control of industry advertising and promotion. There is nothing inherently flawed in the concept of self-regulation. Indeed, when it works well, it can be an efficient and flexible approach (Ayres and Braithwaite, 1992). Unfortunately, in the case of the pharmaceutical industry, persistent and pervasive flaws have been noted, and critics in several countries have made urgent calls for reform (Herxheimer and Collier, 1990; Randall, 1991; Australian Trade Practices Commission, 1992; Chetley and Mintzes, 1992; Kawachi, 1992b; Lexchin, 1992; Lexchin, 1994).

In this chapter, we review the common features and problems of government and voluntary self-regulation in the Third World and in several developed countries. We then discuss why self-regulation appears to be the preferred form of regulation despite its numerous documented problems. Finally, we develop a framework for reforming the system drawing on some recent theories of industrial regulation (Ayres and Braithwaite, 1992).

## Regulatory Options

### Self-Regulation – Common Themes

Although all industrialized countries, and many Third World ones, have laws and regulations governing pharmaceutical promotion, in most cases health authorities have ceded practical control to the pharmaceutical industry. In these countries the industry operates under a set of voluntary codes that nominally place certain limits on advertising and promotional practices such as: outlining the kind of training that company sales representatives (detailers) must have; requiring companies to list safety data in advertisements; not allowing companies to purposely misquote studies in their promotional material; and limiting the kinds of gifts or hospitality that companies can provide to practitioners. However, there are certain other features that are also common to voluntary codes: they tend to be reactive, they lack transparency, they omit large areas of concern, and they lack effective sanctions.

Codes in most countries operate under a reactive as opposed to a proactive style of regulation: action is generally taken only upon receipt of complaints, rather than preventing violations in the first place. Organizations such as the Association of the British Pharmaceutical Industry (ABPI) and the Australian Pharmaceutical Manufacturers Association (APMA) claim to monitor compliance with their voluntary codes by scrutinizing a random selection of advertisements in medical journals. However, their procedures are not defined and, despite monitoring, widespread violations have been documented in both countries (Herxheimer and Collier, 1990; Australian Trade Practices Commission, 1992).

Canada is one of the few countries in which proposed print advertisements have to be submitted for clearance prior to their publication. The Canadian Pharmaceutical Advertising Advisory Board (PAAB), which is independent of the pharmaceutical industry, assesses each submission with respect to compliance with its code of advertising practice (PAAB, 1992). Yet even with prescreening, a significant number of advertisements appear that violate the PAAB code (Hagerman, 1992).

A second feature common to many voluntary codes is their lack of transparency. In several countries voluntary monitoring bodies are under no obligation to publish all their deliberations about alleged breaches of their codes. For example, the Canadian PAAB is not required to publicize the results of complaints against advertisements, even when these complaints have been upheld (Lexchin, 1994). In Britain, an undisclosed number of complaints to the Committee are handled informally and internally, and hence are never publicized (Herxheimer and Collier, 1990). In the United States, the Office of the Inspector General identified the lack of public airing of voluntary code breaches as one of the major weaknesses of self-regulation by the Pharmaceutical Research Manufacturers of America (PhRMA, formerly the Pharmaceutical Manufacturers Association) (Anonymous, 1991a).

A further example of the lack of public accountability in self-regulation has been the absence of formal consumer involvement in the monitoring and enforcement of voluntary codes. The latest revision of the APMA voluntary code of conduct now provides for a consumer group representative on its code of conduct complaints subcommittee (Anonymous, 1993c). By contrast, the U.K. ABPI rejected calls to include a consumer/patient representative on its code of practice committee when it made its latest revisions (Anonymous, 1993a).

The third weakness common to voluntary codes is the narrowness of their interpretation and areas that have been entirely omitted. For instance, none of the codes require companies to give the same amount of prominence or space to the adverse aspects of drugs as they do to the benefits of drugs. The almost universal result is that the positive features are presented in large type with bold graphics, and the warnings appear in much smaller type, often separated by many pages from the graphics (Kline, 1992).

Perhaps the most illustrative example of the limitations of voluntary codes comes from an examination of the Code of Pharmaceutical Marketing Practices of the International Federation of Pharmaceutical Manufacturers Associations (IFPMA) (1982). Although the code pledges companies to ensure that information in advertisements is based on an up-to-date evaluation of all the available scientific evidence, it adds a caveat that where a product has been evaluated and registered by an established regulatory authority, this will be accepted as adequate scientific evidence. This loophole was exploited by Organon when it responded to a letter from the Australian-based Medical Lobby for Appropriate Marketing (MaLAM). Organon's Medical Director avoided the issue of scientific evidence because the indications being questioned were endorsed by the Bangladeshi health authorities (Mansfield, 1992b).

A final common finding in voluntary codes is their lack of timely and effective sanctions. In the United Kingdom, for example, until 1993 it typically took up to 18 weeks for a complaint to be processed under the code of procedure set out by the ABPI (Chetley and Mintzes, 1992). In Belgium, complaints about breaches in the Belgian pharmaceutical industry's voluntary code take more than a year to process

(Anonymous, 1991b). By the time complaints are assessed, irrespective of their outcome, many advertisements have run their course and exerted their impact.

Even when complaints have been upheld, the applicable sanctions are often so weak that they have no deterrent effect on repeated breaches. Before the latest revision of its code in 1993, the ABPI had no power to force an offending company to publish a retraction of a misleading advertisement. In Canada, the only sanction applied by the PAAB is modification or withdrawal of a misleading advertisement and the possibility that the PAAB will request letters of retraction or published notices (PAAB, 1992).

In 1983 WEMOS, a Dutch activist group, filed a complaint with the special code commission of the Dutch Association of Pharmaceutical Industries (NEFARMA) about Organon's marketing practices for anabolic steroids in Third World countries. NEFARMA condemned Organon in very strong terms and later that year Organon claimed that "corrective action had been taken already." However, three years later WEMOS was able to document almost identical marketing practices (WEMOS Pharma Group, 1987).

In summary, one of the most consistent and pervasive findings to emerge from international reviews of voluntary regulation is that it does not work. Voluntary codes are breached on a regular basis, and appear to have no influence in deterring repeated offenses (Harvey, 1990; Herxheimer and Collier, 1990; Tomson and Weerasuriya, 1990; Kawachi, 1992b; Wilkes et al., 1992; Herxheimer et al., 1993; Lexchin, 1994). In view of this long history of repeated violations, it is perhaps surprising that governments have allowed self-regulation to continue. We will examine the motivations of both governments and the industry below.

## Government Control of Promotion

The United States is the major exception when it comes to controlling promotion. In 1962, amendments to the Food, Drug and Cosmetic Act gave jurisdiction over prescription drug promotional campaigns and materials to the Food and Drug Administration (FDA) (Kessler and Pines, 1990). The FDA has defined its authority to cover any material issued by or sponsored by a drug manufacturer that falls within the legal definitions of labeling or advertising. Labeling constitutes written, printed, or graphic matter that accompanies a prescription drug, supplements it, or explains it. The FDA views advertising as anything other than labeling that promotes a drug and that is sponsored by a manufacturer (Kessler and Pines, 1990).

The FDA prohibits the advertising of drugs for unlabeled (unapproved) indications, a policy Bristol-Myers Squibb repeatedly violated between 1988 and 1990 with some of its anticancer products. After a series of warning letters from the FDA, the company agreed to send thousands of corrective letters to physicians around the country, explaining the FDA's concerns and "setting the record straight" (Iglehart, 1991). In November 1991, both ICI and Ciba-Geigy were required to take prompt corrective action to counter their promotional claims for unapproved indications for antihypertensive drugs (Anonymous, 1991d; Chetley and Mintzes, 1992).

However, the FDA is beset with its own limitations that undermine its ability to control promotion effectively. So far it has been restricted to making arrangements with individual companies to curb promotional excesses, rather than dealing with problems on an industry-wide basis. The FDA's attempt to enact a comprehensive set of regulations governing industry-supported scientific and medical educational activities is an example of this weakness. It first issued a draft concept paper in late 1991 outlining a stringent and wide-ranging set of standards to distinguish educational activities that could be funded by drug companies and yet avoid regulation as advertising or promotional labeling (Anonymous, 1991c). Despite a softening of the policy's tone in the face of harsh criticism (Food and Drug Administration, 1992), even this revised version has yet to be finalized.

Finally, as a federal agency the FDA is chronically underfunded. For example, the vast majority of promotional material submitted to the FDA's division of drug advertising and labeling is considered false and/or misleading, but the FDA is able to take action in only 5% of cases because of lack of resources (Anonymous, 1989). These limitations were highlighted in a recent review of 109 journal advertisements. The advertisements were evaluated using criteria based on FDA guidelines. Overall, reviewers would not have recommended publication of 28% of the advertisements, and would have required major revisions before publication in 34% (Wilkes et al., 1992).

## Self-Regulation

### The Government Perspective

When self-regulation works well, it is the least burdensome approach from the point of view of both taxpayers and the regulated industry (Ayres and Braithwaite, 1992: 38). There are two major drawbacks to government regulation—one financial, the other practical. Increasingly, fiscal pressures in almost all countries have prevented government agencies from effectively policing pharmaceutical promotion. Government regulatory agencies rarely have the resources to make it economically rational for firms not to cheat (Ayres and Braithwaite, 1992: 103). The other major drawback is a lack of necessary expertise compared to industry (Herxheimer and Collier, 1990).

Voluntary self-regulation seems attractive because it is a more flexible and cost-effective option than government–industry adversariness. Government regulators reason that in a highly competitive industry, the desire of individual companies to prevent competitors from gaining an edge can be harnessed to serve the public interest through a regime of voluntary self-regulation run by a trade association (Ayres and Braithwaite, 1992: 128).

The problem with this analysis is that industry will always be tempted to exploit the privilege of self-regulation by producing a socially suboptimal level of compliance with regulatory goals. Experience has repeatedly demonstrated this in the case of pharmaceutical product marketing (Kawachi, 1992b).

Effective industry control over its own promotional practices reflects a government-industry relationship termed *clientele pluralism*, in which the state actually relinquishes some of its authority to private-sector actors, typically a trade association

(Atkinson and Coleman, 1989). Although the state voluntarily gives up its power, in reality it has little choice because of the imbalance in resources between the state and the private sector.

In these circumstances few trade associations vested with the authority to regulate drug promotion have made systematic efforts either to monitor the advertising practices of their members or to enforce compliance. The problem is that governments and pharmaceutical manufacturers' associations have different missions. The mission of government is to protect public health by encouraging rational prescribing. The mission of trade associations is primarily to increase sales and profit. From the business perspective, self-regulation is mostly concerned with the control of anticompetitive practices. Therefore, when industrial associations draw up their codes of practice they deliberately make them vague or do not cover certain features of promotion in order to allow companies a wide latitude. Self-regulation works well when anticompetitive promotional practices happen to coincide with government regulators' notions of misleading advertising. Most often, however, the fit is imperfect, because far from being anticompetitive, many misleading advertising tactics are good for business. Therefore, from the public health perspective, the results of voluntary self-regulation are suboptimal.

## The Industry Perspective

New drugs introduced by the pharmaceutical industry seldom represent major therapeutic advances (Randall, 1991). After the first new drug in a class appears, follow-on drugs are, at best, usually minor improvements over the originator. For example, over 100 different brands of drugs are available just to treat hypertension (Kawachi, 1992a). In the past, companies marketing drugs that offered little therapeutic gain could expect to earn substantial sales dollars through a combination of promotion and price inflation (Drake and Uhlman, 1993).

While the current situation with respect to product innovation is not much different from that in the past, health care economics is facing a major crisis in most industrialized countries. Governments are no longer willing to tolerate increasing health care budgets, and restraints are being contemplated or applied in most jurisdictions, including the United States. Under these circumstances pharmaceutical companies will have to rely even more on their promotional departments to maintain sales volume and profits. This reality is reflected in the increasing use of aggressive marketing techniques witnessed in recent years.

Speaking at a 1994 Food and Drug Law Institute meeting, Lucy Rose, director of the FDA's Division of Drug Marketing, Advertising and Communications, said that her division has seen a "tremendous change in the willingness of pharmaceutical companies to take risks when it comes to promoting products" (Anonymous, 1994d). She noted that sales representatives were being provided with excessive information about unapproved indications for drugs and that some companies were setting sales goals far higher than the total patient population for which products were approved (Anonymous, 1994d).

With the growth of managed care and the use of formularies, companies have started to emphasize pharmacoeconomic comparisons in their promotional material to convince formulary managers to stock their drugs. In a number of cases the FDA has ruled that cost-effective claims made in promotional literature were false and misleading because they lacked any supporting data. A 1994 example was Eli Lilly's campaign for Axid (nizatidine), which contained no more supporting data than a comparison of drug costs for competing therapies (Anonymous, 1994a).

Companies in the United States have developed a number of methods for avoiding FDA promotional restrictions. These include indirect promotion via the use of educational or scientific symposia and publications; using open-label studies (studies that are uncontrolled, biased, and nonrepresentative) to support efficacy claims; and various methods of promotion targeted directly at the general public (Morris and Banks, 1990). Among these are direct-to-consumer advertising in public media, using video news releases to encourage news stories about products, and product placement in popular television programs or movies dealing with medical themes (Kessler and Pines, 1990). In the United States alone, industry expenditure on direct-to-consumer advertising increased from about $20 million in 1987 to $90 million in 1990 (Anonymous, 1990).

In the past, industry adopted voluntary codes to forestall the threat of direct government intervention or as a reaction to intense criticism of promotional practices. This was the case in Canada with the development of the PAAB (Raison, 1989), and the IFPMA code was developed to avoid the possibility of the World Health Organization (WHO) promulgating an international marketing code (Health Action International, 1987). These same factors help explain why the PhRMA adopted the American Medical Association's guidelines on promotion just days before U.S. Senate Committee hearings on marketing practices in the industry (Randall, 1991).

In view of the need to use increasingly aggressive promotional tactics to maintain sales volume, it is not surprising that the pharmaceutical industry would prefer to retain a voluntary system of self-regulation and keep government intervention to a minimum. Operating under loose, unenforceable voluntary codes permits bigger sales volume and higher profits compared to the alternative of greater government intervention.

From the perspective of the individual firm, it would seem irrational to comply consistently with the industry's voluntary code under every circumstance. The major cost of compliance with the code is loss of market share to rival manufacturers, compared to which the cost of violations (the probability of detection multiplied by the costs of sanctions) is frequently insignificant; hence, codes are routinely violated (Harvey, 1990; Herxheimer and Collier, 1990; Kawachi, 1992b; Lexchin, 1992; 1994). The same situation applies in the United States where government control is more prominent. According to FDA Deputy Commissioner Mary Pendergast, "The potential financial rewards for violative promotional activities . . . are great, and the risks of serious sanction minimal. . . . Enforcement actions are likely to be less costly to the company than foregoing the broader market" (Anonymous, 1994e).

## Checks and Balances

Based on the foregoing analysis, voluntary regulation appears to suit the mutual interests of most governments and the pharmaceutical industry. Who then provides the countervailing power in this arrangement? Certainly not the consumer. Consumers are not supposed to be familiar enough with the indications and contraindications of medicines to judge the contents of advertising. This lack of professional knowledge is presumably one of the reasons why the pharmaceutical industry in several countries (for example, Britain and New Zealand) has excluded consumer representation on the committees that police their voluntary codes.

The medical profession's response to drug promotion has seldom ranged beyond denial and apathy. Many doctors deny altogether that pharmaceutical promotion has any influence on their prescribing behavior. For examples, see the correspondence columns in the *Journal of the American Medical Association* (April 25, 1990: 2177–79) following publication of the article by Chren et al. (1989), and the correspondence columns of the *New England Journal of Medicine* (December 3, 1992: 1686–88) following publication of the article by Waud (1992).

From time to time, various professional bodies, such as the American College of Physicians (Goldfinger, 1990), and the Royal College of Physicians in Britain (Royal College of Physicians, 1986), have issued guidelines to their members regarding ethical relationships with the industry. Regardless of the noble sentiments in these guidelines, their monitoring provisions, enforceability, and sanctions tend to be even weaker than the industry voluntary codes. Furthermore, these bodies have rarely done much more than publish their guidelines and circulate them to their membership. Experience with guidelines in other areas (Lomas et al., 1989) has amply demonstrated that merely distributing them is unlikely to have an effect on behavior.

## Proposals for Reform

We firmly believe, and the evidence backs us up, that pharmaceutical promotion can influence prescribing behavior (Lexchin, 1993) and, more important, that reliance on promotion for prescribing information increases the likelihood of irrational prescribing. The major challenge is to develop ways to encourage rational prescribing, which means that the drug treatment is appropriate, effective, and safe for the symptoms or disease presented, that the prescribed dosage and duration are correct, and that the most cost-effective regimen has been chosen for the presenting symptom or disease (Haayer, 1982). Eliminating misleading drug promotion is just one of the many strategies to increase rational prescribing. However, no strategy would work if the industry increased pressure with ever-more lavish, aggressive, and innovative strategies to promote their products. Looking at the long-term trends in the industry, including increasing competition from generic manufacturers, price restrictions, increasing pressure to prescribe cost-effectively, and managed care, there is every indication that the pressure to market drugs aggressively will continue to mount. Reforms to prevent abuses of advertising and promotion have to be part of the package of strategies to improve prescribing.

It appears that regulators are faced with the choice between only two options by which to reform pharmaceutical promotion—either to step up direct government intervention, or to continue to work within the existing framework of voluntary regulation. However, Ayres and Braithwaite (1992: 133) point to a middle path.

Their proposals center on a form of regulatory delegation that is grounded in two fundamental principles: an explicit pyramid of sanctions; and *tripartism*, the empowering of public interest groups to take part in the regulatory process.

What they are proposing is different from the clientele pluralist relationship that was discussed earlier. In the model suggested by Ayres and Braithwaite, while the government is delegating regulatory tasks such as the monitoring and policing of voluntary advertising codes to private parties—for example, to industry associations, public interest groups, or a mixture of both—the state retains authority to act should delegation fail, whereas in clientele pluralism the state has essentially withdrawn itself from any further involvement. According to Ayres and Braithwaite (1992: 158), "The delegated aspects of responsive regulation hold out the prospect of a regulatory equilibrium that retains many of the important benefits of competition, while the potential for escalating interventions maintains the integrity and pursuit of regulatory goals to correct market failure."

At the outset, we identified four common features of self-regulation that seem to contribute to their present lack of effectiveness: a reactive style, a lack of transparency and public accountability, limitations in code coverage, and absence of effective sanctions. Correcting these deficiencies, we believe, is consistent with Ayres and Braithwaite's notions of responsive regulation.

## The Enforcement Pyramid

Ayres and Braithwaite (1992: 35–39) argue that regulatory agencies are best able to secure compliance from the industry when they display an explicit enforcement pyramid. In Ayres and Braithwaite's analysis, most regulatory action occurs at the base of the pyramid where attempts are initially made to coax compliance by persuasion. The FDA serves as an example of how a government agency can apply a broad range of sanctions if persuasion fails. It uses its power to issue frequent regulatory letters and to apply a sliding scale of corrective actions ranging from immediate discontinuance of misleading advertising, through issuing of corrective letters or advertisements to medical doctors, to fines and probationary arrangements in which companies submit all advertisements to the FDA for clearance. However, according to FDA Deputy Commissioner Mary Pendergast, the agency has, at present, few tools to deter a company from initiating a campaign that will later prove to be in violation (Anonymous, 1994e).

Lack of cooperation is much more likely for a business facing a regulator with only one deterrence option (which is the case with many existing voluntary codes and for many government regulatory agencies), compared to a regulator with an explicit enforcement pyramid. This is true even where the one deterrence option available to the regulator is maximally potent because it becomes politically impossible and morally unacceptable to use it with any but the most extraordinary offenses (Ayres and Braithwaite, 1992: 36). With the exception of the FDA, few regulatory bodies have a pyramid of sanctions.

One pyramid of sanctions applies at the level of the individual firm. However, Ayres and Braithwaite (1992: 38–39) draw attention to a second enforcement pyramid aimed at the entire industry (see Fig. 14-1). In this model, government communicates to industry that it has at its disposal an escalating set of enforcement strategies, ranging from self-regulation all the way up to command regulation with nondiscretionary punishment. The key contention of Ayres and Braithwaite's theory (1992: 39) is that the use of two enforcement pyramids channels most of the regulatory action to the base of the pyramids where regulation is most effective and least resource intensive.

Their analysis (1992: 158–62) suggests that self-regulation can be strengthened in two ways. First, government can communicate its willingness to escalate its enforcement strategies vis-à-vis the industry as the FDA does. Second, the organization that is delegated to enforce self-regulation (for example, the PAAB in Canada, or the ABPI in Britain) ought to be required to demonstrate an explicit pyramid of sanctions and to effectively communicate the application of the pyramid to consumers, professionals, government, and industry.

### Tripartism

*Tripartism* is the term employed by Ayres and Braithwaite (1992: 54) to describe the empowerment of public interest groups to participate in the regulatory process. In most countries, formal regulation of pharmaceutical promotion has been a two-player game, involving government and industry. But one player, government, may be either unwilling or unable to enter the game. Ayres and Braithwaite (1992: 57) point

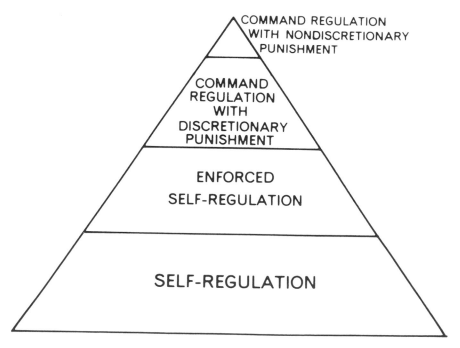

**Figure 14-1.** Example of a pyramid of enforcement strategies. Reproduced with permission from Ayres and Braithwaite (1992: 39).

out that a regulatory process that fosters the evolution of cooperation between two parties also encourages the evolution of capture. Therefore, government officials may be predisposed to cooperate with industry and not rock the boat (Lexchin, 1990). We have already alluded to the observation that a hands-off approach to regulation suits the purposes of many government departments under severe fiscal constraint. Different parts of government may have conflicting agendas with respect to their dealings with the pharmaceutical industry: for example, the primary goal of departments dealing with trade and industry is fostering business growth, which may conflict with the goals of departments charged with protecting and maintaining the public's health.

The goals of tripartism are, then, to grant access to public interest groups to all the information that is available to the regulator, and to give them a seat on the committees or boards that monitor and enforce business self-regulation. Open access to information is a key point for effective consumer representation. To some extent this is already available in the United States through the Freedom of Information Act, but in the United Kingdom the government scuttled a private member's bill that would have provided more transparency in drug licensing (Anonymous, 1993b).

During the Australian Trade Practices Commission (1992) inquiry into the promotion of pharmaceutical products, industry representatives opposed including consumer representation in the regulatory process. However, the Commission noted, "If the public is to have confidence in the scheme, it is important that they have some form of representation and a window on how the scheme operates. A broad-based representative of consumer interest could not only inject a community perspective into the subcommittee's deliberations, but also allow for a reporting back mechanism to a wider constituency" (Australian Trade Practices Commission, 1992).

The APMA has now accepted the need for a consumer representative on its code of conduct complaints subcommittee (Anonymous, 1993c). How to go about picking consumer representatives is a matter that deserves further thought. Ayres and Braithwaite (1992: 57–58) speak in terms of *contestable guardianship*, that is, competition within public interest groups for seats at the negotiating table (or in this case, the monitoring committee). Competition may help prevent consumer representatives from being captured the way that government officials have been. Possibly because no one has challenged the Consumers Association of Canada (CAC) for its seat on the PAAB board, the CAC has changed from an organization that campaigned for the abolition of pharmaceutical advertising in the 1970s to one that lends legitimacy to the weak PAAB code by its acquiescence.

Ayres and Braithwaite (1992: 100) believe that "the realistic aspiration is not for public interest groups to become equal partners with industry and government but for them to be enabled to be credible watchdogs." We are not sure that this analysis would always be accurate but just by having a seat at the table, consumer representatives may be able to strengthen the codes that are used to regulate promotion.

## A Fourth Player

Adding the fourth major player, health care professionals, to the mix could increase industry's willingness to control promotional excesses. It is in the best interest of companies to retain the confidence and good will of prescribers. Once that is lost, there can be disastrous consequences, as Ciba-Geigy found out in the 1970s when Swedish doctors boycotted its products (Hansson, 1989). The model is MaLAM, an independent organization of over 1,000 health care professionals that monitors advertising and engages in a dialogue with companies in an attempt to get them either to justify their claims with solid scientific information or to modify claims that cannot be substantiated. In response to MaLAM's actions a number of companies have either withdrawn drugs or have substantially modified their promotional claims (Mansfield, 1994).

## Conclusion

While we do not believe that the path to achieving meaningful control over pharmaceutical promotion will be easy, we are not entirely pessimistic. There are some indications that the various parties involved are prepared to take action. On the industry side, some companies have progressive internal policies. Ciba-Geigy agrees with the World Health Organization's Ethical Criteria for Medicinal Drug Promotion and would welcome worldwide compliance with the WHO recommendations. Both Glaxo and Bayer have company codes that incorporate the IFPMA code with significant improvements (Mansfield, 1992a).

Some industry associations have made significant modifications to the way they police their codes. The New Zealand code committee is chaired by a practicing judge, solicitor, or a QC (Queen's Counsel—a high-ranking barrister), and a majority of its members come from outside the industry (Anonymous, 1994c). In the United Kingdom the new Prescription Medicines Code of Practice Authority has cut the time taken to assess alleged breaches of the code from 14 to 8-1/2 weeks (Anonymous, 1994b). On the government side, the American FDA is policing promotion with renewed vigor and the Australian government has set up an inquiry to review all aspects of pharmaceutical promotion in that country.

Finally, nongovernmental organizations have achieved some successes. The critical surveys conducted by Milton Silverman and his colleagues of information supplied by companies in drug compendia in the United States and the Third World seem to have produced some measurable changes. In the first survey, conducted in 1974, Silverman found that in Latin America, companies were listing far more indications than in the United States, while the hazards were minimized, glossed over, or totally ignored (Silverman, 1976). By the time of his fourth survey in 1987, most multinational firms were increasingly willing to restrict claims of efficacy for their products to the scientifically justifiable, and to disclose the major hazards of their products (Silverman, Lydecker, and Lee, 1992).

The goal behind regulating promotion is to ensure that when physicians use it for prescribing information, their patients are not going to suffer. All of the reforms that we have advocated will need to be tested in the real world, but we believe that the implementation of tripartism, combined with an explicit enforcement pyramid and watchful health care professionals, has the potential to go a long way to reform current deficiencies in the regulation of pharmaceutical promotion and to help achieve the goal of better pharmaceutical care.

## References

Anonymous (1989) FDA's drug promotion problems. *Scrip* (Feb. 24), No. 1389, p. 14.
Anonymous (1990) Evolving FDA standard on DTC ads. *Scrip* (Oct. 17), No. 1558, p. 19.
Anonymous (1991a) US OIG investigates drug promotion. *Scrip* (Sept. 18), No. 1652, p. 15.
Anonymous (1991b) New Belgian code of practice. *Scrip* (Oct. 16), No. 1660, p. 3.
Anonymous (1991c) FDA concept paper on meetings. *Scrip* (Nov. 8), No. 1667, pp. 16–17.
Anonymous (1991d) FDA warning letters to ICI & Ciba-Geigy. *Scrip* (Dec. 11), No. 1676, p. 13.
Anonymous (1993a) ABPI sets up separate code authority. *Scrip* (Jan. 22), No. 1788, p. 3.
Anonymous (1993b) UK Medicines Information Bill blocked. *Scrip* (May 7/11), No. 1818/ 19, pp. 2–3.
Anonymous (1993c) APMA code breaches in 1992–93. *Scrip* (Sept. 14), No. 1855, pp. 16– 17.
Anonymous (1994a) FDA warns Lilly on Axid promotion. *Scrip* (Aug. 2), No. 1945, pp. 10– 11.
Anonymous (1994b) UK code assessment time cut. *Scrip* (Aug. 16), No. 1949, p. 4.
Anonymous (1994c) New code of practice in New Zealand. *Scrip* (Aug. 16), No. 1949, p. 15.
Anonymous (1994d) Pharmacoeconomics dilemma for FDA. *Scrip* (Sept. 27), No. 1961, p. 10.
Anonymous (1994e) Call for tougher US promotion penalties. *Scrip* (Oct. 28), No. 1970, pp. 18–19.
Atkinson MH and Coleman WD (1989) *The State, Business, and Industrial Change in Canada*. Toronto: University of Toronto Press.
Australian Trade Practices Commission (1992) *Final Report on the Self-Regulation of Promotion and Advertising of Therapeutic Goods*. Canberra: Australian Trade Practices Commission.
Avorn J, Chen M, and Hartley R (1982) Scientific versus commercial sources of influence on the prescribing behavior of physicians. *American Journal of Medicine* 73: 4–8.
Ayres I and Braithwaite J (1992) *Responsive Regulation. Transcending the Deregulation Debate*. New York: Oxford University Press.
Becker MH, Stolley P, Lasagna L, McEvilla J, and Sloane L (1972) Differential education concerning therapeutics and resultant physician prescribing patterns. *Journal of Medical Education* 47: 118–27.
Blondeel L, Cannoodt L, DeMeyeere M, and Proesmans H (1987) Prescription behaviour of 358 Flemish general practitioners. Paper presented at the International Society of General Medicine meeting, Prague.
Chetley A and Mintzes B (eds.) (1992) *Promoting Health or Pushing Drugs?* Amsterdam: Health Action International.
Chren MM, Landefeld CS, and Murray TH (1989) Doctors, drug companies, and gifts. *Journal of the American Medical Association* 262: 3448–51.
Drake D and Uhlman M (1993) *Making Medicine, Making Money*. Kansas City: Andrews and McMeel.
Ferry M, Lamy P, and Becker L (1985) Physicians' knowledge of prescribing for the elderly. A study of primary care physicians in Pennsylvania. *Journal of the American Geriatric Society* 33: 616–21.

Food and Drug Administration (1992) Draft policy statement on industry-supported scientific and educational activities. *Federal Register* 57(229): 58412–14.

Goldfinger SE (1990) Physicians and the pharmaceutical industry. *Annals of Internal Medicine* 112: 624–26.

Greenwood J (1989) *Pharmaceutical Representatives and the Prescribing of Drugs by Family Doctors* [Ph.D. dissertation]. Nottingham, UK: Nottingham University.

Haayer F (1982) Rational prescribing and sources of information. *Social Science and Medicine* 16: 2017–23.

Hagerman M (1992) Prescription drug advertising in Canada: an assessment. Presented to the Deputy Health Ministers Subcommittee on Pharmaceutical Policy Issues. Unpublished.

Hansson O (1989) *Inside Ciba-Geigy*. Penang, Malaysia: International Organization of Consumers Unions.

Harvey K (1990) Pharmaceutical promotion. *Medical Journal of Australia* 152: 57–58.

Health Action International (HAI) (1987) *Promoting Health or Promoting Drugs? A HAI Presentation on Rational Drug Use*. The Hague: HAI.

Healthcare Communications Inc. (1989) *The Effect of Journal Advertising on Market Shares of New Prescriptions*. New York: Association of Independent Medical Publications, Inc.

Herxheimer A and Collier J (1990) Promotion by the British pharmaceutical industry, 1983–1988: a critical analysis of self regulation. *British Medical Journal* 300: 307–11.

Herxheimer A, Lundborg CS, and Westerholm B (1993) Advertisements for medicines in leading medical journals in 18 countries: a 12-month survey of information content and standards. *International Journal of Health Services* 23: 161–72.

Iglehart JK (1991) The Food and Drug Administration and its problems. *New England Journal of Medicine* 325: 217–20.

International Federation of Pharmaceutical Manufacturers Associations (IFPMA) (1982) *IFPMA Code of Pharmaceutical Marketing Practices*. Zurich: IFPMA.

*Journal of the American Medical Association* (1990) Letters to the editor. (April 25) 263: 2177–79.

Kawachi I (1992a) The pressure to treat. In: Davis P (ed.) *For Health or Profit? Medicine, the Pharmaceutical Industry and the State in New Zealand*. Auckland, NZ: Oxford University Press, pp. 162–78.

Kawachi I (1992b) Six case studies of the voluntary regulation of pharmaceutical advertising and promotion. In: Davis P (ed.) *For Health or Profit? Medicine, the Pharmaceutical Industry and the State in New Zealand*. Auckland, NZ: Oxford University Press, pp. 269–87.

Kessler DA and Pines WL (1990) The federal regulation of prescription drug advertising and promotion. *Journal of the American Medical Association* 264: 2409–415.

Kline S (1992) Prescription drug advertising. In: Canadian Public Health Association (CPHA) (ed.) *Communicating Risk, Benefit, and Cost of Pharmaceuticals: Proceedings of an Invitational Workshop*. Vancouver, BC: CPHA, pp. 52–56.

Krupka LR and Vener AM (1985) Prescription drug advertising: trends and implications. *Social Science and Medicine* 20: 191–97.

Lexchin J (1990) Drug makers and drug regulators: too close for comfort. A study of the Canadian situation. *Social Science and Medicine* 31: 1257–63.

Lexchin J (1992) Pharmaceutical promotion in the Third World. *The Journal of Drug Issues* 22: 417–53.

Lexchin J (1993) Interactions between physicians and the pharmaceutical industry: what does the literature say? *Canadian Medical Association Journal* 149: 1401–7.

Lexchin J (1994) Canadian marketing codes: how well are they controlling pharmaceutical promotion? *International Journal of Health Services* 24: 91–104.

Linn LS and Davis MS (1972) Physicians orientation toward the legitimacy of drug use and their preferred source of new drug information. *Social Science and Medicine* 6: 199–203.

Lomas JMA, Anderson GM, Domnick-Pierre K, et al. (1989) Do practice guidelines guide practice? *New England Journal of Medicine* 322: 1306–11.

Mansfield PR (1992a) Drug companies responses to the WHO Ethical Criteria. *MaLAM Newsletter* (April).

Mansfield PR (1992b) Organon, the IFPMA Code and the WHO Ethical Criteria. *MaLAM Newsletter* (December).

Mansfield PR (1994) MaLAM: encouraging trustworthy drug promotion. *Essential Drug Monitor* 17, pp. 6–7.

Mapes R (1977) Aspects of British general practitioners prescribing. *Medical Care* 15: 371–78.

Montgomery DB and Silk AJ (1972) Estimating dynamic effects of market communications expenditures. *Management Science* 18: B-485–501.

Morris LA and Banks DB (1990) New issues in drug advertising and labeling: the five advertising end-runs. *Drug Information Journal* 24: 639–46.

*New England Journal of Medicine* (1992) Letters to the editor. (Dec. 3) 327: 1686–88.

PAAB (Pharmaceutical Advertising Advisory Board) (1992) *PAAB Code of Advertising Acceptance*. Pickering, Ont.: PAAB.

Parsons LJ and Abeele PV (1981) Analysis of sales call effectiveness. *Journal of Marketing Research* 18:107–13.

Raison AV (1989) *The Evolution of Standards for Pharmaceutical Advertising in Canada*. Pickering, Ont.: Pharmaceutical Advertising Advisory Board.

Randall T (1991) Kennedy hearings say no more free lunch—or much else—from drug firms. *Journal of the American Medical Association* 265: 440–42.

Royal College of Physicians (London) (1986) Report of the Working Party. The relationship between physicians and the pharmaceutical industry. *Journal of the Royal College of Physicians of London* 20: 235–57.

Silverman M (1976) *The Drugging of the Americas*. Berkeley: University of California Press.

Silverman M, Lydecker M, and Lee PR (1992) *Bad Medicine: The Prescription Drug Industry in the Third World*. Stanford: Stanford University Press.

Tomson G and Weerasuriya K (1990) Codes and practice: information in drug advertisements—an example from Sri Lanka. *Social Science and Medicine* 31: 737–41.

Walton H (1980) Ad recognition and prescribing by physicians. *Journal of Advertising Research* 20(3): 39–48.

Waud DR (1992) Pharmaceutical promotion—a free lunch? *New England Journal of Medicine* 327: 351–53.

WEMOS Pharma Group (1987) *Organon and Anabolic Steroids*. Amsterdam: WEMOS.

Wilkes MS, Doblin BH, and Shaprio MF (1992) Pharmaceutical advertisements in leading medical journals: experts' assessments. *Annals of Internal Medicine* 116: 912–19.

# 15

## New Approaches to Influencing Physicians' Drug Choices: The Practice-Based Strategy

FLORA M. HAAIJER-RUSKAMP
PETRA DENIG

Prescribing a drug is the most common form of treatment in primary health care. Although considerable differences in international prescribing practices have been described (Kimbel, 1992; Taylor, 1992), two features remain constant—the unbroken rise in levels of drug use since the 1960s and an increasing concern about costs (Haaijer-Ruskamp and Dukes, 1991). Inevitably, policy makers in all industrialized countries are seeking ways of curbing costs, while at the same time striving to maintain the quality of health care. One approach that has wide currency is to try rationalizing drug use.

In this chapter we will look at the effect of different educational approaches on promoting rational prescribing. This concept is often defined solely in terms of the objective characteristics of a drug, such as its efficacy and safety (for example, Dukes, 1990). However, in designing appropriate educational strategies, it is important to consider concepts of rationality from the prescriber's perspective. These concepts are often based on subjective evaluations by the physician and are influenced by a variety of contextual factors. It is the context of prescribing that we consider first.

### The Context of Prescribing

Physicians cannot be viewed as completely autonomous individuals practicing in socially isolated settings. Many relevant contextual factors have been identified in studies investigating variations in drug use (see Table 15-1). While the focus in this chapter is on physicians (level III in the table), the other levels outlined provide the background and context in which doctors work. Factors relevant at the population level refer mainly to the organization of health care. They address the physical and financial availability of drugs for different sections of the population, and issues of drug quality. For the prescribing physician the structure of the health care system determines the range of available options. For example, where access to professional care is poor, self-medication tends to be used as a substitute for prescribed drugs (Leibowitz, 1989). The cultural setting determines the meaning of drug use, such as its social acceptability. Cultural beliefs and attitudes shape the presentation of morbidity, and therefore affect therapeutic choices. Similarly, the physician is part of the same culture and will tend to respond in culturally acceptable ways (Hull and Marshall, 1987; Payer, 1988; Grol et al., 1990a; 1990b).

Some factors at the practice level are demographic, and so are not directly amenable to regulation. This is not true for organizational attributes such as size and structure, which vary greatly cross-nationally (Grol et al., 1993). Apart from demographic factors—with an obvious relevance for morbidity (Forster and Frost, 1991)—the influence of practice attributes is not well understood. The number of GPs in a health center has been shown to correlate with the range of drugs prescribed (McCarthy et al., 1992). Size of practice has been shown to be relevant in some studies (e.g., Hartzema and Christensen, 1983), but not in others (e.g., Cormack

TABLE 15-1.  Contextual Factors Influencing Prescribing

| Level | Relevant factors | Policy instruments |
|---|---|---|
| I. Population | regulation, financing, and availability of medicines and health care; power of the pharmaceutical industry; culture, tradition, beliefs regarding health and illness | legal instruments; requirements of drug registration; health insurance and reimbursement systems for drugs |
| II. Practice | proportion of elderly and female patients; proportion of lower economic class patients (see also IV); urbanization; practice organization and practice size | organization of health care/structure of health care |
| III. Physician | age and gender; attitudes and working style (tendency of physicians to do something instead of wait and see, disease- versus patient-oriented attitude, perceived patient demand); training and education; use of information sources; patient interaction | information and education of physicians |
| IV. Patient | age, gender, social class; social circumstances, expectations, and demands; compliance | patient education, reimbursement system |

*Source*: Dukes, 1985; Cialdella et al., 1991; Haaijer-Ruskamp and Hemminki, 1993.

and Howells, 1992). Workload seems to be primarily determined by demography (McGavock et al., 1993). Financial motives also may be relevant. The degree of urbanization is another factor that has been shown to relate to higher levels of drug use (Haaijer-Ruskamp and Hemminki, 1993), but it remains unclear to what extent this is caused by higher levels of morbidity, presentation of complaints, or availability of other health care services. In summary, for policy makers the modification of practice organization does not present itself as a particularly attractive or effective instrument for the regulation of prescribing.

The patient is a major influence on prescribing. For example, physicians often feel pressured to prescribe by patient demand (Schwarz and Griffin, 1986; Bradley, 1992a; 1992b). In general, physicians overestimate demand (Virji and Britten, 1991). Physicians' estimates of percentages of patients wanting medication range from 20 to 100%, with an average of 50 to 75% (Haaijer-Ruskamp, 1984). In a national study of primary care in The Netherlands, 7.4% of the patients consulting their general practitioners received a drug when they believed they did not need one, while 11.5% did not receive a drug when they thought they needed it (Foets and Sixma, 1991). Some patients are even averse to taking therapeutic drugs (Cartwright and Smith, 1988). Policy makers try to use patient demand to influence prescriber behavior. Charging patients for medication, for example, may decrease patient demand, while lower patient demand is expected to decrease prescribing rates (Soumerai et al., 1993). Advertising prescription-only drugs to the public also makes use of the impact of patient demand on drug use, a practice that is allowed in the United States but prohibited in many countries, including the European Union.

Besides patient demand, compliance issues are of major importance in understanding drug use. For example, improving patient compliance can be a reason for selecting a so-called user-friendly drug, a medication that needs to be taken only once a day, or is easy to administer, or tastes better (Grol, 1992). Particularly when a drug is being selected from a group with similar efficacy and side effects, compliance may be an important consideration in the reckoning of overall cost, as in the case of $H_2$ blockers, for example (Savafi and Hayward, 1992).

Patient-specific factors, though important, do not explain all the variation in prescribing. Physicians' characteristics have been shown to be relevant as well. For example, physicians may choose different therapies for the same patient management problem (Sandvik and Hunskaar, 1990). Age and gender are important factors (Ray et al., 1985; Forrest et al., 1989; Strømme and Botten, 1992). Physicians' attitudes toward medicine and prescribing are also relevant. For example, the doctor's attitude to risk taking is associated with higher prescribing rates; the less willing physicians are to take any risks involved in not treating, the more inclined they are to prescribe (Grol et al., 1990a). Another relevant factor is the extent to which a physician is disease- versus patient-oriented (Grol et al., 1990b).

These factors provide a general understanding of how context may influence physicians' prescribing. However, most of them are not directly amenable to change. One of the central problems is that much remains unclear about how these factors are translated into prescribing decisions; in other words, the actual decision making process is unclear.

## Physicians' Decision Making About Drugs

Decision making about drugs refers, first, to the decision to prescribe and, second, to the selection of a specific medication. After being presented with a health problem, a limited set of solutions comes immediately to the physician's mind; this is the so-called evoked set. For example, a case of simple cystitis might be immediately associated in the doctor's mind with either trimethoprim or co-trimoxazol. Next, a specific therapy must be selected for a specific patient (Denig and Haaijer-Ruskamp, 1992). Each step is obviously subject to different influences. It appears that the evoked set is developed initially during training. This initial set evolves over time as the physician is influenced by the activities of the pharmaceutical industry (advertising, representatives, seeding trials) and by other information and postgraduate education. The influence on the prescribing of general practitioners by hospital specialists is particularly noteworthy (Mugford, Banfield, and O'Hanlon, 1991).

The second step in the decision making process, the choice of a specific therapy from this evoked set for a particular patient, seems either to derive from an active problem solving approach or to be largely a matter of habit. Active problem solving involves the evaluation of expected outcomes for possible treatment options. Relevant decision criteria for choosing a drug treatment include not only biomedical characteristics of the drug, such as efficacy and adverse effects, but also the opinion of colleagues, patient acceptability, and personal experience (McGuire, 1985; Soumerai, McLaughlin, and Avorn, 1989). Cost may be a relevant issue in some instances, but as a rule it is not taken into account much by physicians (Segal and Hepler, 1982; 1985; Chinburapa et al., 1987; Chinburapa and Larson, 1988; 1992; Denig et al., 1993). The recent increase in the prescribing of generics in some countries may indicate that this is changing.

Treatment options for identical problems obviously are not evaluated repeatedly. Rules of thumb are developed that can be explicitly reasoned, developed by trial and error, or copied without any evident reasoning process. In general, 50 to 90% of drug choices can be predicted from expectations about drug treatment and the values attached to these expectations, both indicative of an active problem solving approach (Harrell and Bennet, 1974). Evidence for unreasoned decision routines in drug therapy has also been identified (Hepler et al., 1982).

Increased understanding of the process of drug choice makes it clear that availability of the correct information about drug characteristics is not enough on its own. Such knowledge has to be applied as well. Imaginative educational approaches are needed to address shortcomings not only in the knowledge base but also in its application.

## The Educational Strategy

### Formularies, Guidelines, and Drug Use Review

In the last 10 to 15 years ideas about drug information and strategies to support rational prescribing have changed dramatically. Instead of a one-way stream of data directed at physicians, information is more oriented toward daily medical practice and the requirements of prescribers. This trend can be seen both in university training and in continuing medical education (de Vries, 1993). Drug bulletins, for example, put more emphasis on reviews, often evaluating a whole class of drugs. This orientation to practice requirements is also reflected in the development of formularies that provide a list of preferred drug products, ideally updated on a regular basis to reflect pharmacological improvements.

Guidelines and protocols are the clinical extension of the formulary concept. They provide not only first-choice drugs, but first-choice patient management of a particular disease. A good example of a guideline is the International Consensus on the Treatment of Asthma (NIH, 1992) developed by an international group of experts. The advice given in formularies and guidelines is particularly important in changing physicians' perceptions of acceptable practice. As such they can be a predisposing factor in changing the evoked set. Actual change, however, needs more incentives (Lomas, 1989).

Another relatively recent strategy is drug use review (DUR), sometimes called drug use evaluation. With this approach the use of drugs by individual patients is examined, evaluated for actual or potential problems, corrective actions are proposed or provided, and follow-up measures are instituted. Drug use evaluation is particularly helpful in detecting and preventing possible interactions and adverse effects, redundant drug use (use of several drugs from the same class without apparent justification), high levels of use, and high costs. It can also help provide special care for identified high-risk patients (Armstrong and Terry, 1992). Drug use evaluation is only possible when complete medication histories of patients are available in conjunction with clinical data. This type of data is not usually available for the whole population.

## Educational Approaches

The development of formularies, guidelines, and drug use review are extremely helpful, but are usually not enough in themselves to achieve change; further educational strategies are needed. Over the last decade education about therapeutic drugs has received increasing attention and many different educational approaches have been developed. The main techniques are:

1. The use of printed material on its own
2. Verbal education in face-to-face meetings with the individual prescriber ("academic detailing")
3. Verbal education (mainly carefully targeted lectures) with groups of prescribers
4. Feedback of data to individual prescribers concerning their prescribing patterns, without any advice or comments
5. Feedback of data on individual prescribing patterns combined with group discussions (audit, peer review)
6. Feedback of data concerning individual patients with specific recommendations (DUR)

The first approach consists of the use of printed material such as drug bulletins, drug or disease brochures, and monographs, to improve knowledge and to keep prescribers up-to-date. Adequate knowledge is essential. However, inadequate prescribing is seldom a question of inadequate knowledge alone (Denig, Haaijer-Ruskamp and Zijsling, 1988a). As stated earlier, prescribing decisions are also influenced by the professional environment of the physician, professional norms, patient demand, and prescribers' experiences in the past. In face-to-face meetings one can draw on, and refer back to, the personal experience of the physician and target the message more specifically. The advantage of a group lecture is that it may make use of the professional norm in the group. Though primarily for dissemination of information, group lectures allow for the discussion of norms, decision criteria, and values attached to these criteria. The advantage of individual meetings, as in academic detailing, is that confidentiality may be established more easily; physicians may be more open to discussing their own problems and perceived shortcomings. An individual approach is very time consuming. Often it can only be used in programs oriented to a minority of suboptimal prescribers.

Much prescribing is routine behavior. To change such behavior more reinforcement is needed than simply providing general advice. Auditing programs in peer groups use prescribing data as feedback to show physicians what they actually do and where there is room for improvement. Feedback data can be a motivating trigger and can make physicians aware of problems, particularly in their routine behavior. In some instances feedback data can be provided without comment. In the case of more extensive auditing programs there is an explicit setting of standards, the use of peer review in groups, and feedback about how much physicians adhere to the criteria set.

## Evaluating Educational Interventions

The impact of different approaches on actual prescribing is still not fully understood, partly because of a lack of well-controlled studies. Moreover, most studies have been conducted in the United States; in view of the relevance of contextual factors, one should be careful in trying to extrapolate these results to societies with different cultures and health care systems. Uncontrolled studies seem to overestimate the effect of interventions. Soumerai, McLaughlin and Avorn (1989) identified 44 studies published between 1970 and 1988 evaluating interventions designed to improve prescribing; only 64% were adequately controlled. Of the studies with a well-controlled design, 55% had a positive result, compared with a success rate of 85% in uncontrolled studies. Uncontrolled studies suggest that formularies and guidelines have an effect (Grant, Gregory, and Van Zwannenberg, 1985; Black et al., 1988; Field, 1989), but involvement of physicians in their development, plus additional review, education, and feedback, seem to be necessary for a high level of adherence (Wyatt et al., 1992).

Table 15-2 presents a review of studies evaluating the impact of different educational approaches on prescribing. It builds on the pioneering work of Soumerai et al. (1989), but is limited to studies incorporating adequate controls (in all, 53 randomized or otherwise controlled studies are identified). The introduction of formularies

Table 15-2. Evaluation of Educational Interventions

| | Design | Aimed at | Target Group | Effect on Level K | P | C | O |
|---|---|---|---|---|---|---|---|
| *Printed material* | | | | | | | |
| Watson DS et al. (1975) | CT | 10 topics | 1 | | + | | |
| Sibley JC et al. (1982) | RCT | 18 topics | 1 | + | | | ± |
| Avorn J et al (1983) | RCT | vasodilators, cefalosporines, propoxyfene | 1 | | − | | |
| Schaffner W et al. (1983); Ray WA et al. (1985) | CT | antibiotics | 1 | | − | − | |
| Evans CE et al. (1984; 1986) | RCT | hypertension therapy | 1 | ± | | | − |
| Hershey CO et al. (1988) | RCT | drug costs | 1 | − | | − | |
| Denig P et al. (1990) | CT | IBS/renal colic treatment | 1 | ± | ± | | |
| Angunawela II et al. (1991) | RCT | antibiotics | 1 | | − | | |
| *Face-to-face education in a one-on-one situation* | | | | | | | |
| Stross JK et al. (1980) | CT | antirheumatic | 1 | | + | | |
| McConnell TS (1982) | RCT | tetracycline | 1 | | + | | |
| Schaffner W et al. (1983); Ray WA et al. (1985) | CT | antibiotics | 1 | | ± | ± | |
| Avorn J et al. (1983); Soumerai SB et al. (1986) | RCT | vasodilators, cefalosporines, propoxyfene | 1 | | + | + | |
| Stross JK et al. (1983) | CT | COPD treatment | 1/2 | | + | | − |
| Ray WA et al. (1986) | CT | diazepam | 1 | | ± | | |
| Denig P et al. (1988b) | CT | IBS/renal colic treatment | 1 | + | ± | | |
| Landgren FT et al. (1988) | CT | antibiotics | 2 | | ± | ± | |
| Steele MA et al. (1989) | RCT | drug costs | 1 | | + | | |
| Raisch DW et al. (1990) | CT | antiulcer drugs | 1 | | ± | ± | |
| Font M et al. (1991) | RCT | vasodilators, combination antibiotics, cefalosporines | 1 | | ± | ± | |
| Newton-Syms FAO et al. (1992) | RCT | NSAIDs | 1 | | + | + | |
| Ray WA et al. (1993) | CT | antipsychotic drugs | 2 | | + | | + |
| *Targeted lectures* | | | | | | | |
| Inui T et al. (1976) | RCT | hypertension treatment | 1 | | | | + |
| Klein LE et al. (1981) | CT | antibiotics | 2 | | + | + | |
| White CW et al. (1985) | RCT | myocardial infarction treatment | 2 | + | ± | | |
| Mölstad S et al. (1989) | CT | antibiotics | 1 | | + | | |
| Rutz W et al. (1989; 1990; 1992) | CT | psychotropic drugs | 1 | + | ± | | |

TABLE 15-2. *(Continued)*

| | Design | Aimed at | Target Group | Effect on Level | | | |
|---|---|---|---|---|---|---|---|
| | | | | K | P | C | O |
| Holm M (1990) | RCT | benzodiazepine | 1 | − | | | |
| Angunawela II et al. (1991) | RCT | antibiotics | 1 | | − | | |
| Friis H et al. (1991) | CT | antibiotics | 1 | | + | | |
| *Individual feedback* | | | | | | | |
| Johnson RE et al. (1976) | RCT | all drugs | 1 | − | − | | |
| Koepsell TD et al. (1983) | CT | interactions, redundancies | | | − | | |
| Hershey CO et al. (1986) | RCT | drug costs | 1 | − | | + | |
| Holm M (1990) | RCT | benzodiazepines | 1 | − | | | |
| Meyer TJ et al. (1991) | RCT[a] | all drugs, polypharmacy | 1 | | ± | | |
| Lassen LC et al. (1992) | CT | all drugs | 1 | | − | + | |
| *Audit* | | | | | | | |
| Harris CM et al. (1985) | RCT | all drugs | 1 | | ± | ± | |
| Manheim LM et al. (1990) | RCT | drug costs | 2 | | | + | + |
| Stokx L et al. (1992) | CT | antibiotics, benzodiaze-pines, antiasthmatics, NSAIDS | 1 | | − | | |
| Zijlstra IF et al. (1991) | CT | peptic drugs, hyperten-sives, NSAIDs | 1 | | + | ± | |
| | | | | | ± | | |
| *Drug use review* | | | | | | | |
| McDonald CJ (1976) | CT | drug related events | 2 | − | + | | |
| Herfindal ET et al. (1983) | CT | drugs prescribed by orthopedist | 2 | | | ± | |
| Gehlbach SH et al. (1984) | RCT | drug costs | 1 | | + | | |
| Manning PR et al. (1986) | RCT | several drugs | 1 | | + | | |
| Tierney WM (1986) | RCT | antacids, aspirins, betablockers, anti-depressants, nitrates, metronidazole | 2 | | ± | | |
| Stergachis A et al. (1987) | CT | drug costs | 1 | | ± | − | |
| Tamai IY et al. (1987) | CT | potential drug problems | 1 | | + | | |
| Steele MA et al. (1989) | RCT | drug costs | 1 | | − | | |
| Crischilles EA et al. (1989) | CT | all drugs | 1 | | + | + | |
| Forstrom MJ et al. (1990) | CT | costs of hypertension therapy | 1 | | + | + | |
| Kroenke K et al. (1990) | CT | elderly and polypharmacy | 1 | | + | + | |
| Frazier LM et al. (1991) | RCT | drug costs | 1 | − | | ± | |
| Britton ML et al. (1991) | RCT[a] | all drugs, polypharmacy | 1 | | + | + | |

*(Continued)*

243

TABLE 15-2. Evaluation of Educational Interventions (*Continued*)

| | Design | Aimed at | Target Group | Effect on Level | | | |
|---|---|---|---|---|---|---|---|
| | | | | K | P | C | O |
| Levens Lipton H et al. (1992) | RCT[a] | geriatric prescribing | 2 | | + | | |
| Mason JD and Colley CA (1993) | CT | potential drug therapy problems | 1 | | + | + | |

Design: RCT = randomized controlled trial; CT = controlled trial (non-randomized); [a]patients were divided into intervention and control groups, instead of (groups of) physicians

Aimed at: specific drugs or treatments; reducing costs

Target group: 1 = general practitioners/family physicians/doctors treating outpatients; 2 = physicians treating patients in hospitals

Level of evaluation: K = knowledge of physicians; P = quality of prescribing behavior; C = economic costs; O = patient outcomes or quality of care

Effect: − no significant effect; + significant effect; ± only short-term effects or mixed effects (some positive, some negative)

or guidelines without any additional educational program has only been tested in inadequately controlled studies (see above), and these are not included in the table. In some studies a combination of methods was used, and these have been classified as follows: when verbal education in meetings (lectures) was combined with printed material, the intervention was classified as a targeted lecture; when feedback was combined with group meetings, it was classified as audit, and when it was combined with verbal individual education or individual feedback, it was classified as DUR.

To summarize the material in Table 15-2: printed material appears to be the least effective; face-to-face education (either individually or in small groups) and audit (in peer groups) seem to be more successful; raw feedback data, that is, without any recommendation or discussion with the prescriber, seem to be ineffective; and DUR shows the highest success rates (see Fig. 15-1).

## An Intervention Study—The Area Clinical Pharmacologist

An illustration of a program with mixed results is an experiment with an area clinical pharmacologist (ACP) working alongside GPs and pharmacists to support rational prescribing (Zijlstra, 1991). The study is instructive in highlighting the effort needed to change habits, in indicating why mixed results are so often reported for such interventions, and in suggesting how these outcomes might be improved. The ACP is a clinical pharmacologist working in primary health care, a person with an understanding of clinical medicine as well as drugs. In the Netherlands a national network of local pharmacotherapy counseling groups (PCG) has been in place since 1989. PCGs consist of groups of physician peers, together with the community pharmacist. They meet regularly to exchange information about drug therapy and often work toward local guidelines. The ACP was intended to support existing PCGs and to establish them where none existed. It was believed that the ACP could be important

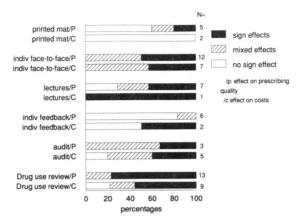

**Figure 15-1.** Impacts of different educational strategies. /P is effect on prescribing quality and /C is effect on cost.

in helping to bridge the disciplinary gap between physicians and pharmacists. Treatment of peptic problems, treatment of hypertension, and choice of NSAIDs were the topics of three separate meetings. For each topic,

1. The ACP presented expert opinion on what the treatment should be
2. A questionnaire about choice of treatment was filled in by the physicians
3. A case history was completed by the physicians
4. Prescribing data indicating actual prescribing patterns of individual physicians were presented

The intervention ended with the same set of recommendations being proffered to each group. This last measure, a set of imposed recommendations, has the advantage of facilitating the comparison of the impact of the ACP across the different groups, but its great disadvantage is that the physicians were not actively involved in its development.

The effect of this program was evaluated for preferred medicine choice, for the number of different medicines used, for volume, and for costs. The results varied for the different therapeutic fields and according to the level of prior involvement with PCGs. The greatest impact was seen in the change of preferred medicine choice for the treatment of peptic problems. Also, physicians who were already used to discussing their prescribing in PCGs changed their behavior most. This suggests that physicians may have to get used to peer groups before they are willing to change their behavior accordingly. On the other hand, it is possible that physicians participating in PCGs before the ACP experiment were early adopters, and therefore more open to change. Most effects were seen after some time had elapsed (at least six months after the intervention), indicating that physicians need time to adjust their prescribing habits.

One of the reasons why a greater impact was not detected could be that the physicians did not always agree with the ACP's recommendations. This became clear in the course of the experiment. In some cases the disagreement was due to inadequate knowledge, while in others advantages and disadvantages were weighed differently by some physicians. This highlighted a general weakness of the program — it was primarily directed to the transfer of knowledge alone. Insufficient attention was paid to the decision making process, an understanding of which is important in learning how to apply the knowledge that has been transferred.

## Conclusion

Policy makers have become increasingly interested in the education of physicians about drug therapy. The last 10 to 15 years have seen a number of new initiatives, many of which have been evaluated. Of these, drug use review seems to be the most effective, judged on both quality of outcome and cost containment. It has to be remembered, however, that such programs need high-quality clinical and medication data about individual patients. Such data may not be available in many settings, particularly in outpatient clinics. Moreover, privacy considerations may hinder the full exploitation of all the technological possibilities. Furthermore, it is not certain whether DUR produces sustained behavioral change once it is discontinued.

Regarding the more educational approaches, the fact that many studies have had mixed results leaves many questions unanswered. The impact of education, for example, seems to be influenced by the message itself; other aspects, such as the credibility and attractiveness of the information and of the messenger, play a role, as well as perceived barriers and the potential for implementing the recommendations (McGuire, 1985). Credibility and attractiveness are particularly important when considering printed material. Although some researchers have argued that printed material is only successful in changing knowledge and not actual prescribing behavior (Soumerai and Avorn, 1984), aspects such as attractiveness, clarity, credibility, and the efficiency of distribution have nevertheless been shown to be important for the successful transmission of information (Lipowski and Becker, 1992).

Regularly distributed bulletins, and bulletins in educational settings, seem to be more effective than material that has been developed for a specific intervention project (Plumridge and Berbatis, 1989). As far as we know, the introduction of formularies and guidelines seems to be moderately successful, but most of these studies have been inadequately controlled (e.g., Feely et al., 1990; Kane et al., 1990). Involvement of the prescriber in the development of the formulary or guidelines, as well as additional review, education, and feedback, seem to be necessary in maintaining a high level of adherence (Harvey et al., 1983; Baker, Lant and Sutters, 1988). Strong involvement of the physician is an important factor in explaining the success of the individual face-to-face education and auditing programs.

Developments within pharmacotherapy will continue to make drug education necessary for practicing physicians. The number of medicines available and the deepening of our understanding of pathophysiology and of the various types of active mechanisms involved have made drug prescribing a complicated matter. It is clear that traditional ways of education are not sufficient. In that respect the development of more practice-oriented approaches is hopeful. In a society requiring a high quality of health care that is also cost effective, policy makers would do well to support successful programs of educational intervention in the practice environment.

## References

Angunawela II, Diwan VK, and Tomson G (1991) Experimental evaluation of the effects of drug information on antibiotic prescribing: a study in outpatient care in an area of Sri Lanka. *International Journal of Epidemiology* 20: 558–64.

Armstrong EP and Terry AK (1992) Impact of drug use evaluation upon ambulatory pharmacy practice. *Annals of Pharmacotherapy* 26: 1546–53.

Avorn J and Soumerai SB (1983) Improving drug-therapy decisions through educational outreach. A randomized controlled trial of academically based "detailing." *New England Journal of Medicine* 308: 1457–63.

Baker JA, Lant AF, and Sutters CA (1988) Seventeen years' experience of a voluntarily based drug rationalisation programme in hospital. *British Medical Journal* 297: 465–69.

Black J, Griffin T, Beisel NW, and Bartels MD (1988) Implementation of an outpatient prescription drug formulary in a managed care system. *American Journal of Hospital Pharmacy* 45: 561–65.

Bradley CP (1992a) Uncomfortable prescribing decisions: a critical incident study. *British Medical Journal* 304: 294–96.

Bradley CP (1992b) Factors which influence the decision whether or not to prescribe: the dilemma facing general practitioners. *British Journal of General Practice* 42: 454–58.

Britton ML and Lurvey PL (1991) Impact of medication profile review on prescribing in a general medicine clinic. *American Journal of Hospital Pharmacy* 48: 265–70.

Cartwright A and Smith C (1988) *Elderly People, their Medicines and their Doctors*. London: Routledge.

Chinburapa V and Larson LN (1988) Predicting prescribing intention and assessing drug attribute importance using conjoint analysis. *Journal of Pharmaceutical Marketing and Management* 3: 3–18.

Chinburapa V and Larson LN (1992) The importance of side effects and outcomes in differentiating between prescription drug products. *Journal of Clinical Pharmacology and Therapeutics* 17: 333–42.

Chinburapa V, Larson LN, Lyle Bootman J, McGhan WF, and Nichloson G (1987) Prescribing intention and the relative importance of drug attributes. A comparative study of HMO and fee-for-service physicians. *Journal of Pharmaceutical Marketing and Management* 2: 89–105.

Cialdella P, Figon G, Haugh MC, and Boissel J (1991) Prescription intentions in relation to therapeutic information: a study of 117 French general practitioners. *Social Science and Medicine* 33: 1263–74.

Cormack MA and Howells E (1992) Factors linked to the prescribing of benzodiazepines by general practice principals and trainees. *Family Practice* 9: 466–71.

Crischilles EA, Helling DK, and Aschoff CR (1989) Effect of clinical pharmacy services on the quality of family practice physician prescribing and medication costs. *DICP Annals of Pharmacotherapy* 23: 417–21.

Denig P and Haaijer-Ruskamp FM (1992) Therapeutic decision making of physicians. *Pharmaceutisch Weekblad Scientific edition* 14: 9–15.

Denig P, Haaijer-Ruskamp FM, Wesseling H, and Versluis A (1993) Towards understanding treatment preferences of hospital physicians. *Social Science and Medicine* 36: 915–24.

Denig P, Haaijer-Ruskamp FM, and Zijsling DH (1988a) How physicians choose their drugs. *Social Science and Medicine* 27: 1381–86.

Denig P, Haaijer-Ruskamp FM, and Zijsling DH (1988b) *Arts en geneesmiddeleninformatie* (Physician and drug information). Groningen, The Netherlands: Styx Publications.

Denig P, Haaijer-Ruskamp FM, and Zijsling DH (1990) The impact of a drug bulletin on knowledge, drug evaluation and prescribing of physicians. *Drug Intelligence and Clinical Pharmacy* 24: 87–93.

de Vries ThPGM (1993) *Presenting Clinical Pharmacology and Therapeutics*. Groningen, The Netherlands: Styx Publications.

Dukes MNG (1985) *The Effects of Drug Regulation*. Lancaster, UK: MTP Press.

Dukes MNG (1990) Rational use of drugs: an overview. In: Muller NF and Hekster YA (eds.) *Progress in Clinical Pharmacy 1989. Rational Use of Drugs*. The Hague: Amsterdam Medical Press BV Noordwijk/SDU Publishers, pp. 3–18.

Evans CE, Haynes RB, Gilbert JR, Taylor DW, Sackett DL, et al. (1984) Educational package on hypertension for primary care physicians. *Canadian Medical Association Journal* 130: 719–22.

Evans CE, Haynes RB, Birkett NJ, Gilbert JR, Taylor DW, et al. (1986) Does a mailed continuing education program improve physician performance? *Journal of the American Medical Association* 255: 501–4.

Feely J, Chan R, Cocoman L, Mulpeter K, and O'Connor P (1990) Hospital formularies: need for continuous intervention. *British Medical Journal* 300: 28–30.

Field J (1989) How do doctors and patients react to the introduction of a practice formulary? *Family Practice* 6: 135–40.

Foets M and Sixma H (1991) *Een nationale studie van ziekten en verrichtingen in de huisartsprak-tijk. Basisrapport: gezondheid en gezondheidsgedrag in de praktijkpopulatie* (A national study of diseases and treatment in general practice. First report: health and health behaviour in the GP population). Utrecht, The Netherlands: Nivel.

Font M, Madridejos R, Catalan A, Jimenez J, Argimon JM, et al. (1991) Mejorar la prescrip-tion de farmacos en atencion primaria: un estudio controlado y aleatorio sobre un metodo educativo (Improving drug prescription in primary care: a controlled and randomized study of an educational method). *Medicinca Clinica* (Barcelona) 96: 201–5.

Forrest JM, McKenna M, Stanley IM, Boaden NT, and Woodcock GT (1989) Continuing education: a survey among general practitioners. *Family Practice* 6: 98–107.

Forster DP and Frost CEB (1991) Use of regression analysis to explain the variation in prescribing rates and costs between family practitioner committees. *British Journal of General Practice* 41: 67–71.

Forstrom MJ, Reid LD, Stergachis AS, and Corliss DA (1990) Effect of a clinical pharmacist program on the cost of hypertension treatment in an HMO family practice clinic. *DICP Annals of Pharmacotherapy* 24: 304–9.

Frazier LM, Brown JT, Divine GW, Fleming GR, Philips NM, et al. (1991) Can physician education lower the cost of prescription drugs? A prospective, controlled trial. *Annals of Internal Medicine* 115: 116–21.

Friis H, Bro F, Mabeck CE, and Vejlsgaard R (1991) Changes in prescription of antibiotics in general practice in relation to different strategies for drug information. *Danish Medical Bulletin* 38: 380–82.

Gehlbach SH, Wilkinson WE, Hammond WE, Clapp NE, Finn AL, et al. (1984) Improving drug prescribing in a primary care practice. *Medical Care* 22: 193–201.

Grant GB, Gregory DA, and Van Zwanenberg TD (1985) Development of a limited formu-lary for general practice. *Lancet* 1: 1030–32.

Grol R (1992) Implementing guidelines in general practice care. *Quality Health Care* 1: 184–91.

Grol R, Whitfield M, de Maeseneer J, and Mokkink H (1990a) Attitudes to risk taking in medical decision making among British, Dutch and Belgian general practitioners. *British Journal of General Practice* 40: 134–36.

Grol R, de Maeseneer J, Whitfield M, and Mokkink H (1990b) Disease-centred versus patient-centred attitudes: comparison of general practitioners in Belgium, Britain and The Netherlands. *Family Practice* 7: 100–103.

Grol R, Wensing M, Jacobs A, and Baker R (eds.) (1993) *Quality Assurance in General Practice; The State of the Art in Europe*. Utrecht, the Netherlands: WONCA European Working Party on Quality in Family Practice (EQuiP)/Dutch College of General Practitioners.

Haaijer-Ruskamp FM (1984) *Het voorschrijfgedrag van de huisarts*. (Prescribing behavior of the General Practitioner) Dissertation. University of Groningen, The Netherlands.

Haaijer-Ruskamp FM and Dukes MNG (1991) *Drugs and Money; The Problem of Cost Containment*. Groningen, The Netherlands: Styx Publications.

Haaijer-Ruskamp FM and Hemminki E (1993) The Social Aspects of Drug Use. In: Dukes MNG (ed.) *Drug Utilization Studies – Methods and Uses*. WHO Regional Publications, European Series 45: 97–124.

Harrell G and Bennet P (1974) An evaluation of the expectancy value model of attitude measurement for physician prescribing behaviour. *Journal of Marketing Research* 8: 269–78.

Harris CM, Fry J, Jarman B, and Woodman E (1985) Prescribing – a case for prolonged treatment. *Journal of the Royal College of General Practitioners* 35: 284–87.

Hartzema AG and Christensen DB (1983) Nonmedical factors associated with the prescribing volume among family practitioners in an HMO. *Medical Care* 21: 990–1000.

Harvey K, Stewart RB, Hemming M, and Moulds R (1983) Use of antibiotic agents in a large teaching hospital. The impact of antibiotic guidelines. *Medical Journal of Australia* 2: 217–21.

Hepler CD, Clyne KE, and Donta ST (1982) Rationales expressed by empiric antibiotic prescribers. *American Journal of Hospital Pharmacy* 39: 1647–55.

Herfindal ET, Bernstein LR, and Kishi DT (1983) Effect of clinical pharmacy services on prescribing on an orthopaedic unit. *American Journal of Hospital Pharmacy* 40: 1945–51.

Hershey CO, Goldberg MI, and Cohen DI (1988) The effect of computerized feedback coupled with a newsletter upon outpatient prescribing charges. *Medical Care* 26: 88–94.

Hershey CO, Porter DK, Breslau D, and Cohen DI (1986) Influence of simple computerized feedback on prescribing charges in an ambulatory clinic. *Medical Care* 24: 472–81.

Holm M (1990) Intervention against long-term use of hypnotics/sedatives in general practice. *Scandanavian Journal of Primary Health Care* 8: 113–17.

Hull FM and Marshall T (1987) Sources of information about new drugs and attitudes towards drug prescribing. *Family Practice* 4: 123–27.

Inui T, Yourtec EL, and Williamson JW (1976) Improved outcomes in hypertension after physician tutorials: a controlled trial. *Annals of Internal Medicine* 84: 646–51.

Johnson RE, Campbell WH, Azevedo D, and Christensen DB (1976) Studying the impact of patient drug profiles in an HMO. *Medical Care* 14: 799–807.

Kane MP, Briceland LL, Garris RE, and Favreau BN (1990) Drug-use review program for concurrent histamine H2-receptor antagonist-sucralfate therapy. *American Journal of Hospital Pharmacy* 47: 2007–10.

Kimbel KH (1992) Drug prescribing patterns in Europe. *International Journal of Clinical Pharmacology, Therapy and Toxicology* 30: 450–61.

Klein LE, Charache P, and Johannes RS (1981) Effect of physician tutorials on prescribing patterns of graduate physicians. *Journal of Medical Education* 56: 504–11.

Koepsell TD, Gurtel AL, Diehr PH, Temkin NR, Helfand KH, et al. (1983) The Seattle evaluation of computerized drug profiles: effects on prescribing practices and resource use. *American Journal of Public Health* 73: 850–55.

Kroenke LTCK and Pinholt EM (1990) Reducing polypharmacy in the elderly. A controlled trial of physician feedback. *Journal of the American Geriatric Society* 38: 31–36.

Landgren FT, Harvey KJ, Mashford ML, Moulds RFW, Guthrie B, et al. (1988) Changing antibiotic prescribing by educational marketing. *Medical Journal of Australia* 149: 595–99.

Lassen LC and Kristensen FB (1992) Peer comparison feedback to achieve rational and economical drug therapy in general practice: a controlled intervention study. *Scandinavian Journal of Primary Health Care* 10: 76–80.

Leibowitz A (1989) Substitution between prescribed and over-the-counter medications. *Medical Care* 27: 85–94.

Levens Lipton H, Bero LA, Bird JA, and McPhee SJ (1992) The impact of clinical pharmacists' consultations on physicians' geriatric drug prescribing – a randomized controlled trial. *Medical Care* 30: 646–58.

Lipowski EE and Becker M (1992) Presentation of drug prescribing guidelines and physician response. *Quality Review Bulletin* 18: 461–70.

Lomas J, Anderson GM, Domnick-Pierre K, et al. (1989) Do practices guidelines guide practice? The effect of a consensus statement on the practice of physicians. *New England Journal of Medicine* 321: 1306–311.

Manheim LM, Feinglass J, Hughes R, Martin GJ, Conrad K, et al. (1990) Training house officers to be cost conscious. Effects of an educational intervention on charges and length of stay. *Medical Care* 28: 29–40.

Manning PR, Lee PV, Clintworth WA, Denson TA, Oppenheimer PR, et al. (1986) Changing prescribing practices through individual continuing education. *Journal of the American Medical Assocation* 256: 230–32.

Mason JD and Colley CA (1993) Effectiveness of an ambulatory care clinical pharmacist: a controlled trial. *Annals of Pharmacotherapy* 27: 555–59.

McCarthy M, Wilson-Davis K, and McGavock H (1992) Relationship between the number of partners in a general practice and the number of different drugs prescribed by that practice. *British Journal of General Practice* 42: 10–12.

McConnell TS, Cushing AH, Bankhurst AD, Healy JL, McIlvenna PA, et al. (1982) Physician behaviour modification using claims data: tetracycline for upper respiratory infection. *Western Journal of Medicine* 137: 448–50.

McDonald CJ (1976) Protocol-based computer reminders, the quality of care and the non-perfectibility of man. *New England Journal of Medicine* 295: 1351–55.

McGavock H, Wilson-Davis K, and Milligan E (1993) Completing the triangle – relationship between practice demography, general practitioner workload and prescribing. *Pharmacoepidemiology and Drug Safety* 2: 133–43.

McGuire WJ (1985) Attitudes and attitude change In: Lindzey G and Aronson E (eds.) *Handbook of Social Psychology*. New York: Random House, pp. 233–46.

Meyer TJ, Van Kooten D, Marsh S, and Prochazka AV (1991) Reduction of polypharmacy by feedback to clinicians. *Journal of General Internal Medicine* 6: 133–36.

Mölstad S and Hovelius B (1989) Reduction in antibiotic usage following an educational programme. *Family Practice* 6: 33–37.

Mugford M, Banfield P, and O'Hanlon M (1991) Effects of feedback of information on clinical practice: a review. *British Medical Journal* 303: 398–402.

Newton-Syms FAO, Dawson PH, Cooke J, Feely M, Booth TG, et al. (1992) The influence of an academic representative on prescribing by general practitioners. *British Journal of Clinical Pharmacology* 33: 69–73.

NIH (National Institutes of Health) (1992) *International Consensus Report on Diagnosis and Treatment of Asthma.* Bethesda, MD: National Institutes of Health.

Payer L (1988) *Medicine and Culture.* New York: Henry Holt and Co.

Plumridge R and Berbatis CG (1989) Drug bulletins: effectiveness in modifying prescribing and methods of improving impact. *DICP Annals of Pharmacotherapy* 23: 330–34.

Raisch DW, Bootman JL, Larson LN, and McGhan WF (1990) Improving antiulcer agent prescribing in a Health Maintenance Organization. *American Journal of Hospital Pharmacy* 47: 1766–73.

Ray WA, Blazer DG, Schaffner W, and Federspiel CF (1986) Reducing long-term diazepam prescribing in office practice. *Journal of the American Medical Association* 256: 2536–39.

Ray WA, Fisk R, Schaffner W, and Federspiel CF (1985) Improving antibiotic prescribing in outpatient practice. *Medical Care* 23: 1307–13.

Ray WA, Schaffner W, and Federspiel CF (1985) Persistence of improvement in antibiotic prescribing. *Journal of the American Medical Association* 253: 1774–76.

Ray WA, Taylor JA, Meador KG, Lichtenstein MJ, Griffin MR, et al. (1993) Reducing antipsychotic drug use in nursing homes. A controlled trial of provider education. *Archives of Internal Medicine* 153: 713–21.

Rutz W, Von Knorring L, Walinder J, and Wistedt B (1990) Effect of an educational program for general practitioners on Gotland on the pattern of prescription of psychotropic drugs. *Acta Psychiatrica Scandinavica* 82: 399–403.

Rutz W, Von Knorring L, and Walinder J (1992) Long-term effects of an educational program for general practitioners given by the Swedish Committee for the Prevention and Treatment of Depression. *Acta Psychiatrica Scandinavica* 85: 83–88.

Rutz W, Walinder J, Eberhard G, Holmberg G, Von Knorring A-L, et al. (1989) An educational program on depressive disorders for general practitioners on Gotland: background and evaluation. *Acta Psychiatrica Scandinavica* 79: 19–26.

Sandvik H and Hunskaar S (1990) Doctors' characteristics and practice patterns in general practice: an analysis based on management of urinary incontinence. *Scandinavian Journal of Primary Health Care* 8: 179–82.

Savafi KT and Hayward RA (1992) Choosing between apples and apples: physicians' choices of prescription drugs that have similar side effects and efficacies. *Journal of General Internal Medicine* 7: 32–37.

Schaffner W, Ray WA, Federspiel CF, and Miller WO (1983) Improving antibiotic prescribing in office practice. A controlled trial of three educational methods. *Journal of the American Medical Association* 250: 1728–32.

Schwartz S and Griffin T (1986) *Medical Thinking. The Psychology of Medical Judgment and Decision Making.* New York: Springer-Verlag.

Segal R and Hepler CD (1982) Prescribers' beliefs and values as predictors of drug choices. *American Journal of Hospital Pharmacy* 39: 1391–97.

Segal R and Hepler CD (1985) Drug choice as a problem solving process. *Medical Care* 23: 967–76.

Sibley JC, Sackett DL, Neufeld V, Gerrard B, Rudnick KV, et al. (1982) A randomized trial of continuing medical education. *New England Journal of Medicine* 306: 511–15.

Soumerai SB and Avorn J (1984) Efficacy and cost-containment in pharmacotherapy. *Milbank Memorial Fund Quarterly* 62: 447–74.

Soumerai SB and Avorn J (1986) Economic and policy analysis of university based drug-detailing. *Medical Care* 24: 313–31.

Soumerai SB, McLaughlin TJ, and Avorn J (1989) Improving drug prescribing in primary care: a critical analysis of the experimental literature. *Milbank Quarterly* 67: 268–317.

Soumerai SB, Ross-Degnan D, Fortess EE, and Abelson J (1993) A critical analysis of studies of state drug reimbursement policies. Research in need of discipline. *Milbank Quarterly* 71: 217–52.

Steele MA, Bess DT, Franse VL, and Graber SE (1989) Cost effectiveness of two interventions for reducing outpatient prescribing costs. *DICP Annals of Pharmacotherapy* 23: 497–500.

Stergachis A, Fors M, Wagner FH, Dewayne D, and Penna P (1987) Effects of clinical pharmacists on drug prescribing. *American Journal of Hospital Pharmacy* 44: 525–28.

Stokx LJ, Gloerich ABM, and Kersten TJJMT (1992) *Kostenbesparing door kwaliteitsbevordering Evaluatie van een programma van deskundigheidsbevordering voor huisartsen* (Cost saving through quality improvement. Evaluation of an educational program for GPs) Utrecht, The Netherlands: Nivel.

Strømme HK and Botten G (1992) Factors relating to the choice of antihypertensive and hypnotic drug treatment in old patients. A study of a sample of Norwegian general practitioners. *Scandinavian Journal of Primary Health Care* 10: 301–5.

Stross JK and Bole GG (1980) Evaluation of a continuing education program in rheumatoid arthritis. *Arthritis and Rheumatism* 23: 846–49.

Stross JK, Hiss RG, Watts CM, Davis WK, and MacDonald R (1983) Continuing education in pulmonary disease for primary-care physicians. *American Review of Respiratory Disease* 127: 739–46.

Tamai IY, Rubenstein LZ, Josephson KR, and Yamauchi JA (1987) Impact of computerized drug profiles and a consulting pharmacist on outpatient prescribing patterns: a clinical trial. *Drug Intelligence Clinical Pharmacy* 21: 890–95.

Taylor D (1992) Prescribing in Europe—forces for change. *British Medical Journal* 304: 239–42.

Tierney WM, Hui SL, and McDonald CJ (1986) Delayed feedback of physician performance versus immediate reminders to perform preventive care. *Medical Care* 24: 659–66.

Virji A and Britten N (1991) A study of the relationship between patients' attitudes and doctors' prescribing. *Family Practice* 8: 314–19.

Watson DS, Stenhouse NS, and Jellet LB (1975) General practitioner prescribing habits: the Western Australian experience. *Medical Journal of Australia* 2: 946–47.

White CW, Albanese MA, Brown DD, and Caplan RM (1985) The effectiveness of continuing medical education in changing the behaviour of physicians caring for patients with acute myocardial infarction. *Annals of Internal Medicine* 102: 686–92.

Wyatt TD, Reilly PM, Morrow NC, and Passmore CM (1992) Short-lived effects of a formulary on anti-infective prescribing—the need for continuing peer review? *Family Practice* 9: 461–65.

Zijlstra IF (1991) *De regionaal klinisch farmacoloog; farmacotherapie overleg met huisarts en apotheker* (The area clinical pharmacologist; pharmacotherapy counseling with GP and pharmacist). Dissertation. University of Groningen, The Netherlands.

# Conclusion:
# Policy Scenarios for
# Prescription Drugs

## HUBERT LEUFKENS
## PETER DAVIS

Prescription medicines are therapeutic products that harness the powerful and potentially liberating technology of pharmacological treatment. The technical features of
prescription drugs, however, have not been the focus of this book. Rather, the
overriding concern has been with the policy environment of pharmaceuticals; that is,
with the social and cultural context of medicine use, the underlying market and
industrial structure, and the wider regulatory and policy setting.

Why a book on prescription medicines should be devoted almost exclusively to
the policy environment is plain enough; it is a field that is openly and vigorously
contested, and raises a wide range of analytically challenging issues that remain
largely unresolved. While the scientific and technical foundations of pharmacological
treatment are hardly immune from controversy (for example, see Chapter 1), the
really serious debate begins with the introduction of this technology into people's
lives; issues of safety, social impact, cost, innovation, and control arise as soon as a
personal technology such as prescription drugs moves off the laboratory bench and
into the real-world setting for active use.

Pharmaceuticals, like other personal technologies, are ubiquitous, potent, costly,
and, apparently, a prerequisite to the good life. If, as we maintain, prescription
medicines are an instructive example, then there is an opportunity to consider some

of the more general policy questions raised by the impact of technology on society. This is the focus of this concluding chapter.

Initially we argue that controversies of the kind canvassed in this book need not be seen as merely polemical and divisive in their outcomes. Instead, they can be highly productive, as long as they are the stimulus for new ideas and the systematic exploration and development of policy options. One analytical method designed to facilitate such a process is the technique known as scenario planning. We illustrate the application of this technique to prescription medicines, drawing on a recently published study (Leufkens et al., 1994). We then consider its relevance in bringing together the threads of argument identified in this book.

## Technological Change and Policy Planning

If one thing is clear from the preceding chapters it is that the policy environment of the prescription medicines is a disputed one. There is a diversity of perceptions, interests, and values in the pharmaceutical marketplace, which is reflected in a constantly changing political kaleidoscope of issue and debate (Anonymous, 1991; Dukes, 1991). The image of technology as a neutral entity—an instrument, a means to an end—is deceptive (Foote, 1987). Technology—and medicines are exemplary in this respect—has both benign and potentially threatening dimensions (Schwarz and Thompson, 1990). Furthermore, there are rivalries and conflicts that reflect the interests of the different parties associated with technology and its diffusion in society (Bijker and Law, 1992). The chapters in this book have charted a range of drug policy issues. Inevitably, such issues present starkly contrasting policy choices that are inseparable from their social and political context (Grabowski, 1982; Griffin, 1991).

Controversies are an intrinsic part of the dynamics of technological change. Indeed, Rip (1986) has stressed the value of controversies of just the kind that have been canvassed in this book, seeing in them a powerful vehicle for the stimulation of public debate and problem-solving activity. Rip's concept of constructive technology assessment reflects a strategy both for reconciling the duality of facts and values and for ultimately yielding creative solutions for policy making.

Controversies can assist in several ways in strategic planning. With the systematic analysis of such turbulent events we can identify cyclical movements, some of which determine how the world looks for decades, while others are much more short-lived. Observation of past shifts enables us to determine a range of what is plausible and to construct pictures of what the world ahead might look like. These are *scenarios*. The value of such scenarios lies in the stimulation of thinking and debate about the future; users should be prompted to think in ways that help prepare for what the future might hold.

The purpose of scenario analysis, therefore, is to identify problems and dilemmas and discover the interactions between the various factors that ultimately determine the shape of the future. Controversies provide analytical food for thought; they encourage us to leave familiar paths and prepare for new situations. The kind of approach used here involves selecting a small number of plausible stories of the future (in our case, four). Various sets of assumptions are made, and from them plausible scenarios are constructed; in other words, they *could* happen (Wack, 1985a; 1985b).

Scenarios must be critical in their content; the worlds they depict must differ from one another in crucial respects. It is the compilers' task to make a carefully considered choice of what these crucial contrasts are. That choice follows from an analysis of driving forces (or "drivers"), the trends and developments likely to shape the future in relevant respects. Analysis of these drivers ultimately leads to the selection of the critical elements that form the building blocks of the scenarios. Thus, the uncertainties surrounding the future of medicines in health care need not engender an attitude of defeatism or cynical relativism. Scenarios are intended to promote innovative thinking by helping the reader break free from familiar mental maps. Preparing for plausible futures helps us generate the knowledge and mental equipment needed for these eventualities (Sanders, 1987; Schwartz, 1991).

## Four Scenarios of the Future of Medicines

For more than a decade The Netherlands has maintained a Steering Committee on Future Health Scenarios to develop analyses for health policy. One such analysis concerned the role of medicines in health care (Leufkens et al., 1994). The scenario planners undertaking this study applied concepts and techniques that have been widely used in the business world, particularly in large corporations such as Shell, but that have been employed relatively little in the process of setting public policy goals (although see Pannenborg, 1986).

A total of six driving forces ("megatrends") were identified that seemed likely to play a role in shaping the future of medicines. These were demographic change, the process of internationalization, scientific and technological developments, socioeconomic change, developments in informatics, and the rise of consumerism.

1. The impact of demographic trends on drug consumption is unambiguous: there will be a steady rise, driven mainly by the growing burden of disease associated with an aging population.
2. In the case of internationalization, there is likely to be a split between a supply side with an increasingly international focus on production and licensing, and a demand side, still dominated by political, economic, and cultural factors at the national level.
3. A growing synergy between the basic sciences and associated technologies – information technology (IT), materials, biotechnology – is also predicted. This increases the likelihood of breakthroughs in drug treatment.
4. On the socioeconomic side, the effect of trends in resource availability could be to jeopardize the commitment to social solidarity that underpins the principle of universal access to health care.
5. The spread of IT facilitates risk monitoring (and hence the technological resolution of risk-related problems), accelerates the spread of knowledge, and enables monitoring of the actions of health care providers.
6. Finally, there are the implications of the rise of consumerism. Safety is a major concern of the patient movement, yet the growing value attached to patient autonomy implies an acceptance of some measure of personal – including financial – risk.

It is clear, however, that even if these six key forces were the only specific determinants of the future, the outcome of their interaction might take quite different and sometimes paradoxical forms. One can predict, for example, a growing trust in market forces (driven by international developments, consumerism, and increasing technological possibilities), while at the same time equal access to health care services, cost containment, and the fear of health hazards all call for more coordination and control.

The relative influence of these six determinants has been captured in two major dimensions (called "scenario drivers"): one represents the range of possible regulatory responses, from an emphasis on market forces to an attachment to coordination and control, while the other reflects the polarity of attitudes about medical technology, ranging from aversion to enthusiastic acceptance.

On the basis of these two drivers, a set of four alternative scenarios was constructed (see Table 16-1). While the Risk Avoidance and Technology on Demand scenarios represent polar opposites in prevailing attitudes about medical technology, Sobriety in Sufficiency and Market Unfettered encapsulate contrasting orientations to the social and economic regulation of prescription medicines.

## Conclusion and Synthesis

Scenarios are intended to confront and to stimulate reflection, although provocative scenarios can be rejected as extremely unlikely, or even irrational. Critics of the medicalization of everyday life (Kawachi and Conrad, Chapter 2), for instance, will hardly feel comfortable with the scenario Technology on Demand, while players in the pharmaceutical industry whose job it is to develop new drugs (Kaitin, Chapter 7) will have difficulty accepting the implications of Sobriety in Sufficiency. Furthermore, the chapters in Part III are good examples of how contrasting regulatory trends affect drug policies in unpredictable ways: the liberalization of the availability of medicines—the switch to OTC (Vaillancourt Rosenau and Thoer, Chapter 12)—can,

TABLE 16-1. Sections of the Book Across Four Different Scenarios on the Future of Medicines

| Sections of Book | Four Scenarios on the Future of Medicines | | | |
| --- | --- | --- | --- | --- |
| | Risk Avoidance | Sobriety in Sufficiency | Technology on Demand | Free Market Unfettered |
| Social and cultural context | mistrust, defensive, technophobia | social solidarity, restraint, moral transition | technological optimism, pragmatic | consumption-oriented, accept inequality |
| Industry and market | crisis, risk avoidance, liability culture | improve existing drugs, generics, managed care | high-tech, innovative, medicines as cost-effective | competitive, pluralist, short-term orientation |
| Regulatory and policy setting | chaos, irrational weighing | added value, essential drugs, protocols | technology push, professional dominance | free-market driven, little control |

for example, go along with a plea for the greater control of marketing (Lexchin and Kawachi, Chapter 14) and physician drug choice (Haaijer-Ruskamp and Denig, Chapter 15).

In Table 16-1 the three parts of this book are cross-tabulated against the four policy scenarios. Major themes are highlighted in the body of the table. These attempt to capture the significant contrasts across each scenario. Hence, to take the first row and concentrate on attitudes toward technology, the social and cultural context shows a range from mistrust (under Risk Avoidance), to restraint (Sobriety in Sufficiency), optimism (Technology on Demand), and consumption orientation (Free Market Unfettered). In the second row the crucial contrasts are: liability culture, improvement of existing drugs, high-tech innovative, and competitive pluralistic. Finally, for regulation and policy, the continuum on the management of drugs stretches from irrational weighing to essential drugs and protocols, professional control, and market forces.

Given this format, and given the range of issues depicted in Table 16-1, what conclusions can we draw from the material covered in the preceding chapters about likely future policy scenarios in prescription medicines? Taking first the treatment of issues of social and cultural context in Part I, the overall balance can be called one of caution. We could hardly characterize the chapters as strongly optimistic or consumerist. Nor could they be seen as mistrustful or technophobic. The mood in these first five chapters is perhaps best represented as somewhere between Risk Avoidance and Sobriety in Sufficiency. This contrasts with the chapters on industry and market. These were much closer to accepting the competitive and pluralistic model (column four). Finally, as canvassed in the chapters in Part III, the thrust of international innovation in regulation seems to represent something of a mix of Sobriety in Sufficiency (essential drugs, protocols) — and Technology on Demand (professional dominance).

Judging from the preceding chapters, therefore, the most likely future scenario is not one that falls easily into any of the four developed from the planning study outlined above. Instead, we get a mixed model that emphasizes respect for social solidarity and caution about excessive use, but that at the same time is prepared to countenance the use of market mechanisms in the interests of innovation and consumer choice — albeit within the context of professionally determined principles of regulation and control. Perhaps the closest identifiable policy model from the recent literature is the concept of market solidarity developed by Redwood (1992) as one attempt to reconcile market principles of efficiency and social goals of distributive justice.

A variant of the market solidarity model has the potential to be a viable policy alternative in the current range of options. It would, however, require a certain flexibility on the part of the industry and the modification of what many perceive to be its siege mentality. Governments and insurers simply cannot contemplate major budget deficits with equanimity. Only a commitment by the industry to partnership and joint responsibility in addressing problems of cost, safety, and inappropriate usage will yield long-term and durable solutions.

What the future will bring remains uncertain. Will it be a variant of one of the four scenarios identified above, or will it be a mix like the market solidarity model? At this stage it is impossible to predict. Nevertheless, by trying to break open mental maps, scenarios may be an important tool in learning and in planning to steer society toward this uncertain future. At the very least, they provide one technique by which the material from the preceding chapters can be systematically marshalled to address the analytical issues uncovered in this book. While the policy environment remains inherently contested, we trust that the scenario approach will contribute to the systematic, informed, and strategic thinking required if we are to make real advances in public policy on prescription medicines.

## Acknowledgment

Much of the work on scenarios originated in numerous discussions with others. Among all those we would like to thank Albert Bakker, Graham Dukes, Flora Haaijer-Ruskamp and Hank Schut.

## References

Anonymous (1991) European drug regulation—anti-protectionism or consumer protection? *The Lancet* 337: 1571–72.

Bijker WE and Law J (eds.) (1992) *Shaping Technology/Building Society. Studies in Sociotechnical Change*. Cambridge, MA: MIT Press.

Dukes MNG (1991) Drug policies: the need for constructive criticism. *Post Marketing Surveillance* 5: 231–35.

Foote SB (1987) Assessing medical technology assessment: past, present, and future. *Milbank Quarterly* 65: 59–80.

Grabowski H (1982) Public policy and innovation: the case of pharmaceuticals. *Technovation* 1: 157–89.

Griffin MT (1991) AIDS drugs and the pharmaceutical industry: a need to reform. *American Journal of Law and Medicine* 17: 363–410.

Leufkens H, Haaijer-Ruskamp F, Bakker A, and Dukes G (1994) Scenario analysis of the future of medicines. *British Medical Journal* 309: 1137–40.

Pannenborg, CO (1986) Scenarios as a method of exploring the future of health care. In: WHO Regional Office for Europe (ed.) *Health Projections in Europe. Methods and Applications*. Copenhagen: WHO Regional Office for Europe, pp. 236–51.

Redwood, H (1992) *The Dynamics of Drug Pricing and Reimbursement in the European Community*. Suffolk, UK: Oldwicks Press Ltd.

Rip A (1986) Societal processes of technology assessment. In: Becker HA and Porter AL (eds.) *Impact Assessment Today*. Utrecht, The Netherlands: Jan van Arkel, pp. 415–33.

Sanders R (1987) Penetrating the fog of technology's social dimensions. *Technology in Society* 9: 163–80.

Schwarz M and Thompson M (1990) *Divided We Stand. Redefining Politics, Technology and Social Choice*. New York: Harvester Wheatsheaf.

Schwartz P (1991) *The Art of the Long View. Planning for the Future in an Uncertain World*. New York: Bantam Books.

Wack P (1985a) Scenarios: uncharted waters ahead (Part I). *Harvard Business Review* (September–October) 73–89.

Wack P (1985b) Scenarios: shooting the rapids (Part II). *Harvard Business Review* (November–December) 139–50.

# Index